Cardiology Words and Phrases

Second Edition

Cardiac Imaging
Cardiac Surgery
Cardiopulmonary
Cardiothoracic
Cardiovascular
Pediatric Cardiology

Health Professions Institute • Modesto, California • 1995

Cardiology Words and Phrases
Second Edition

Sally Crenshaw Pitman
Editor & Publisher
Health Professions Institute
P. O. Box 801
Modesto, CA 95353
Phone (209) 551-2112
Fax (209) 551-0404

Printed by
Parks Printing & Lithograph
Modesto, California

ISBN 0-934385-63-7
Last digit is the print number: 9 8 7 6

With love and gratitude
to our mothers

Loraine Crenshaw
Louise Adams
Marion Campbell

Preface

Cardiology Words and Phrases, second edition, is an update of the 196-page quick-reference guide we published in the summer of 1989. This new book, however, with nearly 50,000 entries in 570 pages, is far more than a mere revision of the earlier book.

When we decided to update the cardiology book in 1994, we thought it would be useful to include pulmonary, thoracic, and vascular words since many references to the heart, lungs, and chest appear in cardiology dictation. We wanted terminology from cardiac imaging and surgery of the heart, lungs, circulatory system, and chest, as well as pediatric cardiology.

After a year of research we had tripled the number of entries in the earlier edition, and we simply had to stop and go to press. Although this edition is by no means an exhaustive list of words and phrases in these specialties, we are confident that we have gathered the most relevant and useful words and phrases in cardiology and cardiopulmonary medicine, as well as imaging and cardiac, cardiopulmonary, cardiothoracic, and cardiovascular surgery.

We've culled words and phrases from hundreds of transcripts of cardiology and pulmonary medical and surgical dictation, as well as textbooks, scholarly journals, and other references.

The research and editing for this edition were done primarily by Ellen Drake and Sally Pitman. The first edition of *Cardiology Words and Phrases* was mainly the work of Susan M. Turley and Linda Campbell and the staff of Health Professions Institute, although we had help from many of our medical transcription colleagues as well.

Invaluable assistance in verifying the accuracy of entries and reconciling discrepancies from various authoritative references was provided by John H. Dirckx, M.D., medical editorial consultant, Dayton, Ohio, and Bron Taylor, an experienced medical transcriptionist and researcher in San Francisco.

My warmest gratitude to all.

Sally Crenshaw Pitman, M.A.
Editor & Publisher

How to Use This Book

The words and phrases in this book are alphabetized letter by letter of all words in the entry, ignoring puntuation marks and words in parentheses. The possessive form (*'s*) is omitted from eponyms for ease in alphabetizing. Numbers are alphabetized as if written out, with the exception of subscripts and superscripts which are ignored.

Eponyms may be located alphabetically as well as under the nouns they modify. For example, *Jatene arterial switch procedure* and *Jatene-Macchi prosthetic valve* may be found under *Jatene* as well as under *operation* and *valve*.

The main entry *drug-related terms* includes descriptive terms related to drugs, not the names of pharmaceuticals. The names of hundreds of medications (generic and brand names) used in cardiology and pulmonary medicine appear under the main entry *medications*.

The main entries *artery* and *vein* include phrases and descriptive terms related to arteries and veins as they are dictated in patient reports, rather than the names of anatomical terms readily available in medical dictionaries. Physicians dictate many abbreviations, especially for anatomical groups, and those terms frequently abbreviated in medical dictation are listed as main entries with their translations and as subentries.

In medical dictation physicians arbitrarily refer to a diagnostic, therapeutic, or operative procedure (both invasive and noninvasive) as an *approach*, *method*, *operation*, *procedure*, *repair*, or *technique*, or by the type of procedure, such as *angioplasty*. Thus, all procedures are listed alphabetically by the eponym or noun as well as under the type of procedure and under the main entry *operation*.

Instruments used in operative, therapeutic, and diagnostic procedures may also be referred to variously as an *apparatus*, *device*, *instrument*, *system*, or a particular type of device, such as a *catheter*. Thus, instruments are listed under the type when there are many examples given, and those devices or instruments or machines that do not fit neatly under their own categories are listed under the general term *device* or *system*.

A few main entries with extensive subentries include the following:

angina	catheter	graft	prosthesis
aorta	clamp	heart	pulse
artery	contrast medium	infarction	sign
asthma	defect	lead	sound
atrioventricular	disease	lung	stenosis
beat	echocardiogram	murmur	syndrome
block	electrocardiogram	operation	tachycardia
bronchitis	electrode	pacemaker	test
bypass	embolism	pain	valve
cardiac	emphysema	pneumonia	vein
cardiomyopathy	endocarditis	pressure	ventricle

A, a

"a" (augment)(ed)
AA (ascending aorta)
AA curve; A_1A_2 curve
AA interval; A_1A_2 interval
AAA ("triple A") (abdominal aortic aneurysm)
AACD (abdominal aortic counterpulsation device)
AAI pacemaker (atrial demand inhibited)
AAI pacing mode
AAI rate-adaptive mode
AAI rate-modulated mode
AAI rate-responsive mode
AAIR pacemaker syndrome
AAIR pacing (atrial rate adaptive)
AAMI (Advancement of Medical Instrumentation)
AAMI validation criteria
a/A ratio
Aase syndrome
AAT pacemaker (atrial demand triggered)
A bands of sarcomere
Abbott artery
Abbott radioimmunoassay kit
Abbreviated Injury Scale

abbreviated interval
A-B-C (airway, breathing, circulation) sequence (cardiopulmonary resuscitation)
abdomen, protuberant
abdominal aneurysm
abdominal aorta, infrarenal
abdominal aorta thrombosis
abdominal aortic aneurysm (AAA)
abdominal asthma
abdominal bruit
abdominal coarctation
abdominal heterotaxy
abdominal left ventricular assist device (ALVAD)
abdominal mass
    nonpulsatile
    pulsatile
abdominal respirations
abdominojugular reflux
ABE (acute bacterial endocarditis)
aberrant conduction
aberrant coronary artery
aberrant depolarization of ventricular muscle
aberrant left pulmonary artery
aberrantly conducted beats

1

aberrant QRS complex
aberrant vascular channels
aberration
    intraventricular
    metabolic
    nonspecific T wave
    ventricular
ABG, ABGs (arterial blood gas)(es)
    (see *blood gas)*
ABI (ankle-brachial index)
ability, cardiac pumping
Abiomed biventricular support (BVS)
    system
Abiomed cardiac device
ablated myocardium
ablation
    accessory conduction (ACA)
    accessory pathway
    atrioventricular nodal
    bundle of His
    continuous wave
    cryosurgical
    direct current (DCA)
    electrode catheter
    endocardial
    endocardial catheter
    His bundle
    intracoronary ethanol
    intraoperative laser
    Kent bundle
    laser
    myocardial
    percutaneous radiofrequency
        catheter
    pulsed laser
    radiofrequency (RFA)
    transaortic radiofrequency
    transapical endocardial
    transcatheter His bundle
    transcoronary chemical
    transseptal radiofrequency
    transvenous

ablation of arrhythmogenic areas in
    myocardium
ablation of myocardium
ablation of pathway, surgical
ablation surgery in congenital vascular
    defect
ablation therapy arrhythmia
ablative device
Ablatr temperature control device for
    radiofrequency catheter ablation
abnormal airways stretch
abnormal bleeding
abnormal chest cage
abnormal gradient
abnormal heart sound
abnormal hemoglobin
abnormal physiologic splitting
abnormal pulmonary venous drainage
abnormalities of platelet function
abnormalities of small blood vessels
abnormality, abnormalities
    akinetic wall motion
    baseline ST segment
    brisk wall motion
    conduction
    ectopic wall motion
    exercise-induced wall motion
    focal wall motion
    global
    intraventricular conduction
    LV (left ventricular) wall motion
    nonspecific T wave
    occult circulatory
    perfusion
    persistent wall motion
    regional wall motion
    segmental perfusion
    subsegmental perfusion
    transient wall motion
    wall motion
abnormality of arch of aorta
abnormally loud first heart sound

abolished by breath-holding
abolition of ventricular tachycardia
abortive shock capability
abrade
Abrahams sign
Abramo-Fiedler syndrome
Abrams needle
abrupt onset
abrupt tapering
abrupt vessel closure
abscess
    aortic root
    blood-streaked
    foul-smelling
    lung
    metastatic
    putrid
    subphrenic
abscess drainage
abscess formation
absence
    congenital pericardial
    partial pericardial
absence of left side of pericardium
absence of sweating
absence of ventricular activity
absent aortic knob on chest x-ray
absent apex pulse
absent apical impulse
absent breath sounds
absent bronchial cartilage
absent pericardium, congenital
absent peripheral veins
absent pulmonary valve syndrome
absent P waves
absent respirations
absent runoff
absent tactile fremitus
absolute artery dimensions
absolute blood eosinophil count
absolute cardiac dullness (ACD)
absolute eosinophilia

absolute neutrophilia
absolute refractory period (ARP)
absorbable suture
abundant collateral circulation
AC (aortic closure) interval
ACA (accessory conduction ablation)
ACAD (atherosclerotic carotid artery
    disease)
accelerated atherosclerosis
accelerated atrioventricular conduction
accelerated atrioventricular junctional
    rhythm
accelerated ejection
accelerated hypertension
accelerated idioventricular rhythm
    (AIVR)
accelerated respirations
acceleration
acceleration map
acceleration of ventricular tachycardia
accelerator globulin (AcG) blood
    coagulation factor
Accent-DG balloon
accentuated pulmonic component
accentuated second pulmonic sound
accentuation
accessible lesion
accessory atrioventricular conduction
accessory atrioventricular pathway
accessory blood supply
accessory hemiazygos vein
accessory muscles of respiration
accessory pathway (AP)
    ablation of
    concealed
accessory pathway potentials
accessory pathway reentrant PSVT
    (paroxysmal supraventricular
    tachycardia)
accessory respiratory muscle activity
accessory sinuses
acid-base balance

accident
  cardiovascular (CVA)
  cerebrovascular (CVA)
accordioning of the stent coils
Accucap CO_2/O_2 monitor
Accucom cardiac output monitor
Accufix pacemaker lead
Acculith pacemaker
accumulation
  dependent extracellular fluid
  fluid
  lactic acid
accumulation of air in interlobar spaces
accumulation of gas under serous tunic
  of intestine
Accutorr monitor
ACD (Active Compression-
  Decompression) Resuscitator
ACE (angiotensin-converting enzyme)
ACE challenge
ACE inhibitor
ACE (asymptomatic complex ectopy)
ACE fixed-wire balloon catheter
ace of spades sign on angiogram
acetaminophen overdose
AcG (accelerator globulin) blood
  coagulation factor
ACG (apexcardiogram, -graphy)
achalasia of thoracic esophagus
  (also called cardiospasm)
Achiever balloon dilatation catheter
Achromobacter
acid
  arachidonic
  epsilon-aminocaproic
  gadolinium-diethylenetriamine–
    pentaacetic
  glycyrrhetinic
  hydrocyanic
  lactic
  nicotinic

acid *(cont.)*
  omega-3 fatty
  paraaminosalicylic
acid aspiration pneumonitis
acid-base equilibrium
acid-base imbalance
acid-base status
acidemia
  metabolic
  moderate respiratory
acid-fast bacilli (AFB) stain
acid-fast culture
acid lipase deficiency
acid maltase deficiency
acidosis
  metabolic
  respiratory
acidotic
acid phosphatase, histamine
acid pulmonary aspiration syndrome
acid reflux
acid regurgitation
acid release, hydrocyanic vanillylmandelic
acineresis/dyskinesis
Acinetobacter baumannii
aCL (anticardiolipin) antibody
Acland-Banis arteriotomy set
ACLS (advanced cardiac life support)
  protocol
acme, pain
Acorn nebulizer
Acosta (or D'Acosta) syndrome
acoustic backscatter characteristics of
  blood
acoustic impedance
acoustic quantification, left ventricular
  ejection fraction
acoustic shadowing
acoustic window
acquired aneurysm

acquired bronchiectasis
acquired disease
acquired heart murmur
acquired hemolytic anemia
acquired lesion
acquired lymphedema
acquired mitral stenosis
acquired prolonged Q-T interval
acquired tracheobronchomalacia
acquired unilateral hyperlucent lung
acquired ventricular septal defect
  (AVSD)
acquisition, data
acquisition technique
acrocyanosis
acromegalic
acromegaly
acroparesthesia
  Schultze
  simple
acrylates in vaso-occlusive angiotherapy
ACS (Advanced Catheter Systems;
  Cardiovascular Systems)
ACS angioplasty Y connector
ACS guide wire
ACS Indeflator
ACS JL4 (Judkins left 4) French
  catheter
ACS LIMA guide
ACS Mini catheter
ACS RX coronary dilatation catheter
ACS SULP II balloon
ACT (activated clotting time) protocol
ACTH (adrenocorticotropic hormone)
ACTH hypersecretion
ACTH secretion
Actinobacillus endocarditis infection
actinomycete, thermophilic
actinomycosis
actinomycotic pericarditis
action potential, cardiac

action potential duration (APD)
action, prolonged
activated clotting time (ACT)
activated partial thromboplastin time
  (APTT)
activation
  complement
  Hageman factor
  inappropriate (of ICD)
activation of fibrinolysin
activator
  plasminogen
  recombinant tissue type plasmino-
    gen (rt-PA)
  tissue plasminogen (t-PA)
active bleeding site
Active Compression-Decompression
  (ACD) Resuscitator
active congestion
active emptying fraction (left atrium)
active fixation lead
active hyperemia
active mode
Activitrax variable rate pacemaker
activity
  breathlessness after
  ectopic atrial
  inappropriately elevated plasma
    renin
  inotropic
  pulseless electrical
  sympathomimetic
  triggered
activity sensor modulated atrial rate
  adaptive pacing (AAIR)
actocardiotocograph fetal heart monitor
actuator component
actuator, double-acting
Acuson computed sonography
Acuson echocardiographic equipment
acute alveolar hypoperfusion
acute aortic regurgitation syndrome

acute aortic thrombosis
acute arteritis
acute attack of bronchospasm
acute bacterial endocarditis (ABE)
acute benign pericarditis
acute blood loss
acute bronchitis
acute cerebrovascular insufficiency
acute compression triad
acute coronary insufficiency
acute coronary syndrome
acute eosinophilic pneumonia
acute exacerbation
acute febrile mucocutaneous lymph
  node syndrome (MCLS)
acute heart failure
acute hemodynamic overload
acute idiopathic pericarditis
acute infectious bronchitis
acute inhalation injury
acute interstitial myocarditis
acute intramural hematoma
acute irritative bronchitis
acute laryngotracheal bronchitis
acute left heart failure
acute massive lung collapse
acute mediastinitis
acute mesenteric artery occlusion
acute mountain sickness
acute myocardial infarction (AMI)
acute nonspecific pericarditis
acute pancreatitis
acute pericarditis
acute pharyngitis
acute pleurisy
acute pneumonitis
acute pulmonary edema
acute renal failure
acute respiratory arrest
acute respiratory center paralysis
acute respiratory failure (ARF)
acute rheumatic endocarditis (ARE)

acute rheumatic fever (ARF)
acute rheumatic myocarditis (ARM)
acute rheumatic pericarditis (ARP)
acute tracheitis
acute tracheobronchitis
acute traumatic rupture of aortic
  isthmus
acute tuberculosis
acute type B aortic dissection
acute ventilatory failure
acute vessel closure
a, c, v (positive) waves on jugular
  pulse wave tracing
acyanosis
acyanotic congenital heart disease
acyl coenzyme A deficiency
acyl-CoA dehydrogenase, deficiency
  of long chain
AD (aortic diameter)
Adamkiewicz artery
Adams-DeWeese vena caval clip
Adams-Stokes disease
Adams-Stokes syncope
Adams-Stokes syndrome
adapter
  butterfly
  side-arm
  sleeve
adaptive burst pacing
adaptive hypertrophy
adductor magnus muscle
adenocarcinoma
adenoma
  adrenal cortical
  aldosterone-producing
  bronchial
adenomatoid malformation
adenomatous polyp
adenopathy
  axillary
  hilar
  mediastinal

adenopathy *(cont.)*
  symmetrical mediastinal
adenosine diphosphate (ADP) platelet
  adhesiveness
adenosine echocardiography
adenosine triphosphate (ATP)
adenosquamous carcinoma
adenovirus
adequate air exchange
adequate cardiac output
adequate collateral circulation
adequate coronary perfusion
adequate heparinization
adequate stroke volume
ADH (antidiuretic hormone) secretion
adherent pericardium, rheumatic
adherent thrombus
adhesion, adhesions
  fibrous pleural
  freeing up of
  inflammatory
  lysed
  pericardial
  pericardial diaphragmatic
  pleural
  pleuropulmonary
  probe (to vessel wall)
  taking down of
adhesion-inducing agent
adhesions between lung and
  pericardium
adhesive pericarditis
adhesive phlebitis
adhesive pleurisy
adhesiveness, platelet
ad hoc (improvised)
"a" dip on echocardiogram
adjunctive biological glue
adjunctive technique
adjunctive therapy
adjunctive treatment
adjuvant chemotherapy

adjuvant therapy
administration
  heparin
  volume
admixture, obligatory (of systemic
  venous and pulmonary venous
  blood)
Adolph's Salt Substitute
ADP (adenosine diphosphate)
ADR Ultramark 4 ultrasound
adrenal cortical adenoma
adrenal disease
adrenal gland hyperfunction
adrenal gland hypofunction
adrenal hyperplasia, congenital
adrenal medulla
adrenal steroidogenesis
adrenal steroids
adrenal vein sampling
adrenal venous aldosterone level
adrenalectomy
adrenalin
adrenergic blockade
adrenergic drive
adrenergic receptor
adrenocortical hyperplasia
adrenocorticotropic hormone
adrenomedullary triad
Adriamycin cardiotoxicity
Adson forceps
Adson hook
Adson maneuver
Adson test
adult fibroelastosis
adult-onset reactive airways disease
adult respiratory distress syndrome
  (ARDS)
adult sudden death
adult tuberculosis
advanced cardiac life support (ACLS)
advanced cardiogenic shock

advanced tuberculous constrictive
  pericarditis
adventitia
  thickened
  tunica
adventitial cystic disease
adventitious breath sounds
adventitious heart sounds
adventitious lung sounds
adverse complications
adverse event
AEC (aortic ejection click)
AECG (ambulatory ECG)
AED (automatic external defibrillator)
Ae-H interval
AEI (atrial escape interval)
A_2 equal to P_2
Aequitron pacemaker
aeration disturbances
aerobic exercise
aerobic gram-positive bacilli
Aerobicycle (powered treadmill)
aerobullosis
Aerochamber face mask
Aerodyne bicycle
aeroembolism
aerogenic tuberculosis
Aeropent (aerosolized pentamidine)
aerophagia
aerosol
  metered-dose
  radioactive
aerosol therapy
aerosolized lidocaine
aerosolized pentamidine
Aero Tech II nebulizer
AET (automatic ectopic tachycardia)
AF (aortic flow)
AF (atrial fibrillation)
A_2, false
AFB (acid-fast bacilli) stain
AFBG (aortofemoral bypass graft)

afferent conduit
afferent nerve stimulation syncope
A fib (atrial fibrillation) pattern
AFl (atrial flutter)
AFP pacemaker
African trypanosomiasis
after-depolarizations
afterload
  cardiac
  increased ventricular
  left ventricular
  ventricular
afterload agent
afterload reduction
Afzelius syndrome
AG (anion gap)
Agar-IF (immunofixation in agar) of
  blood serum
agenesis
  lung
  pulmonary artery
agent
  afterload
  antiarrhythmic
  antiplatelet
  beta-adrenergic receptor blocking
  beta-adrenoceptor blocking
agglutination factor
  Duffy
  Kell
  Kidd
  Lewis
  Lutheran
agglutinins, febrile
aggravated by deep inspiration
aggregated eosinophil granules
aggregation, platelet
aggressive interstitial infiltrate
aggressive perivascular infiltrate
aggressive pulmonary toilet
agitation
agonal (or agony) clot

agonal phase, bradycardic
agonal tracing (on EKG)
agonist, beta
agony thrombus
agraphia
A_2 greater than P_2
ague
AHA (American Heart Association)
AHA low-fat diet
AHC (apical hypertrophic cardio-
  myopathy)
A-H curve
A_2 heart sound (aortic valve closure)
AH:HA ratio
AHG (antihemophilic globulin)
AHI (apnea/hypopnea index)
A-H interval
"ahn mahs" (en masse)
AHT (arterial hypertension)
AI (aortic insufficiency) pacing
AICA (anterior inferior communicating
  artery)
AICD (automatic implantable
  cardioverter defibrillator)
AICD pacemaker
AICD plus Tachylog
AICD shocks
AICD-B and AICD-BR pacemaker
AID (automatic implantable or
  internal defibrillator)
AID-B pacemaker
A_2 incisural interval
AIOD (aortoiliac obstructive disease)
air boluses
air bronchogram
air cell
air column, corrugated
air-conditioner lung
air-driven artificial heart
air embolism or embolus
air exchange

air-filled lungs
air-fluid level
air hunger
air in lung connective tissue
air in pleural cavity on x-ray
air interface on x-ray
air leak
airless lung
airlessness, alveolar
airless state
air pocket
air-powered nebulizer
air, room
air sac
air space
  apical (on x-ray)
  terminal
air trapping
airway, airways
  artificial
  asthmatic
  clear
  dynamic compression of
  emergency
  esophageal obturator
  hypertonic
  large
  natural
  oral
  oropharyngeal
  reactive
  small
airway caliber
airway collapse
airway conductance and resistance
airway control
airway constriction
airway epithelial irritant receptors
airway hyperresponsiveness
airway ischemia
airway narrowing (asthma)

airway obstruction caused by:
  asthma
  chronic bronchitis
  cystic fibrosis
  emphysema
  mucoviscidosis
airway opening pressure
airway pressure release ventilation
airway resistance (R_{AW})
airway responsiveness
airway sensitivity
airways stretch, abnormal
AIVR (accelerated idioventricular
  rhythm)
AK (atrial kick)
akinesia
  apical
  global
  inferior wall
  lateral wall
  regional
  septal
  wall
akinesis
akinetic left ventricle
akinetic mutism
akinetic posterior wall
akinetic segmental wall motion
Akutsu III TAH (total artificial heart)
alae nasi, flaring of the
Alagille syndrome
alar chest
alar flaring
alba dolens, phlegmasia
Albini nodule
Albright disease
albumin concentration
albumin solution
Albuminar blood volume expander
albuminized woven Dacron tube graft
albuminoid sputum

albuterol bronchodilator
ALCAPA (anomalous origin of left
  coronary artery from the pulmonary
  artery) syndrome
Alcock catheter plug
alcohol ablation therapy for arrhythmias
alcoholic cardiomegaly-emphysema
alcoholic cardiomyopathy
alcoholic cardiomyopathy with beriberi
alcoholic dilated cardiomyopathy
alcoholic heart
aldosterone
  circadian rhythm of plasma
  postural stimulation of
aldosterone level
  adrenal venous
  circulating
aldosterone production, autonomous
aldosterone secretion, autonomous
aldosterone secretion rate
aldosterone-producing adenoma (APA)
aldosteronism
  primary
  pseudoprimary
  secondary
Aldrete needle
Aldrich-Mees line
Aldrich syndrome
ALEC (artificial lung-expanding
  compound)
Alexander rib raspatory
Alexander rib stripper
Alexander syndrome
Alexander-Farabeuf rib rasp
alexia
Alfred M. Large vena cava clamp
algorithm
aliasing phenomenon in Doppler
  studies
A-line (arterial line)
aliquot dose

alkaline phosphatase
alkalosis
  acapnial
  compensated
  hypokalemic
  metabolic
  respiratory
alkaptonuria
allantoic vessel thrombosis
Allen test prior to radial artery
  cannulation
Allen-Brown criteria
Allen circulatory test
allergen
allergen extract, lyophilized
allergenic exposure
allergen-induced bronchial hyperresponsiveness
allergen-induced bronchial reaction
allergic alveolitis
allergic alveolitis syndrome
allergic angiitis
allergic angiitis and granulomatosis
allergic asthma
allergic bronchopulmonary
  aspergillosis
allergic bronchopulmonary fungal
  disease
allergic exposure
allergic granulomatosis
allergic myocardial granulomatous
  disease
allergic reaction
  type I (atopic or anaphylactic)
  type II (cytotoxic)
  type III (immune-complex-
    mediated)
  type IV (cell-mediated or delayed)
allergic respiratory disease
allergic rhinitis
allergies to pollen, dust, molds
allergy, bronchopulmonary

alleviated
alligator pacing cable
Allis grasping forceps
Allis-Adair clamp
Allison lung retractor
allogeneic transplantation
allograft
  cardiac
  cryopreserved human aortic
  lung
allograft coronary artery disease
allograft reaction
allotransplantation
ALMD (asymptomatic left main
  disease)
Aloka color Doppler system for blood
  flow imaging
Aloka echocardiograph machine
AL-1 catheter
$alpha_1$ or alpha-1
$alpha_1$-adrenergic blocking agent
alpha-adrenoreceptor blockers
alpha-adrenoreceptor stimulant
alpha-agonists, central
$alpha_1$ antitrypsin
$alpha_1$ antitrypsin deficiency
alpha-blockade
alpha-galactosidase A deficiency
$alpha_1$ proteinase inhibitor (a_1PI)
  deficiency
alpha receptor
alpha-stat strategy
alpha thalassemia
Alport syndrome
ALT (alanine aminotransferase),
  elevated
alteration, ST segment
altered consciousness
alternans
  electrical
  pulsus
  total

alternating blue and white mattress
    sutures
alternating current
alternative modality
alternatives, feasible
altitude anoxia
altitude sickness
AL-II guiding catheter
aluminosis of lung
aluminum oxide inhalation
Alupent breathing treatments via
    machine
ALVAD (abdominal left ventricular
    assist device)
alveolar airlessness
alveolar-arterial oxygen pressure
    difference
alveolar atrophy
alveolar capillaries
alveolar capillary block syndrome
alveolar-capillary membrane
alveolar carcinoma
alveolar cell (type I or II)
alveolar cell carcinoma
alveolar cell ghosts
alveolar cell tumor
alveolar collapse
alveolar consolidation
alveolar cysts
alveolar dilatations of lung tissue
alveolar distention
alveolar duct emphysema
alveolar ducts
alveolar edema
alveolar emphysema
alveolar eosinophilia
alveolar exudate
alveolar gas
alveolar glands
alveolar hypocarbia
alveolar hypoplasia
alveolar hypoventilation, primary

alveolar microlithiasis
alveolar necrosis
alveolar overventilation
alveolar pneumonopathy
alveolar proteinosis, pulmonary
alveolar pulmonary edema
alveolar rupture
alveolar sac
alveolar septa
    scarred
    thickened
alveolar septal inflammation
alveolar stability
alveolar underventilation with
    hypercapnia
alveolar ventilation, reduced
alveolar volume
alveolar wall edema
alveolar wall tension
alveolar-arterial oxygen tension
    gradient
alveolar-capillary block
alveolar-capillary membrane damage
alveoli (pl. of alveolus)
alveoli pulmonis (also pulmonum)
alveolitis
    allergic
    cryptogenic fibrosing
    desquamative
    extrinsic allergic
    fibrosing
    generalized
    lymphoid
    neutrophil
    T-helper lymphocyte
alveolitis with honeycombing
alveolitis with hyaline membrane
alveolocapillary membrane
alveolus (pl. alveoli), pulmonary
Alzate catheter
AMA-Fab (antimyosin monoclonal
    antibody with Fab fragment)

AMA-Fab scintigraphy
Amato body
amaurosis fugax
amber-colored pulmonary secretions
Amberlite particles
ambient ozone exposure
ambiguus, situs
Ambrose criteria for thrombotic lesions
Ambu bag
ambued, ambuing (slang)
ambulant
ambulatory electrocardiogram, -graphy
ambulatory equilibrium angiocardiography
ambulatory monitoring (Holter)
ambulatory status
AMC needle
amebiasis pericarditis
amenable to surgery
amenable to wedge resection
American Heart Association (AHA) classification of stenosis
American Heart Association (AHA) diet for hypercholesterolemia
American Optical oximeter
Amershan radioimmunoassay kit
AMI (acute myocardial infarction)
AMI (anterior myocardial infarction)
aminocaproic acid
aminoglycosides
Amipaque contrast material
AML (anterior mitral leaflet)
ammonium chloride
amniotic fluid embolism (embolus)
A-mode echocardiography
amp (amplitude)
amphoric breath sounds
amphoric breathing
amphoric respirations
Amplatz cardiac catheter
Amplatz dilator
Amplatz femoral catheter

Amplatz right coronary catheter
Amplatz Super Stiff guide wire
Amplatz technique
Amplatz torque wire
Amplatz tube guide
amplitude
   aortic
   apical IVS (interventricular septum)
   C-A mitral valve
   cardiac signal
   D-E
   decreased P wave
   diminished wave
   EKG wave
   low
   mid-IVS (interventricular septum)
   posterior LV (left ventricular) wall
   precordial impulse
   pulse
   QRS complex
   R wave
   S_1
   septal
   valve opening
   variance
amplitude of motion
amputation sign
AMR (acute rheumatic myocarditis)
AMS (automatic mode switching) in pacemaker
AMVL (anterior mitral valve leaflet)
A_2/MVO interval (aortic valve closure to mitral valve opening)
amyloid heart disease
amyloidoma
amyloidosis
   cardiac
   familial
   primary
   senile cardiac
   systemic
amyloidotic cardiomyopathy

ANA (antinuclear antibody) test
anacrotic limb of carotid arterial pulse
anacrotic notch of carotid arterial pulse
anaerobic aspiration
anaerobic lung infection
anaerobic threshold
analogous
analysis (see also *assay, test*)
    arterial blood gas
    Doppler spectral
    Northern blot
    PCR (polymerase chain reaction)
    quantitative
    slot blot
    Southern blot
    Western blot
analyzer, pacemaker system
anaphylactoid reaction
anaphylatoxins
anaphylaxis
anasarca
anastomosis (anatomical or surgical)
    aorta-to-vein
    aortic
    aorticopulmonary or aorto-
        pulmonary
    arterio-arterial
    arteriolovenularis
    arteriovenous
    ascending aorta to pulmonary artery
    Baffe
    beveled
    bidirectional cavopulmonary
    Blalock-Taussig
    Cabrol I
    caval-pulmonary artery
    cavopulmonary
    cobra-head
    Cooley intrapericardial
    Cooley modification of Waterston
    diamond
    diamond-shaped

anastomosis *(cont.)*
    distal
    end-to-end
    end-to-side
    end-to-side portacaval
    Glenn
    glomeriform arteriovenous
    glomeriform arteriovenular
    heterocladic
    homocladic
    intercoronary
    internal mammary artery to
        coronary artery
    Kugel
    laser-assisted microvascular
        (LAMA)
    left pulmonary artery to
        descending aorta
    LIMA (left internal mammary
        artery)
    Martin-Gruber
    mesocaval
    microvascular
    outflow
    portacaval
    portosystemic
    Potts
    Potts-Smith side-to-side
    precapillary
    proximal
    right atrium to pulmonary artery
    right internal mammary artery
    right pulmonary artery to
        ascending aorta
    right subclavian to pulmonary
        artery
    Riolan
    side-to-end
    side-to-side
    simple arteriovenous
    simple arteriovenular
    splenorenal

anastomosis *(cont.)*
  Sucquet-Hoyer
  superior vena cava to distal right
    pulmonary artery
  superior vena cava to pulmonary
    artery
  systemic to pulmonary artery
  systemic-pulmonary artery
  tensionless
  terminoterminal
  tracheal
  vascular
  Waterston-Cooley
  Waterston extrapericardial
anastomotic defect
anastomotic disruption
anastomotic hemorrhage
anastomotic pseudoaneurysm
anastomotic stricture
anastomotica magna, arteria
anatomical dead space
anatomically dominant
anatomic shunt flow
anatomy
  distorted
  left-dominant coronary
  right-dominant coronary
anchor, anchored
ancillary
Ancylostoma braziliense infection
Ancylostoma duodenale infection
Ancylostoma infection
Anderson-Keys method for total serum
  cholesterol
Andral decubitus
Andrews Pynchon suction tube
Andrews suction tip
anecdotal relationship
anecdotal response
anechoic mantle
Anel method

anemia
  achylic
  acquired hemolytic
  acute
  acute posthemorrhagic
  anhematopoietic
  aplastic
  apparent
  aregenerative
  autoimmune hemolytic (AIHA)
  Blackfan-Diamond
  bone marrow replacement
  congenital (of newborn)
  congenital hypoplastic
  congenital pernicious
  Cooley
  cow's milk
  deficiency
  Diamond-Blackfan
  dilution
  drug-induced immune hemolytic
  folic acid deficiency
  hemolytic
  hemorrhagic
  hereditary hemolytic
  hereditary iron-loading
  hereditary sideroblastic
  hypochromic
  hypochromic microcytic
  hypoplastic
  immune hemolytic
  immunohemolytic
  iron-deficiency
  juvenile pernicious
  macrocytic
  Malin
  Mediterranean
  microangiopathic
  microangiopathic hemolytic
  microcytic
  normochromic

anemia *(cont.)*
  normocytic
  nutritional
  nutritional macrocytic
  osteosclerotic
  pernicious
  physiologic
  physiological
  polar
  posthemorrhagic (of newborn)
  progressive
  scorbutic
  sickle cell
  sideropenic
  splenic
  spur-cell
  tropical macrocytic
  vitamin B_{12} deficiency
  X-linked
anemic phlebitis
anergy panel
anesthesia
  angiospastic
  blow-by
  crash induction of
  Dyclone gargle
  epidural
  hypotensive
  induction of
  mask
aneuploidy
aneurysm
  abdominal
  abdominal aortic (AAA)
  acquired
  ampullary
  aortic
  aortic arch
  aortic sinus
  aortic sinusal
  aortoiliac
  arterial

aneurysm *(cont.)*
  arteriosclerotic
  arteriovenous
  arteriovenous pulmonary
  ascending
  ascending aortic
  atherosclerotic
  atrial septal
  axillary
  bacterial
  berry
  berry intracranial
  bland aortic
  brain
  cardiac
  carotid artery
  cerebral
  Charcot-Bouchard
  circumscript
  cirsoid
  compound
  congenital
  congenital aortic sinus
  congenital cerebral
  coronary artery
  coronary vessel
  Crawford technique for
  cylindroid
  DeBakey technique for
  debulking of the
  descending thoracic
  dissecting
  dissecting aortic
  distal aortic arch
  ductal
  ectatic
  embolic
  false
  fusiform
  hernial
  imperforate
  infected

aneurysm *(cont.)*
  innominate
  intracranial
  intramural coronary artery
  isthmus
  juxtarenal aortic
  late false
  lateral
  left ventricular
  luetic aortic
  mesh-wrapping of aortic
  miliary
  mixed
  mural
  mycotic
  mycotic suprarenal
  nodular
  orbital
  pararenal aortic
  Park
  pelvic
  postinfarction ventricular
  Potts
  pulmonary arteriovenous
  pulmonary artery compression
    ascending aorta
  pulmonary artery mycotic
  racemose
  Rasmussen
  renal
  renal artery
  Richet
  Rodriguez
  ruptured
  ruptured atherosclerotic
  sacciform
  saccular
  sacculated
  serpentine
  Shekelton
  sinus of Valsalva
  spindle-shaped

aneurysm *(cont.)*
  spontaneous infantile ductal
  spurious
  suprasellar
  syphilitic
  thoracic
  thoracic aorta
  thoracoabdominal
  traumatic
  true
  tubular
  Valsalva sinus
  varicose
  venous
  ventricular
  ventricular septal
  verminous
  windsock
  worm
  wrapping of abdominal aortic
aneurysmal bruit
aneurysmal bulging
aneurysmal cough
aneurysmal dilatation
aneurysmal hematoma
aneurysmal phthisis
aneurysmal rupture, contained
aneurysmal sac, wrapped
aneurysmal varix
aneurysmal wall, sliver of
aneurysm cavity
aneurysm clipping
aneurysmectomy
  apicoseptal
  left ventricular
aneurysmoplasty, Matas
aneurysmorrhaphy, popliteal artery
aneurysm resection
ANF (atrial natriuretic factor)
AngeLase combined mapping-laser
  probe
Angell-Shiley bioprosthetic valve

Angell-Shiley xenograft prosthetic
  valve
Angelman syndrome
angel wing sign
AngeMed Sentinel ICD device
Anger-type scintillation camera
angiitis
  hypersensitivity
  necrotizing
  necrotizing granulomatous
angina (angina pectoris)
  accelerated
  atypical
  bandlike
  chronic stable
  classic
  clinical
  cold-induced
  coronary spastic
  coronary vasospastic
  crescendo
  crescendo-decrescendo
  de novo
  eating-induced
  effort
  emotional
  esophageal
  esophageal spasm mimicking
  excruciatingly painful
  exercise-induced
  exertional
  focal
  gradual onset of
  Heberden
  hypercyanotic
  intractable
  Ludwig
  new onset
  nocturnal
  pacing-induced
  post-AMI (acute myocardial
    infarction)

angina (cont.)
  postinfarction
  postprandial
  preinfarction
  Prinzmetal variant
  progressive
  recurrent
  refractory
  rest
  rest-related
  retrosternal heaviness with
  Rougnon-Heberden
  stable
  sudden onset of
  treadmill-induced
  typical
  typical effort
  unstable
  variable threshold
  variant
  vasomotor
  vasospastic
  vasotonic
  walk-through
angina after meals
angina at low work load
angina at rest
angina cordis
angina cruris
angina decubitus syndrome
angina, descriptions of
  brought on or precipitated by,
    anxiety
    cold weather
    eating a heavy meal
    emotional stress or upset
    exercise
    exertion
    exposure to cold
    heavy meals
    sexual intercourse
    smoking

angina *(cont.)*
 straining at the stool
 stress
 worry/anxiety
 burning feeling
 crushing chest pain
 elephant on chest feeling
 feeling of impending doom
 gradual onset
 heartburn-type feeling
 heaviness in chest
 indigestion-like feeling
 pinching chest pain
 precordial chest pain
 pressure-like sensation
 radiation down/into arm
 radiation down/into epigastrium
 radiation down/into fingers
 radiation down/into left arm
 radiation down/into scapula
 radiation up/into jaw
 radiation up/into left shoulder
 radiation up/into neck
 referred chest pain
 retrosternal burning; heaviness
 smothering sensation
 squeezing chest discomfort
 substernal burning
 sudden onset
 suffocating chest pain
 tightness of chest
angina equivalent
angina-equivalent dyspnea
angina intermedia syndrome
angina inversa
anginal episode
anginalike
anginal spell
anginal syndrome
angina of first effort
angina pectoris (see *angina*)

angina pectoris sine dolore
angina pectoris variant
angina precipitated by exertion
angina provoked by ergonovine
 maleate
angina relieved by rest
angina syndrome
angina unrelieved by nitroglycerin
angina vasomotoria
angina with recent increase in
 frequency
anginosa, syncope
anginosus, status
angiocardiographically
angiocardiography (see *angiogram*)
 ambulatory equilibrium
 equilibrium radionuclide
 first-pass radionuclide exercise
 gated equilibrium radionuclide
 transseptal
angiocatheter
 Deseret
 Eppendorf
 Mikro-tip
Angiocath PRN flexible catheter
Angio-Conray contrast medium
Angiocor prosthetic valve
angiodysplasia
angiodysplastic lesion
angioedema
 hereditary
 Milton
angiogram, -graphy
 (also angiocardiogram)
 adrenal
 aortic root
 balloon occlusion pulmonary
 biplane left ventricular
 biplane orthogonal
 blood-pool radionuclide
 Brown-Dodge method for

angiogram *(cont.)*
  cardiac
  carotid
  celiac
  cerebral
  cine
  contrast
  coronary
  digital subtraction pulmonary
  dobutamine thallium
  DSA (digital subtraction)
  electrocardiogram-synchronized
    digital subtraction
  equilibrium radionuclide
  first-pass nuclide rest and exercise
  first-pass radionuclide
  fluorescein
  gated blood pool
  gated nuclear
  gated radionuclide
  IDIS (intraoperative digital
    subtraction)
  intra-arterial DSA
  intravenous DSA
  Judkins coronary
  left ventricular
  mesenteric
  postangioplasty
  post-tourniquet occlusion
  PTCA coronary
  pulmonary
  pulmonary artery wedge
  pulmonary vein wedge
  pulmonary wedge
  radionuclide (RNA)
  rest and exercise gated nuclear
  selective coronary cine
  single plane
  sitting-up view
  transvenous digital subtraction
  ventricular

angiogram (or angiography) suite
angiographically occult vessel
angiography (see *angiogram*)
angiohemophilia
angioid streaks, retinal
angiokeratoma corporis diffusum
angiokeratoma corporis diffusum
  universale
Angio-Kit catheter
angiolithic degeneration
angioma arteriale racemosum
angioma cavernosum
angioma venosum racemosum
angiomata, spider
angiomatosis arteritis
Angiomedics catheter
angioneurotic edema
angio-osteohypertrophy syndrome
angiopathy, peripheral
angioplastiable
angioplasty
  balloon
  boot-strap two-vessel
  coronary artery
  coronary balloon
  Dotter-Judkins technique for
    percutaneous transluminal
  Gruentzig balloon catheter
  iliac artery
  LAIS excimer laser for coronary
  laser
  laser balloon
  laser thermal coronary
  laser-assisted balloon (LABA)
  microwave thermal balloon
  multilesion
  multivessel
  one-vessel
  patch
  patch-graft
  percutaneous laser

angioplasty *(cont.)*
  percutaneous transluminal (PTA)
  percutaneous transluminal coronary
    (PTCA)
  peripheral
  peripheral laser (PLA)
  single-vessel
  supported
  synthetic patch
  transluminal
  transluminal balloon
  transluminal coronary artery
  vein patch
angioplasty catheter, high-speed
  rotation dynamic
angioplasty laser, Lastec System
angioplasty sheath
angioplasty technique, Gruentzig
angioreticuloendothelioma of heart
angiosarcoma, cavernous
angiosarcoma of heart
angioscope
  flexible
  Mitsubishi
  Olympus
angioscope for in situ bypass
angioscopy
  fiberoptic
  percutaneous intracoronary
angiotensin-converting enzyme (ACE)
  inhibitor
angiotensin II antagonist
angiotripsy
angle
  cardiodiaphragmatic
  cardiohepatic
  cardiophrenic
  costal
  costophrenic
  duodenojejunal
  Ebstein

angle *(cont.)*
  infrasternal
  Louis
  Ludovici
  Ludwig
  nail-to-nailbed (clubbing)
  phase
  phrenopericardial
  Pirogoff
  QRST
  sternal
  sternoclavicular
  substernal
  venous
  xiphoid
angled pleural tube
angle of the jaw, jugular venous
  distention to the
angor pectoris (variant of angina
  pectoris)
angry appearance
angulated lesion
angulated segment
anhidrosis
Anichkov (or Anitschkow)
Anichkov cell
Anichkov myocyte
Animal House fever
anion gap (AG)
anisotropic reentry
anisoylated plasminogen streptokinase
  activator complex (APSAC)
anistreplase thrombolysis
ankle-arm index (AAI)
ankle-brachial index (ABI)
ankle-brachial systolic pressure index
ankle swelling
ankylosing spondylitis
anniversary phenomenon
annular abscess
annular calcification

annular cartilage, bronchial
annular constriction
annular dilatation
annular disruption
annular foreshortening
annular fracture
annular hypoplasia
annular placement of sutures
annular plication
annuli fibrosi cordis
annuloaortic ectasia
annulocuspid hinge
annuloplasty or anuloplasty
   anterior
   Carpentier
   De Vega
   Kay
   mitral
   patch graft
   prosthetic ring
   septal
   subcommissural suture
   tricuspid valve
   Wooler
annuloplasty ring
   Puig Massana-Shiley
   Sculptor flexible
annulorrhaphy
annulus or anulus
   aortic valve
   atrioventricular
   calcified
   friable
   mitral; mitral valve
   pulmonary
   pulmonary valve
   redundant scallop of posterior
   septal tricuspid
   tricuspid valve
   valve
annulus fibrosus
annulus ovalis

annulus overriding the ventricular
   septum
annulus plication
anodal block
anodal patch electrode, anterior
anode, transvenous
anomalous accessory pathway
anomalous atrioventricular conduction
   pathways
anomalous atrioventricular excitation
anomalous conduction
anomalous distribution
anomalous drainage
anomalous origin of left coronary
   artery
anomalous pathway
anomalous pulmonary artery and
   vascular sling
anomalous pulmonary origin of the
   coronary artery
anomalous pulmonary venous
   connection
      partial
      total
anomalous pulmonary venous drainage
anomalous pulmonary venous return
anomalous retroesophageal right
   subclavian artery
anomalous vein of scimitar syndrome
anomalous vessel
anomaly
   aortic arch
   cardiac
   congenital cardiac
   conotruncal congenital
   cutaneous vascular
   Ebstein
   extracardiac
   Freund
   May-Hegglin
   Shone
   Taussig-Bing

anomaly *(cont.)*
  tricuspid valve
  Uhl
anorexia
anoxia
  altitude
  cerebral
anoxic arrest
ANP (atrial natriuretic polypeptide)
Anrep effect
ansa subclavia
antacids, relieved by
antagonist
  angiotensin II
  beta
  calcium
  calcium channel
antagonist therapy, vitamin K
antecedent history
antecubital approach for cardiac
  catheterization
antecubital approach for catheter
  insertion
antecubital fossa
antecubital fossa cutdown
antecubital space
antecubital vein
antegrade (forward)
antegrade blood flow
antegrade conduction
antegrade fashion, catheter advanced in
antegrade fast pathway
antegrade filling of vessels
antegrade flow
antegrade perfusion
antegrade refractory period
antemortem clot
anterior annuloplasty (Konno
  procedure)
anterior anodal patch electrode
anterior aorta transposition of great
  arteries

anterior aortic sinus
anterior axillary line
anterior basal bronchi
anterior basal segment
anterior border of lung
anterior border of sternocleidomastoid
  muscle
anterior bowing of sternum
anterior bronchi
anterior cardiac vein
anterior chest wall syndrome
anterior chest wall thrombophlebitis
anterior commissure
anterior coronary plexus (of heart)
anterior cusp
anterior descending artery, superdominant left
anterior fascicular block
anterior inferior communicating artery
  (AICA)
anterior intercostal artery
anterior internodal pathway
anterior internodal tract of Bachman
anterior interventricular groove
anterior leaflet prolapse
anterior magna, arteria radicularis
anterior mediastinal compartment
anterior mediastinum
anterior mitral valve leaflet
anterior motion
  palpable
  visible
anterior motion of posterior mitral
  valve leaflet
anterior papillary muscle
anterior parasternal motion, sustained
anterior/posterior (AP)
anterior pulmonary plexus
anterior rectus sheath divided
  transversely
anterior semilunar valve
anterior septal myocardial infarction

anterior table
anterior tracheal displacement
anterior wall dyskinesis
anterior wall myocardial infarction
anteroapical wall myocardial infarction
anterograde conduction
anterolateral incision
anterolateral muscle-sparing lateral
  thoracotomy
anterolateral wall myocardial infarction
anteroposterior diameter
anteroseptal commissure
anteroseptal wall myocardial infarction
anteverted nares
anthelminthic therapy
anthracosilicosis
anthracosis
anthracyclines
anthraquinones
anthrocotic tuberculosis
Anthron heparinized antithrombogenic
  catheter
antiadrenergic agent
antiaggregant, platelet
antianginal agent
antianginal drug
antianginal therapy
antiarrhythmia agent
antiarrhythmic drugs, classes I-V
antiarrhythmics
antibacterial therapy
antibiotic
  perioperative
  postoperative
  preoperative
  prophylactic
  quinolone
antibiotic solution
antibiotic therapy
antibody, antibodies
  anticardiolipin (aCL)
  antimyosin

antibody *(cont.)*
  antimyosin monoclonal (with Fab
    fragment) (AMA-Fab)
  antinuclear (ANA)
  antiphospholipid
  heterophile
  IgM anti-human parvovirus
  indium
  indium-labeled antimyosin
  OKT3 monoclonal
  monoclonal
  polyclonal anticardiac myosin
  precipitating
  7E3 monoclonal antiplatelet
  sheep antidigoxin Fab
  SS-A (Ro)
  SS-B (La)
  teichoic acid
  whole blood monoclonal
antibody-antigen complex
anticardiolipin (aCL) antibody
anticoagulant
  coumarin-type
  hirudin (recombinant desulfato-
    hirudin)
  oral
anticoagulant drugs
anticoagulant prophylaxis
anticoagulant therapy
anticoagulation
  long-term
  oral
  systemic heparin
anticoronary diet
antidepressants, tricyclic
antidiuretic hormone (ADH)
antiDNAse B
antidromic AV (atrioventricular)
  reciprocating tachycardia
antidromic circus movement
  tachycardia
antidromic conduction

antidromic tachycardia
antiembolic stockings
antifibrin antibody imaging
antifibrinolytic drugs
antifiliarial drug
antigen
    Aspergillus
    autogenous
    histocompatibility
    HLA-B27
    human leukocyte, B27
    serum cryptococcal
antigen challenge, nasal
antihemophilic blood coagulation factor
antihemophilic globulin (AHG)
antihistamines
antihyperlipidemic drug
antihypertensive drug
antihypertensive therapy
anti-inflammatory drug
anti-ischemic
antilymphocyte globulin
antimicrobial drugs
antimicrobial therapy
antimony
antimyosin antibodies
antineutrophilic cytoplasmic antibody
antinuclear antibody (ANA)
antiphospholipid (aPL) antibody
antiphospholipid syndrome (APS)
antiplatelet agent
antiplatelet drug
antirejection regimen
antiseptic drug
antispasmodic drug
antistreptolysin O
antitachycardia pacemaker
antitachycardia pacing therapy
antithrombin III (ATnativ)
antithrombin III antigen
antithrombin III deficiency

antithymocyte globulin
antitubercular
antituberculosis drugs
antitussives
antiviral drugs
antiviral therapy
antritis, acute
Antyllus method
anuloplasty (see *annuloplasty*)
anulus, anular (see *annulus*)
anuria
anxiety and insomnia
anxiety, profound
anxiolytic
anxious
Ao, AO (aorta)
AO (aortic opening)
AO/AC (aortic valve opening/aortic
    valve closing) ratio
AOC (aortic opening click)
aorta
    abdominal
    arch of
    ascending (AA)
    biventricular origin of
    biventricular transposed
    calcified
    central
    cervical
    coarctation of
    coarcted
    cross-clamping of
    D-malposition of
    descending
    descending thoracic
    dextroposed
    dextropositioned
    double-barreled
    dynamic
    elongation of
    incision of

aorta *(cont.)*
  infrarenal abdominal
  kinked
  L-malposition
  overriding
  palpable
  pericardial
  porcelain
  preductal coarctation of
  recoarctation of the
  reconstruction of
  root of
  sclerosis of
  small feminine
  supraceliac
  supradiaphragmatic
  terminal
  thoracic
  thoracoabdominal
  transposed
  unwinding of
  ventral
aorta abdominalis
aorta ascendens
aorta clamped cephalad to aneurysm
aorta idiopathic necrosis
aorta-iliac-femoral bypass
aorta-renal bypass
aorta sacrococcygea
aorta-subclavian-carotid bypass
aorta-to-vein anastomosis
aortic allograft
aortic anastomosis
aortic annular region
aortic annulus
aortic arch
  congenital interruption of
  double
  penetrating injury to
aortic arch anomaly
aortic arch arteritis
aortic arch atresia

aortic arch calcification-osteoporosis-
  tooth-buds hypoplasia syndrome
aortic arch hypoplasia syndrome
aortic arch interruption
aortic arch lesion
aortic arch obstruction
aortic arch syndrome
aortic arteritis
aortic atherosclerosis
  juxtarenal
  pararenal
aortic atresia
aortic bifurcation
aortic bifurcation graft, Edwards
  woven Teflon
aortic bifurcation syndrome
aortic bulb
aortic "button" technique
aortic cannulation
aortic cartilage
aortic clamp
aortic closure (AC)
aortic coarctation, juxtaductal
aortic coarctation-related hypertension
aortic coarctation syndrome
aortic component of murmur
aortic configuration of cardiac shadow
  on x-ray
aortic cross-clamp
aortic cusp
  perforated
  ruptured
aortic cusps' separation
aortic diameter (AD)
aortic diastolic murmur
aortic dilatation
aortic dissection
  DeBakey classification of
  thoracic
  type B
aortic ejection click (AEC)
aortic ejection sound, palpable

aortic elongation
aortic hiatus
aortic homograft
aortic impedance
aortic incisura
aortic incompetence
aortic insufficiency (AI)
aortic insult
aortic isthmus, hypoplasia of
aortic knob, blurring of
aortic knob contour
aortic knuckle
aortic leaflets, redundant
aortic-left ventricular pressure
    difference
aortic-left ventricular tunnel
aortic nipple sign
aortic opening (AO)
aortic opening click (AOC)
aorticopulmonary anastomosis
aorticopulmonary defect
aorticopulmonary septal defect
aorticopulmonary shunt
aorticopulmonary trunk
aorticopulmonary window
aorticopulmonary window operation
aortic orifice
aortic override
aortic oxygen saturation
aortic paravalvular leak
aortic pressure
aortic pseudoaneurysm
aortic pullback
aortic-pulmonary shunt
aortic regurgitation (AR)
    congenital
    massive
    syphilitic
aortic resection
aortic root angiogram
aortic root dilatation

aortic root, dilated
aortic root enlargement
aortic root homograft
aortic root perfusion needle
aortic root pressure
aortic root ratio
aortic root replacement
aortic run-off
aortic rupture
aortic second sound
aortic segment
    intradiaphragmatic
    intramuscular
aortic shag
aortic sinus
aortic sinus aneurysm
aortic sinus to right ventricle fistula
aortic sound
aortic spindle
aortic stenosis (AS)
    calcific
    congenital
    congenital subvalvular
    congenital valvular
    hypercalcemia-supravalvular
    supravalvar
    supravalvular (SAS, SVAS)
    uncomplicated supraclavicular
aortic stenosis secondary to bicuspid
    aortic valve
aortic stiffness
aortic stump blow-out
aortic subvalvular ring
aortic-superior mesenteric bypass
aortic systolic murmur
aortic thrill
aortic thromboembolism
aortic thrombosis, terminal
aortic tract complex
aortic tract complex hypoplasia
aortic transection, traumatic

aortic tube graft
aortic valve
  bicommissural
  bicuspid
  composite
  native
  unicommissural
aortic valve annulus
aortic valve area
aortic valve atresia
aortic valve calcification
aortic valve disease
aortic valve endocarditis
aortic valve incompetence
aortic valve insufficiency
aortic valve leaflet
aortic valve obstruction
aortic valve pressure gradient
aortic valve prosthesis (see *prosthesis*)
aortic valve regurgitation
aortic valve repair
aortic valve replacement (AVR)
aortic valve stenosis
  acquired
  congenital
aortic valve thickening
aortic valvotomy, closed transventricular
aortic valvular incompetence
aortic valvular insufficiency
aortic valvulotomy
aortic vasa vasorum
aortic vent suction line
aortic vestibule
aortic vestibule of ventricle
aortic window node
aortic wrap
aortitis
  Döhle-Heller (or Doehle)
  giant cell
  luetic
  nummular

aortitis *(cont.)*
  rheumatic
  syphilitic
  Takayasu
aortoarteritis (types I-IV)
  nonspecific
  nonspecific inflammatory
aortobifemoral bypass graft
aortobifemoral reconstruction
aortobiprofunda bypass graft
aortocarotid bypass
aortocaval fistula
aortoceliac bypass
aortocoronary saphenous vein bypass
  graft
aortocoronary snake graft
aortocoronary valve
aortoduodenal
aortoenteric
aortoenteric fistula
aortoesophageal
aortofemoral arteriography with
  run-off views
aortofemoral bypass graft (AFBG)
aortogastric
aortogram or aortography
  abdominal
  arch
  biplanar
  contrast
  digital subtraction supravalvular
  flush
  retrograde
  retrograde femoral
  retrograde transaxillary
  supravalvular
  thoracic
  thoracic arch
  translumbar
  ultrasonic
aortogram with distal runoff
aortoiliac aneurysm

aortoiliac bypass
aortoiliac disease
aortoiliac obstruction
aortoiliac obstructive disease (AIOD)
aortoiliac occlusive disease
aortoiliac thrombosis
aortoiliac-popliteal bypass
aortoiliofemoral arteries
aortoiliofemoral bypass
aortoiliofemoral endarterectomy
aortomegaly, diffuse
aorto-ostial "Y" saphenous vein graft
aorto-ostium
aortopathy, idiopathic medial
aortoplasty
    balloon
    patch-graft
    posterior patch
    subclavian flap
aortoplasty with patch graft
aortopopliteal bypass
aortopulmonary anastomosis
aortopulmonary collaterals
aortopulmonary fistula
aortopulmonary shunt
aortopulmonary tunnel
aortopulmonary window
aortopulmonary window operation
aortorrhaphy
aortosclerosis
aortotome, Goosen
aortotomy
    circular
    curvilinear
    longitudinal
    transverse
    trapdoor-type
aortovelography, transcutaneous (TAV)
aortoventriculoplasty
AoV (aortic valve)
Ap (apical)
AP (accessory pathway)

AP (anterior/posterior)
APA (aldosterone-producing adenoma)
APB (atrial premature beat)
APC (atrial premature complex)
APC (atrial premature contraction)
APD (action potential duration)
Apert syndrome
aperture
apex (pl. apices)
    cardiac
    displaced left ventricular
    heart
    left ventricular
    lung
    systolic retraction of
    uptilted cardiac
apex beat
apexcardiogram, -graphy (ACG)
apex cordis (of heart)
apex of heart
apex of Koch triangle
apex of left ventricle
apex of lung
apex of ventricle
apex pulse, absent
apheresis of autoantibodies
apheresis of cold precipitable serum
    proteins
apheresis of erythrocytes
apheresis of leukocyte fractions
apheresis of plasma
apheresis of platelets
aphonic pectoriloquy
API (ankle-arm pressure index)
apical air space (on x-ray)
apical and subcostal four-chambered
    view
apical aortic valved conduit
apical beat, displaced
apical beat displacement, inferolateral
apical cap sign
apical four-chamber view

apical hypertrophic cardiomyopathy
apical hypoperfusion on thallium scan
apical impulse
    absent
    double systolic
    downward displacement
    hyperdynamic
    sustained
apical impulse displaced to the left
apical infiltrate
apical-lateral wall myocardial
    infarction
apical midsystolic click
apical posterior artery
apical posterolateral region of left
    ventricle
apical pulse
apical scar
apical scarring
apical segment
apical short-axis slice
apical surface of heart
apical thrust
apical tissue
apical two-chamber view
apical window
apices (pl. of apex)
apicoabdominal bypass
apicoaortic (abdominal) conduit
apicoaortic shunt
apicoaortic valved conduit
apicoposterior bronchi
apicoseptal aneurysmectomy
aPL (antiphospholipid) antibody
aplasia
    red cell
    right ventricular myocardial
aplasia of the deep veins
aplastic anemia
APM (anterior papillary muscle)
apnea
    central
    idiopathic obstructive sleep

apnea *(cont.)*
    obstructive sleep
    transient
apnea/hypopnea index (AHI)
apneic episodes, intermittent
apneustic breathing
Apo A1 LDL-cholesterol subfraction
Apo A2 LDL-cholesterol subfraction
Apo B LDL-cholesterol subfraction
Apogee CX 200 echo system (ablation)
A point
apolipoprotein
aponeurosis, bicipital
apoplectiform
apoplexy
    pulmonary artery
    pulmonary vein
apoprotein (A-E)
apparatus
    breathing
    enlarged valve
    mitral
    tensor
    valvular
appearance
    angry
    beavertail (of balloon profile)
    bullneck
    coarse
    cobra-head
    cushingoid
    fine-speckled
    fish-flesh
    Florence flask
    frondlike
    ground-glass
    heterogeneous
    homogeneous
    lobulated saccular
    plucked chicken
    reticulogranular
    shocky
    string-of-beads

appearance *(cont.)*
 toxic
 trilayer
 whorled
appearance and exclusion, normal
appendage
 atrial
 left atrial (LAA)
 right atrial (RAA)
 truncated atrial
 wide-based blunt-ended right-sided
  atrial
applesauce sign
appliance, removable Herbst
appose
apposition
apposition of leaflets
apprehension
apprehensive
approach
 axillofemoral
 brachial
 cephalic
 deltopectoral
 external jugular
 femoral venous
 femorofemoral
 groin
 internal jugular
 left subcostal
 median sternotomy
 percutaneous transfemoral
 retrograde femoral arterial
 retroperitoneal
 subclavicular
 subcostal
 subxiphoid
 thoracoabdominal
 transaortic
 transatrial
 transdiaphragmatic
 transpectoral

approach *(cont.)*
 transperitoneal
 transthoracic
 transtricuspid
 transvenous
 transventricular
 transxiphoid pacemaker lead
 umbilical venous
approximate, loosely
approximated
approximation
approximator
 Lemmon sternal
 Pilling Wolvek sternal
 rib
 Wolvek sternal
APSAC (anisoylated plasminogen
 streptokinase activator complex)
APTT (activated partial thromboplastin
 time)
Apt test
APUD (amine precursor uptake and
 decarboxylation) cell
apudoma
AR (atrial rate)
AR (aortic regurgitation)
arachidonic acid cascade
araldehyde-tanned bovine carotid
 artery graft
araneus, nevus
Arani double loop guiding catheter
Arantii, ductus
Arantius body
Arantius canal
arborization, Purkinje
arc
ARC (argon beam electrocoagulator)
 laser
arcade
 mitral
 septal
arcade of collaterals

arch
 aortic
 bifid aortic
 distal aortic
 double aortic
 hypoplastic
 mid aortic
 right aortic
 right-sided
 transverse
 transverse aortic
 Zimmerman
arch and carotid arteriography
arch hypoplasia
Archer syndrome
arching of mitral valve leaflet
architecture
 lung
 mural
arch of aorta
arch repair, concomitant
Arco pacemaker
Arco lithium pacemaker
arcuate arteries
arcuate vessels
arcus, corneal
arcus senilis
arc welder's lung
ARDS (adult respiratory distress
 syndrome)
ARE (acute rheumatic endocarditis)
area
 aortic
 aortic valve (AVA)
 arrhythmogenic
 artery
 Bamberger
 body surface (BSA)
 cardiac frontal
 cross-sectional (CSA)
 echo-free
 effective balloon dilated (EBDA)

area *(cont.)*
 Erb
 hilar
 luminal cross-sectional
 midsternal
 mitral valve (MVA)
 perihilar
 peroneal
 pulmonic
 sonolucent
 stenosis
 subglottic
 tricuspid
 valve
area-length method for ejection fraction
areas of denudation
areolar tissue
ARF (acute respiratory failure)
ARF (acute rheumatic fever)
arginine vasopressin
argon laser
Argyle chest tube
Argyle Sentinel Seal chest tube
Argyle Turkel safety thoracentesis
 system
Argyll Robertson pupils
arm ergometry stress test
armour heart
arm-to-tongue time
Army-Navy retractor
Arneth syndrome
arousal, episodic
ARP (absolute refractory period)
ARP (acute rheumatic pericarditis)
array electrode
arrest
 anoxic
 asystolic cardiac
 bradyarrhythmic cardiac
 cardiac
 cardioplegic
 cardiopulmonary

arrest *(cont.)*
  cardiorespiratory
  circulatory
  cold cardioplegia
  cold potassium solution-induced
    cardiac
  deep hypothermic circulatory
  electrical circulatory
  heart
  hypothermic
  hypothermic circulatory
  hypothermic fibrillating
  intermittent sinus
  profound hypothermic circulatory
    (PHCA)
  recurrent cardiac
  respiratory
  sinus
  transient sinus
arrested circulation
arrhythmia
  atrioventricular junctional
  AV (atrioventricular) nodal
    Wenckebach
  baseline
  complex atrial
  continuous
  drug-refractory
  exercise-aggravated
  exercise-induced
  extrasystolic
  high-density ventricular
  inducible
  intermittent
  juvenile
  lethal
  life-threatening
  malignant
  malignant ventricular
  nodal
  nonlethal
  nonrespiratory sinus

arrhythmia *(cont.)*
  pacing-induced termination of
  paroxysmal supraventricular
  perpetual
  phasic
  postmalignant
  postperfusion
  reentrant
  reperfusion
  respiratory sinus
  sinus
  spontaneous
  stress-related
  supraventricular
arrhythmia circuit
arrhythmia classification
arrhythmia detection
arrhythmia focus
arrhythmia-induced syncope
Arrhythmia Net arrhythmia monitor
arrhythmogenic area of ventricle
arrhythmogenic area in myocardium
arrhythmogenic border zone
arrhythmogenic disease
arrhythmogenic right ventricular
  cardiomyopathy
arrhythmogenic right ventricular
  dysplasia (ARVD) syndrome
arrhythmogenic scar
arrhythmogenic site
arrhythmogenic ventricular activity
  (AVA)
Arrow-Berman balloon angioplasty
  catheter
ArrowGard Blue Line catheter
ArrowGard central venous catheter
arrowhead-shaped
Arrow-Howes multilumen catheter
Arrow pneumothorax kit
Arrow pulmonary artery catheter
Arrow Twin Cath multilumen
  peripheral catheter

arteria anastomotica magna
arterial-alveolar CO_2 tension difference
arterial aneurysm
arterial avulsion
arterial blood gases (ABGs) (see
   blood gas)
arterial blood gases on 100% oxygen
arterial blood gases on room air
arterial blood pressure (BP)
arterial brachiocephalic trunk
arterial bruit, interscapulovertebral
arterial cannula, peripheral
arterial cannulation
arterial capillaries
arterial circulation
arterial cutoff
arterial degenerative disease
arterial dilatation and rupture
arterial embolectomy catheter
arterial endothelium
arterial fibromuscular dysplasia
arterial fibromuscular hyperplasia
arterial gradient
arterial hyperemia
arterial hypertension
arterial hypocarbia
arterial hypoplasia
arterial hypoxemia
arterial hypoxia
arterial intima, diffuse thickening of
arterial ischemia index
arterialization of venous blood
arterial line (A-line)
arterial lumen
arterial malformation (AM)
arterial obstruction
arterial oxygen content
arterial oxygen saturation (SaO_2)
arterial oxygen unsaturation
arterial partial pressure of CO_2
   (mm Hg) ($PaCO_2$)

arterial partial pressure of O_2 (mm Hg)
   (PaO_2)
arterial patency
arterial peak systolic pressure
arterial pressure
arterial pulsation
arterial recoil
arterial return, central
arterial runoff
arterial rupture and dilatation
arterial sclerosis
arterial segment
arterial sheath
arterial spasm
arterial spasm adjacent to plaque
arterial steal
arterial supply of parietal pleura
arterial switch operation
arterial thrombosis
arterial topography
arterial tree
arteria lusoria
arteria magna
arterial varices
arterial wall dynamics
arterial wall thickness, preacinar
arterial wedge pressure, pulmonary
arteria radicularis anterior magna
arterio-arterial anastomosis
arteriocapillary sclerosis
arteriogram, -graphy
   aorta and runoff
   aortofemoral (with run-off views)
   arch
   balloon occlusion
   biplane pelvic
   biplane quantitative coronary
   bronchial
   carotid
   celiac
   cine

arteriogram *(cont.)*
  coronary
  delayed phase of
  intraoperative
  Judkins selective coronary
  left coronary cine
  thrombotic pulmonary (TPA)
arteriolar sclerosis
arterioplasty
arteriorenal
arteriosclerosis
  calcific
  cerebral
  coronary
  generalized
  hyaline
  hypertensive
  intimal
  infantile
  intimal
  medial
  Mönckeberg (Moenckeberg)
  obliterative
  peripheral
  presenile
  pulmonary
  senile
arteriosclerosis obliterans (ASO)
arteriosclerotic cardiovascular disease
  (ASCVD)
arteriosclerotic dementia
arteriosclerotic deposits
arteriosclerotic heart disease (ASHD)
arteriosclerotic lining of narrowed
  arteries
arteriosclerotic peripheral vascular
  disease
arteriosclerotic plaques
arteriostenosis
arteriosubmammary incision

arteriosum, ligamentum
arteriosus
  persistent truncus
  pseudotruncus
  true truncus
  truncus
arteriotomy
  brachial
  longitudinal
  transverse
arteriovenous (AV)
arteriovenous aneurysm
arteriovenous fistula (AVF), coronary
arteriovenous fistula of lung
arteriovenous malformation (AVM)
arteriovenous microshunt
arteriovenous nicking
arteriovenous oxygen content
  difference
arteriovenous oxygen difference
  (AVD O$_2$)
  pulmonary
  systemic
arteriovenous pressure gradient
arteriovenous shunt defects
arteriovenous varix
arteritis
  acute
  aortic
  aortic arch
  brachiocephalic
  cerebral
  coronary
  cranial
  giant cell
  granulomatous
  Horton giant cell
  infantile
  infectious
  innominate artery

arteritis *(cont.)*
  localized visceral
  necrotizing
  obliterative
  para-arterial angiomatosis
  pulmonary
  rheumatic
  supra-aortic Takayasu
  syphilitic
  Takayasu
  temporal
  tuberculous
  young female aortic arch
arteritis obliterans
arteritis umbilicalis
artery, arteries (see also branch)
  Abbott
  aberrant coronary
  aberrant left pulmonary
  Adamkiewicz
  anomalous origin of
  anterior descending branch of left
    coronary
  anterior inferior communicating
    (AICA)
  aortoiliofemoral
  apical posterior
  arcuate
  atrioventricular node
  AV (atrioventricular) nodal
  beading of
  brachial
  brachiocephalic
  calcified
  celiac
  cerebral
  circumflex (circ, CF, CX)
  coronary
  circumflex groove
  common carotid (CCA)
  common femoral
  common iliac

artery *(cont.)*
  conus
  corduroy
  coronary
  descending septal
  diagonal branch of
  diagonal branch of left anterior
    descending coronary
  diagonal coronary
  dilated
  distal circumflex marginal
  dominant coronary
  dominant left coronary
  dominant right coronary
  Drummond marginal
  eccentric coronary
  epicardial coronary
  external carotid
  external iliac
  familial fibromuscular dysplasia of
  first diagonal branch
  first obtuse marginal
  gastroepiploic
  high left main diagonal
  hilar
  hypogastric
  inferior mesenteric
  infragenicular popliteal
  infrageniculate
  innominate
  intercostal
  intermediate coronary
  internal carotid (ICA)
  internal iliac
  internal mammary (IMA)
  internal thoracic
  intraacinar pulmonary
  Kugel
  LAD (left anterior descending)
    coronary
  LCA (left coronary)
  LCF or LCX (left circumflex)

artery *(cont.)*
   left anterior descending
   left circumflex coronary
   left common femoral
   left coronary (LCA)
   left internal mammary (LIMA)
   left main coronary (LMCA)
   left pulmonary (LPA)
   LIMA (left internal mammary)
   LMCA (left main coronary)
   main pulmonary (MPA)
   mainstem coronary
   mammary
   marginal branch of left circumflex
     coronary
   marginal branch of right coronary
   marginal circumflex
   medial plantar
   musculophrenic
   native coronary
   obtuse marginal (OM) coronary
   overriding great
   PDA (posterior descending)
   perforating
   peripancreatic
   peroneal
   phrenic
   pipestem
   plaque-containing
   popliteal
   posterior descending (PDA)
   posterior descending branch of
     right coronary
   posterior descending coronary
   posterior inferior communicating
     (PICA)
   posterior intercostal
   profunda femoris
   proximal anterior descending
   proximal left anterior descending
   proximal popliteal
   pulmonary (PA)

artery *(cont.)*
   radicular
   ramus intermedius
   ramus medialis
   reperfused
   resilient
   retroesophageal right subclavian
   right coronary (RCA)
   right femoral
   right pulmonary (RPA)
   right ventricular branch of right
     coronary
   septal perforator
   sinoatrial node
   sinus nodal
   stenotic coronary
   subclavian
   subcostal
   superficial femoral (SFA)
   superior epigastric
   superior genicular
   superior intercostal
   superior mesenteric
   superior thyroid
   temporal
   thyroid
   truncal
   vertebral
   weakened
artery (arterial) patency
artery system, iliac
artery takeoff
artery-vein-nerve bundle
arthralgias and myalgias
arthritis
   acute rheumatic
   chronic post-rheumatic fever
   Jaccoud
   rheumatoid
   subacute rheumatic
arthropathy-camptodactyly syndrome
articular capsule

articular rheumatism
articulation of thorax
artifact
  acoustic
  attenuation
  baseline
  catheter
  catheter impact
  catheter tip motion
  catheter tip position
  catheter whip
  end-pressure
  linear
  mirror image
  mosaic
  motion
  muscle
  pacemaker
  pacing
artifact due to body contour orbit
artifact due to partial volume effect
artifact image
artifacts mimicking intimal flaps
artifactual
artificial blood
  Fluosol plasma expander
  100% O_2 + fluorocarbons
  recombinant hemoglobin (rHb1.1)
  SFHB (stroma-free hemoglobin,
    pyridoxilated)
artificial cardiac pacemaker
artificial cardiac valve
artificial heart (see also *heart*)
  air-driven
  Akutsu III total (TAH)
  ALVAD (intra-abdominal left
    ventricular assist device)
  Baylor total
  electromechanical
  Jarvik VII or Jarvik-7
  Liotta total (TAH)

artificial heart *(cont.)*
  Symbion J-7 70-mL ventricle
  Symbion Jarvik-7
  University of Akron
  Utah total (TAH)
artificial left ventricular assist device
  (LVAD)
artificial lung
artificial lung-expanding compound
  (ALEC)
artificial lung, IVOX (intravascular
  oxygenator)
artificial pacemaker
artificial pneumothorax
artificial respiration
artificial ventilation
AR 2 diagnostic guiding catheter
ARVD (arrhythmogenic right ventricular dysplasia)
Arvidsson dimension-length method
  for ventricular volume
Arzco pacemaker
Arzco TAPSUL pill electrode
AS (aortic stenosis)
ASA (American Society of Anesthesia)
  risk classification (I-IV)
ASA (asthma, nasal polyps, aspirin)
  triad
asbestos
asbestos bodies
asbestos exposure
asbestos-induced pleural fibrosis
asbestosis
asbestos pleural plaques
asbestos-related pleural disease
Ascaris infection
Ascaris lumbricoides infection
Ascaris suum infection
ASCD (aborted sudden cardiac death)
ascending aneurysm replacement
ascending aorta (AA)

ascending aorta-abdominal aorta
bypass graft
ascending aorta hypoplasia
ascending aortic aneurysm
ascending contrast phlebography
ascending hypoplasia of aorta
ascending phlebography
ascertain, ascertained
Aschner phenomenon
Aschoff body
Aschoff cell
Aschoff node
Aschoff nodules
Aschoff-Tawara node
ascites, chylous
ascites, massive
ascorbate dilution curve
ASCVD (arterio- or atherosclerotic
cardiovascular disease)
ASD (atrial septal defect)
ASD, transcatheter occlusion of (with
button device)
aseptic myocarditis of newborn
aseptic technique
ASH (asymmetric septal hypertrophy)
ASHD (arteriosclerotic heart disease)
ashen
Ashman beat
Ashman index
Ashman phenomenon
Ask-Upmark kidney
ASM (atrial systolic murmur)
ASO (arteriosclerosis obliterans)
ASO (antistreptolysin-O) titer test
aspartate aminotransferase (AST)
aspartylglycosaminuria
aspergillosis, allergic broncho-
pulmonary
Aspergillus antigen
Aspergillus fumigatus
Aspergillus precipitins, serum
Aspergillus terreus

asphyxia, neonatal
asphyxial membrane
asphyxiating thoracic dystrophy
aspirate
aspirated acid vomitus
aspirated debris
aspirated foreign body
aspiration
anaerobic
CT-guided
foreign-body
percutaneous (of pericardial cyst)
percutaneous transthoracic
percutaneous transtracheal
pericardial fluid
pulmonary
tracheal
transtracheal
ultrasound-guided transthoracic
needle
aspiration biopsy
aspiration of air
aspiration of blood from pleural cavity
aspiration of foreign body
aspiration of pus from pleural cavity
aspiration of serous fluid from pleural
cavity
aspiration pneumonia
aspiration pneumonitis
aspirin challenge, inhalation
aspirin inhalation provocation
aspirin, prophylactic use of
aspirin therapy
aspirin-intolerant asthmatic
aspirin-precipitated asthma
aspirin-sensitive asthmatic
asplenia
ASPVD (atherosclerotic pulmonary
vascular disease)
assay (see also *test, analysis*)
endotoxin
enzyme-linked immunosorbent

assay *(cont.)*
   limulus amebocyte lysate
   three-antigen recombinant
      immunoblot
assessment
   invasive
   noninvasive
   regional wall motion
assist
   mechanical cardiac
   mechanial respiratory
assistance
   extracorporeal hepatic
   ventilatory
assisted breathing
assisted circulation
assisted ventilation
Assman focus
assumed Fick method for cardiac
   output
AST (aspartate aminotransferase)
asthenia
   neurocirculatory
   neuroregulatory
asthenic habitus
asthma
   abdominal
   allergic
   alveolar
   aspirin-intolerant
   atopic
   bacterial
   bronchial
   bronchitic
   cardiac
   cat
   catarrhal
   childhood
   cotton-dust
   cutaneous
   detergent
   diisocyanate

asthma *(cont.)*
   dust
   Elsner
   emphysematous
   eosinophilic
   essential
   exercise-induced
   extrinsic
   food
   grinder's
   hay
   Heberden
   horse
   humid
   hypercapnic acute
   infective
   intrinsic
   irritant-induced
   isocyanate
   Kopp
   late-onset
   Millar
   miller's
   miner's
   nasal
   nervous
   nocturnal
   nocturnal worsening of
   nonallergic
   occupational
   platinum
   pollen
   potter's
   red-cedar
   reflex
   refractory
   Rostan
   Sequoia (sequoiosis)
   sexual
   sodium-induced
   spasmodic
   steam-fitter's

asthma *(cont.)*
    stone
    stripper's
    symptomatic
    thymic
    true
    Wichmann
    wood
asthma attack caused by
    allergenic exposure to airborne
        pollens and molds
    allergenic exposure to animal
        danders
    allergenic exposure to house dust
    emotional upset
    exercise
    exposure to specific allergens
    inhalation of cigarette smoke
    inhalation of cold air
    inhalation of fresh paint
    inhalation of gasoline fumes
    inhalation of irritants
    inhalation of noxious odors
    nonspecific factors
    stress
    viral respiratory infection
asthma convulsivum
asthma crystals
asthma-like symptoms
asthma precipitated by aspirin
asthma precipitated by NSAIDs
asthmatic airways
asthmatic bronchitis
asthmatic crisis
asthmaticus, status
asthmatoid respirations
asthmatoid wheeze
Astra lab tests
Astra pacemaker
Astrand treadmill
ASTZ (antistreptozyme) test

ASVIP (atrial synchronous ventricular
    inhibited pacemaker)
asymmetric crying facies
asymmetric hypertrophy of septum
asymmetric pulmonary congestion
asymmetric septal hypertrophy (ASH)
asymmetrical thorax
asymmetry
    facial
    thoracic
asymptomatic
asynchronism
asynchronous pacemaker
asynchrony
asyneresis
asynergic myocardium
asynergy
    infarct-localized
    left ventricular
    regional
    segmental
asystole
    Beau
    cardiac
    complete atrial and ventricular
    ventricular
asystolic cardiac arrest
asystolic pauses
atactic breathing
ataxia
    Friedreich
    spinocerebellar
atelectasis
    absorption
    acquired
    acute
    acute massive
    apical
    basilar
    bibasilar discoid
    chronic

atelectasis *(cont.)*
  compression
  confluent areas of
  congenital
  congestive
  discoid
  disc-like
  initial
  lobar
  lobular
  lower pulmolnary lobe
  middle pulmonary lobe
  obstructive
  patchy
  perpetuation of
  platelike
  primary
  reabsorption
  relaxation
  resorption
  secondary
  segmental
  slowly developing
  subsegmental lower lobe
  upper pulmonary lobe
atelectasis treated by lobectomy
atelectasis treated by segmental
  resection
atelectatic lung
atelectatic rales
atherectomized vessel
atherectomy
  directional
  directional coronary
  percutaneous coronary rotational
    (PCRA)
  retrograde
  rotational
  rotational coronary
  transcutaneous extraction catheter
atherectomy catheter
atherectomy cutter

atherectomy device
  directional
  extraction
  PET balloon Simpson
  rotational
atherectomy technique
  double-wire
  kissing
AtheroCath, Simpson
atheroembolism
atherogenesis
atherogenic LDL cholesterol
atherolytic guide wire
atherolytic reperfusion guide wire
atheroma, coral reef
atheroma formation, exuberant
atheroma molding
atheromata
atheromatous cholesterol crystal
  embolization
atheromatous debris
atheromatous degeneration
atheromatous material
atheromatous embolism
atheromatous plaque
atheromatous plaque breakup by
  balloon catheter
atheromatous stenosis, femoropopliteal
athero-occlusive disease
atherosclerosis
  accelerated
  extracranial carotid artery
  fatty streak
  fibrous plaque
  intimal
  intracranial carotid artery
  juxtarenal aortic
  native
  pararenal aortic
  virulent
atherosclerosis obliterans
atherosclerotic aortic ulcer, penetrating

atherosclerotic cardiovascular disease
(ASCVD)
atherosclerotic carotid artery disease
(ACAD)
atherosclerotic debris
atherosclerotic fatty streaks
atherosclerotic gangrene
atherosclerotic narrowing
atherosclerotic occlusive syndrome
atherosclerotic plaque
atherosclerotic stenosis
atherothrombotic
atherothrombotic brain infarction
athletic heart
athrombia
ATL (anterior tricuspid leaflet)
Atlas LP PTCA balloon dilatation
catheter
Atlas ULP balloon dilatation catheter
atm. (atmospheres)
atmospheres of pressure
ATnativ (antithrombin III)
atopic asthma
atopy
ATP (adenosine triphosphate)
ATP (antitachycardia pacing)
ATPase
Atraloc needle
Atrauclip hemostatic clip
atraumatic Hasson grasper
atraumatic occlusion of vessels
atraumatic vascular clamp
atresia
    aortic
    aortic arch
    aortic valve
    choanal
    esophageal
    familial
    infundibular
    mitral
    mitral valve

atresia *(cont.)*
    pulmonary
    pulmonary valve
    pulmonary vein
    pulmonic
    tricuspid
    valvular
    ventricular
atresic
atretic
atria (pl. of atrium)
atria, situs ambiguus
atrial activation mapping, retrograde
atrial activation time
atrial appendage
atrial arrhythmia
atrial asynchronous pacemaker
atrial baffle
atrial capture
atrial cardioverter-defibrillator,
    implantable automatic
atrial compliance
atrial conduction
atrial couplets
atrial cuff
atrial demand inhibited pacemaker
atrial demand triggered pacemaker
atrial disk
atrial ectopic automatic tachycardia
atrial ectopy
atrial effective refractory period
atrial escape interval
atrial escape rhythm
atrial-femoral bypass
atrial fibrillation (AF)
    chronic
    hyperthyroidism-induced
    paroxysmal
atrial fibrillation with high-rate
    ventricular response
atrial fibrillation with rapid ventricular
    response

atrial flutter (AFl)
atrial focus
atrial gallop
atrial gallop rhythm
atrial gallop sound
atrial infarction
atrial irritability
atrial isomerism
atrialization
atrialized ventricle
atrial kick
atrial lead
atrial myocytes
atrial myxoma
atrial natriuretic factor (ANF)
atrial natriuretic peptide
atrial natriuretic polypeptide (ANP)
atrial overdrive pacing
atrial paced beat
atrial paced cycle length
atrial pacing
atrial pacing stress test
atrial pacing wire, temporary
atrial paroxysmal tachycardia (APT)
atrial partition
atrial premature complex (APC)
atrial premature contractions
atrial premature depolarizations
atrial rate (AR)
atrial reentrant PSVT (paroxysmal
   supraventricular tachycardia)
atrial reentry
atrial repolarization wave
atrial right-to-left shunting
atrial sensed event
atrial septal aneurysm
atrial septal defect (ASD)
atrial septal defect occlusion
   (buttoned device)
atrial septal defect with mitral stenosis
atrial septal umbrella
atrial septectomy

atrial septostomy
   balloon
   transcatheter knife blade
atrial septotomy, balloon
atrial septum
atrial single and double extrastimulation
atrial situs
atrial situs solitus
atrial sound
atrial standstill
atrial suture line
atrial synchronous ventricular
   pacemaker
atrial systole
atrial systolic murmur (ASM)
atrial thrombosis
atrial transposition
Atricor pacemaker
atriocaval junction
atriofascicular tract
atriography, negative contrast left
atrio-His bypass tract
atriohisian (atrio-Hisian)
atrio-Hisian bypass tract
atrio-Hisian fiber
atrio-His pathway
atrioplasty, V-Y
atriopulmonary patch
atrioseptoplasty
atriotomy orifice
atrioventricular (AV)
atrioventricular annulus
atrioventricular block
   congenital
   first-degree
   Mobitz classification of
   Mobitz I and II
   second-degree
   third-degree
atrioventricular bundle
atrioventricular canal

atrioventricular canal defects
atrioventricular concordance
atrioventricular concordant connection
atrioventricular conduction pathways
atrioventricular conduction system
atrioventricular delay
atrioventricular discordance
atrioventricular discordant connection
atrioventricular dissociation,
  isorhythmic
atrioventricular excitation, anomalous
atrioventricular groove
atrioventricular heart block
atrioventricular interval
atrioventricular junction
atrioventricular junctional escape beat
atrioventricular junctional escape junction
atrioventricular junctional pacemaker
atrioventricular junctional premature
  contraction
atrioventricular junctional rhythm
atrioventricular junctional tachycardia
atrioventricular nodal artery
atrioventricular nodal bypass tract
atrioventricular nodal conduction
atrioventricular nodal delay
atrioventricular nodal pathway
atrioventricular nodal reentrant PSVT
  (paroxysmal supraventricular
  tachycardia)
atrioventricular nodal reentry
  tachycardia (AVNRT)
atrioventricular nodal rhythm
atrioventricular nodal tachycardia
  (AVNT)
atrioventricular nodal Wenckebach
  arrhythmia
atrioventricular node artery
atrioventricular node conduction
  abnormality

atrioventricular node mesothelioma
atrioventricular node reentry
  tachycardia
atrioventricular orifice
atrioventricular ostium
atrioventricular reciprocating
  tachycardia
atrioventricular ring
atrioventricular septal defect
atrioventricular septum
atrioventricular sequential pacing
atrioventricular synchrony
atrioventricular tachycardia,
  reciprocating
atrioventricular time
atrioventricular valves (mitral and
  tricuspid)
atrioventriculare commune, ostium
Atri-pace I bipolar flared pacing
  catheter
atrium (pl. atria)
  common
  giant left
  high right
  left (LA)
  low septal right
  nontrabeculated
  oblique vein of left
  pulmonary
  right (RA)
  single
  thin-walled
  trabeculated
Atrium Blood Recovery System
atrium cordis
atrium dexter/sinister cordis
atrium pulmonale
atrium sinistrum
atrophic emphysema
atrophic rhinitis
atrophic thrombosis

atrophy
  alveolar
  brown
  lobular lung
  multiple system (MSA)
  vascular
atrophy of alveoli
atropine flush
atropine via endotracheal tube
attachment
  commissural
  intimate (of diseased vessel)
  vascular
attack
  Adams-Stokes
  heart
  Morgagni-Adams-Stokes
  Stokes-Adams
  syncopal
  transient ischemic (TIA)
  vagal
  vasovagal
attenuate
attenuated image
attenuation
  aortic
  breast
  expiratory
attenuation artifact (on x-ray)
attenuation by breast tissue
attenuation by hemidiaphragm
attenuation scan
atypical angina
atypical aortic valve stenosis
atypical chest pain
atypical coarctation
atypical interstitial pneumonia
atypical mycobacteriosis
atypical subisthmic coarctation
atypical tuberculosis infection
atypical verrucous endocarditis
audibility

audible breath sounds
audible expiratory splitting of S_2
audible splitting
audible S_3
audible wheezing
audible wheezing without a stethoscope
Auenbrugger sign
augment
augmentation
  inspiratory
  mechanical
  pressure
augmented bipolar limb leads
augmented cardiac output
augmented EKG leads
augmented filling of right ventricle
augmented stroke volume
augmented V waves
auricle
  left
  right
auricular rate
Aurora dual-chamber pacemaker
Aurora pulse generator
Ausculscope
auscultation and percussion
auscultation of lungs
auscultation, pulmonary
auscultatory cadence, rhythmic
auscultatory crackles
auscultatory findings
auscultatory gap
auscultatory sounds
Austin Flint murmur
Austin Flint phenomenon
Austin Flint respirations
Austin Flint rumble (murmur)
Autima II dual-chamber cardiac
  pacemaker
Autima II pacemaker
autoantibodies to phospholipid
autoclave

autoclaved, steam
autoclot
autoerythrocyte sensitization syndrome
autoerythrophagocytosis
autogenous antigen
autogenous blood transfusion
autogenous graft
autogenous saphenous vein graft
autograft
Autohaler, Maxair
autoimmune
autoimmune disorder
autoimmune hemolytic anemia (AIHA)
autoimmunity
autologous blood transfusion
autologous clot
autologous fibrin glue
autologous graft
autologous patch graft
autologous pericardium
autologous reversed vein graft
autologous vein graft
automated border detection by echocardiography
automatic atrial tachycardia
automatic external defibrillator (AED)
automatic implantable cardioverter defibrillator (AICD)
automatic implantable defibrillator (AID)
automatic interval limit
automatic mode switching (AMS) in pacemaker
automatic pacemaker
automatic tachycardia, atrial ectopic
automaticity
  enhanced
  pacemaker
  sinus node
  triggered
autonomic dysfunction

autonomic insufficiency
autonomic nerves
autonomic neuropathy
autonomous production of aldosterone
autonomous secretion of aldosterone
Autoplex Factor VIII inhibitor bypass product
autopsy request granted
autopsy request not granted
autoregulation of cerebral blood flow
autosomal dominant ectopia lentis
autosuture
Auto Suture Premium TA 55 surgical stapler
Auto-Suture surgical stapler
autotransfusion system
autotransfusor, Cell-Saver
AVA (aortic valve area)
AVA (arrhythmogenic ventricular activity)
AV (aortic valve) repair
AV (arteriovenous) (see *arteriovenous*)
AV (arterial/venous) oxygen difference
AV (atrioventricular) (see *atrioventricular*)
avascularity
AVCO aortic balloon
AVD (aortic valvular disease)
AVD (atrioventricular dissociation)
AVDH (atrioventricular delay hysteresis)
AVDI (atrioventricular delay interval)
AVD O$_2$ (arteriovenous oxygen difference)
Avenue insertion tool
AVF (arteriovenous fistula)
aVF (augmented lead, left foot) EKG lead
AVG (aortic valve gradient)
avian tuberculosis (transmissible to humans)

Avitene topical hemostatic material
avium-intracellulare, Mycobacterium
(MAI)
Avius sequential pacemaker
aVL (augmented lead, left arm) EKG
lead
AVM (arteriovenous malformation)
AVNR (atrioventricular nodal rhythm)
AVNRT (atrioventricular nodal
reentrant tachycardia)
AVNT (atrioventricular nodal tachycardia)
AVP (ambulant venous pressure)
AV-Paceport thermodilution catheter
AVR (aortic valve replacement)
aVR (augmented lead, right arm) EKG
lead
AVRT (atrioventricular reciprocating
tachycardia)
AVSD (acquired ventricular septal
defect)
avulsion
   arterial
   iatrogenic
   venous
awareness of heart beat
a wave (jugular venous pulse)
   cannon
   giant
   intermittent cannon
A wave (on EKG)
A wave larger than V wave
A wave of cardiac apex pulse
A wave pressure on atrial catheterization
axillary-axillary bypass graft
axillary-brachial bypass graft
axillary electrode

axillary-femoral bypass graft
axillary-femorofemoral bypass graft
axillary vein traumatic thrombosis
axillobifemoral bypass graft
axillofemoral approach
axillofemoral bypass graft
Axiom DG balloon angioplasty
   catheter
axis (pl. axes)
   arterial
   clockwise rotation of electrical
   electrical
   heart
   indeterminate
   J point electrical
   junctional
   left
   mean electrical
   mean QRS
   normal
   normal QRS
   P wave
   QRS vertical
   right
   superior QRS
   twisting on the electrical
   variable
axis deviation on EKG
   horizontal
   left
   vertical
axis of EKG lead
axis of heart
Ayerza-Arrillaga disease
Ayerza disease or syndrome
azygos lobe of lung
azygos system of veins
azygos vein

B, b

Baader syndrome
Babcock grasping forceps
Babesia bovis
Babesia divergens
Babesia, intraerythrocytic
Babesia microti
babesiosis
BABYbird respirator
Baccelli sign of pleural effusion
Bachmann
    anterior internodal tract of
    pathway of
Bachmann bundle of fibers
Bachmann bundle reentry
bacillary embolism
bacillary epithelioid angiomatosis
    (BEA)
bacille Calmette-Guérin (BCG)
bacilli, enteric gram-negative
bacitracin-kanamycin solution
back-bleeding
backflow
backflow from arterial line
backflow of blood into atria
backrush of blood into left ventricle
backscatter characteristics of blood
back stroke volume

backup of blood
backward flow
backward heart failure
Bactec culture test
bacteremia
    catheter-induced
    cryptogenic
    pulmonary artery catheter-related
bacteremic shock
bacterial bronchitis
bacterial endocarditis, subacute (SBE)
bacterial endotoxins, gram-negative
bacterial infection, chronic indolent
bacterial myocarditis
bacterial pericarditis
bacterial pneumonia or pneumonitis
bacterial vegetation
bactericidal drugs
bacteriostatic drugs
Bacteroides fragilis
Bacteroides intermedius
"bad" cholesterol
Baffe anastomosis
baffle
    atrial
    construction of intra-atrial
    hemi-Mustard pericardial

baffle *(cont.)*
  interatrial
  intra-atrial
  intracardiac
  Mustard
  pericardial
  Senning type of intra-atrial
baffled tunnel
baffle leak
bag
  Ambu
  Douglas
  Lahey
  manual resuscitation
bagasse (sugar cane) worker's
  syndrome
bagassosis
bagged (ventilated)
bagging
bagpipe sign
Bahnson aortic clamp
Bailey aortic clamp
Bailey aortic valve cutting forceps
Bailey-Gibbon rib contractor
Bailey-Glover-O'Neill commissur-
  otomy knife
Bailey rib approximator
Bailey rib contractor
Bailey rib spreader
bailout catheter
bailout valvuloplasty
Baim pacing catheter
Baim-Turi cardiac device
Baim-Turi monitoring/pacing catheter
Bainbridge reflex
BAL (bronchoalveolar lavage)
BALF (bronchoalveolar lavage fluid)
Balke protocol for cardiac exercise
  stress testing
Balke treadmill exercise protocol
Balke-Ware treadmill exercise (stress
  testing) protocol

ball and seat valve
ballistocardiography
ball-occluder valve
balloon
  ACS SULP II
  AVCO aortic
  bifoil
  Blue Max
  Extractor three-lumen retrieval
  Fogarty
  Grüntzig (Gruentzig)
  Hartzler angioplasty
  intra-aortic (IAB)
  kissing
  Kontron intra-aortic
  LPS
  Mansfield
  Percor DL-II (dual-lumen)
    intra-aortic
  Percor-Stat intra-aortic
  PET
  pulsation
  Sci-Med Express Monorail
  self-positioning
  slave
  Soto USCI
  Stack autoperfusion balloon
  trefoil
  waist in the
balloon and blade septostomy
balloon and coil embolization
balloon aortoplasty
balloon atrial septostomy
balloon atrial septotomy
balloon catheter fenestration
balloon catheter, Monorail
balloon counterpulsation
balloon embolization (therapeutic)
balloon-expandable flexible coil stent
balloon-expandable intravascular stent
balloon fenestration procedure
balloon-flotation pacing catheter

balloon inflation
  sequential
  simultaneous
balloon into left atrium during systole
balloon (verb) mitral valve leaflets
balloon mitral valvotomy
balloon mitral valvuloplasty
balloon occlusion
balloon occlusion arteriography
balloon occlusion pulmonary angiography
Balloon-on-a-Wire cardiac device
balloon pump
balloon septostomy
balloon sizing
balloon-tipped catheter
balloon-tipped, dual-channel fiberoptic
  bronchoscope
balloon-tipped end-hole catheter
balloon-tipped flow-directed
  pulmonary artery catheter
balloon valvotomy
balloon valvuloplasty
ball poppet of prosthetic valve
ball valve thrombus
ball-valve-type valve prosthesis
ball-wedge catheter
Bamberger sign
bamboo bodies
band
  CPK-MB
  intercaval
  moderator
  parietal
  septal
  septum
bandage, Esmarch
bandbox sound
band cell
banding, pulmonary artery
band-1
Bannister angioedema disease

barbed epicardial pacing lead
Barbero-Marcial method of truncus
  arteriosus repair
Bard arterial cannula
Bard cardiopulmonary support pump
Bard cardiopulmonary support system
Bard Clamshell Septal Umbrella
Bard CPS system
Bard guiding catheter
Bardic cannula
Bardic cutdown catheter
Bard nonsteerable bipolar electrode
Bard PDA Umbrella
Bard percutaneous cardiopulmonary
  support system
Bard-Parker knife
barium-impregnated poppet
barking cough
Barlow syndrome
baroreceptor, carotid
baroreceptor-mediated response
baroreceptor sensitivity
baroreflex
  carotid
  sinoatrial
baroreflex sensitivity
barotrauma, pulmonary
barrel-chested appearance
barrel-shaped chest
barrier, blood-brain
Bartter syndrome
basal chordae
basal crepitation
basal movements (on x-ray)
basal short-axis slice
basal systolic murmur
basal temperatures
basal tuberculosis
basal zone
basal-lateral wall myocardial infarction
base deficit
base excess

base of heart
base of lung
baseline artifact
baseline EKG
baseline, return to
baseline ST segment abnormality
baseline standing blood pressure
baseline standing pulse rate
basement membrane
base of heart
base of lung
basic blood pressure (BP)
basic cardiac life support (BCLS)
basic cycle length (BCL)
basic drive cycle length (BDCL)
basic rate
basilar artery insufficiency
basilar artery syndrome
basilar carotid murmur
basilar infiltration
basilar intracerebral hemorrhage
basilar rales
basilar zone infiltration
basilic vein
Basix pacemaker
basket cell
basket, pericardial
basketlike calcification
basting stitch or suture
bat's wing shadow (on x-ray)
Batten disease
battery
    external pacemaker
    pacemaker
    test
battery voltage
Baumgarten portal hypertension variant
bauxite fibrosis of lung
bauxite lung
bauxite pneumoconiosis
Baxter catheter
Baxter mechanical valve

Bayes theorem in exercise stress testing
Bayliss effect
Baylor total artificial heart
Bazett formula
Bazin disease
Bazin erythema induratum
BBB (bundle branch block)
BBBB (bilateral bundle branch block)
BBR (bundle branch reentry)
B bump on echocardiogram
BCL (basic cycle length)
BCLS (basic cardiac life support)
BDCL (basic drive cycle length)
BEA (bacillary epithelioid angiomatosis)
beading of artery
Beale ganglion cell
Beall circumflex artery scissors
Beall disk valve prosthesis
Beall mitral valve prosthesis
Beall prosthetic mitral valve
Beall-Surgitool ball-cage prosthetic
    valve
Beall-Surgitool disk prosthetic valve
bean bag was placed over the incision
Bear Cub ventilator
beat, beats (see also *heartbeat*)
    aberrantly conducted
    apex
    apical
    Ashman
    asynchronous
    atrial escape
    atrial fusion
    atrial paced
    atrial premature (APB)
    atrioventricular (AV) junctional
        escape
    automatic
    captured
    coupled
    coupled premature

beat *(cont.)*
  downward displaced apical
  Dressler fusion
  dropped
  echo
  ectopic
  ectopic ventricular
  entrained
  escape
  forced
  fusion
  interpolated
  junctional escape
  malignant
  missed
  missing
  paced
  paired
  postectopic
  premature atrial (PAB)
  premature ventricular (PVB)
  pseudofusion
  reciprocal
  skipped
  summation
  sustained ventricular apex
  triplet
  twinned
  ventricular paced
  ventricular ectopic (VEB)
  ventricular escape
  ventricular fusion
  ventricular premature (VPB)
beating at a fixed rate
beating heart, empty
beats per minute (BPM or bpm)
beat-to-beat variability
Beatty-Bright friction sound
Beau asystole
Beau disease
Beaver blade
Beaver knife

beavertail appearance of balloon profile
Beck clamp
Becker disease
Becker muscular dystrophy
Becker sign
Becker syndrome
Beckman O_2 analyzer
Beckman retractor
Beck miniature aortic clamp
Beck-Potts clamp
Beck triad
Beck vascular clamp
Becton-Dickinson introducer
Becton-Dickinson Teflon-sheathed
  needle
bed
  capillary
  monitor
  pulmonary
  pulmonary vascular
  vascular
bedside commode
beef-lung heparin
beefy red color
beep-o-gram
beer and cobalt syndrome
beer-drinker's syndrome
beer-drinker's cardiomyopathy
behavioral changes
Behçet syndrome
bell of stethoscope
ball sound
below-knee popliteal to distal peroneal
  reversed vein graft
bend, hand-shaped
bends (noun)
Benestent
Bengolea arterial forceps
benign hypertension
benign idioventricular rhythm runs
benign pericarditis, acute
benign pneumoconiosis

Bentall inclusion technique
Bentall operation for coronary ostial
  revascularization
Bentall wrap-inclusion composite valve
  graft procedure
Bentley Duraflo II extracorporeal
  perfusion circuit
Bentley oxygenator
Bentley transducer
Bentson guide wire
beriberi cardiomyopathy
beriberi with alcoholic cardiomyopathy
Berman angiographic catheter
Berman aortic clamp
Bernard-Soulier disease or syndrome
Bernheim syndrome
Bernheim-Schmincke syndrome
Bernoulli formula (equation) of
  velocity
Bernoulli theorem
Bernstein acid infusion test
Bernstein catheter
Bernstein study
berry aneurysm, intracranial
Berry sternal needle holder
berylliosis
beryllium disease
beta-adrenergic blockade
beta-adrenergic blocker therapy
beta-adrenergic blocking agent
beta-adrenergic reception blockade
beta-adrenergic receptor
$beta_1$-adrenergic receptor
$beta_2$-adrenergic receptor
beta-adrenergic receptor blocking agent
beta-adrenoreceptor blocking agent
beta agonist
beta antagonist
beta-blockade
beta blocker
Betadine prep (preparation)
beta lipoprotein fraction

$beta_2$-microglobulin level
beta thalassemia
beta-thromboglobulin plasma level
Bethea sign
Bethune rib shears
Bethune rongeur
Better Breathing HEPA-tech half-mask
  respirator
Beuren syndrome
bevel
beveled anastomosis
beveled thin-walled needle
beveled transection
beveling
Bezold-Jarisch reflex
Bianchi nodules
Bianchi valve
biatrial myxoma
biatriatum, cor triloculare
bibasilar crackles
bibasilar discoid atelectasis
bibasilar rales
bibeveled
BICAP unit
bicaval cannulation
Biceps bipolar coagulator
Bichat fat pad
Bichat membrane
bicipital aponeurosis
bicommissural aortic valve
bicuspid aortic valve
bicuspid atrioventricular valve
bicuspid valvular aortic stenosis
bicycle
  Aerobicycle
  Aerodyne
  Collins
  Siemens-Albis
  Tredex powered
bicycle ergometer exercise test
bicycle ergometry (exercise stress
  testing)

bicycle exercise radionuclide ventriculography
bicycle exercise test
bidirectional cavopulmonary anastomosis
bidirectional Glenn procedure
bidirectional lead configuration
bidirectional ventricular tachycardia
Biermer change of sound
Biermer sign
bifascicular heart block
bifid precordial impulse
bifoil balloon
bifurcate
bifurcated graft
bifurcated J-shaped tined atrial pacing and defibrillation lead
bifurcation
    aortic
    carotid
    iliac
    patent
    pulmonary artery
bifurcation graft
bifurcation lesion
bifurcation of pulmonary trunk
bifurcation of trachea
bigeminal rhythm
bigeminus, pulsus
bigeminy
    atrial
    atrioventricular nodal
    escape-capture
    nodal
    reciprocal
    ventricular
bigeminy bisferious pulse
bilateral anterior chest bulge
bilateral anterior thoracotomy
bilateral interstitial pulmonary infiltrates
bilateral saphenous varices

bilateral staged thoracotomies
bilateral upper lobe cavitary infiltrates
bilateral venous engorgement
bile acid sequestrants
bilharziasis
    cardiopulmonary
    protopulmonary
billowing mitral valve
bilobectomy
BIMA (bilateral internal mammary artery) reconstruction
binomial distribution
Binswanger dementia (or disease)
biodegradable stent
Biograft stabilized human umbilical vein
bioimpedance, thoracic electrical (TEB)
biological tissue valve
BioMedicus pump
Biomer (segmented polyurethane)
Bionit vascular prosthesis
biophysical profile (BPP)
BioPolyMeric graft for femoropopliteal bypass
bioprosthesis (see *prosthesis*)
biopsy
    aspiration
    bronchial
    closed lung
    closed pleural
    CT-scan directed needle
    drill
    endomyocardial
    excision(al)
    fine needle
    incisional
    lung
    needle
    open
    open lung
    percutaneous endomyocardial
    percutaneous pericardial

biopsy *(cont.)*
  pericardial
  pleural
  right ventricular endomyocardial
  scalene node
  transbronchial
  transbronchial lung
  transthoracic needle aspiration
  transvenous endomyocardial
biopsy and washings
biopsy cup forceps
biopsy forceps
bioptome
Caves-Schulz
Kawai
King
Konno
Olympus
Stanford left ventricular
Biorate pacemaker
Biot breathing
Biot respirations
Biot sign
Biotrack coagulation monitor
Biotronik pacemaker
biphasic complex on EKG
biphasic electrical shock
biphasic P wave
biphasic shock
biplanar aortography
biplane area-length method (echocardiography)
biplane left ventricular angiogram
biplane fluoroscopy
biplane orthogonal views
biplane pelvic arteriography
biplane pelvic oblique study
biplane transesophageal echocardiography (TEE)
bipolar atrial pacing
bipolar coagulation

bipolar endocardial lead
bipolar generator
bipolar lead
bipolar limb lead
bipolar pacemaker
bipolar sensing, integrated
bipolar temporary heartwire
bipolar temporary pacemaker catheter
bird breeder's lung
bird fancier's lung
bird fancier's syndrome
bird handler's lung
Bird respirator
Bird sign
bird's nest percutaneous IVC filter
bird's nest vena caval filter,
  Gianturco-Roehm
birthmark, varicosities, and limb
  enlargement
bisferiens pulse
bisferiens, pulsus
bisferious pulse
bishop's nod
Bisping electrode
bites, suture
biventricular assist device (BVAD)
biventricular global systolic
  dysfunction
biventricular hypertrophy
biventricular support system, Abiomed
biventricular transposed aorta
biventricularly
Bivona tracheostomy tube
bizarre QRS complexes
Björk-Shiley aortic valve prosthesis
Björk-Shiley floating disc prosthesis
Björk-Shiley monostrut valve
Björk-Shiley valve prosthesis
black lung disease
Blackfan-Diamond syndrome
blackout

blade
  Bard-Parker
  Beaver
  electrosurgical
  knife
blade atrial septostomy
Blalock-Hanlon atrial septectomy
Blalock-Hanlon operation
Blalock-Niedner clamp
Blalock pulmonary clamp
Blalock running horizontal mattress
  suture
Blalock shunt
Blalock-Taussig anastomosis
Blalock-Taussig procedure for "blue
  baby" syndrome
Blalock-Taussig shunt
blanch
blanching, skin
bland aortic aneurysm
bland edema
bland embolism
Bland-Garland-White syndrome
blanket
  circulating water
  cooling
  hypothermia
blast chest
blastomycosis endocarditis
BLB mask
bleb
  emphysematous
  ruptured emphysematous
  subpleural
bleed (noun)
bleeding
  abnormal
  excessive
  intrapericardial
  massive intracranial
bleeding control

bleeding diathesis
bleeding disorder
bleeding site, active
bleeding tendency
bleeding time (see also *time*)
  Duke
  Ivy
blind dimple in floor of left atrium
blind endarterectomy
blind nasal intubation
blind percutaneous puncture of subclavian vein
blind pouch
blind tibial outflow tracts
blindness, transient monocular
bloater, blue
block (see also *heart block*)
  acquired symptomatic AV
  air
  alveolar-capillary
  anodal
  anterior fascicular
  anterograde
  arborization
  atrioventricular (AV) heart
  AV (atrioventricular)
  AV Wenckebach heart
  BBB (bundle branch)
  BBBB (bilateral bundle branch)
  bifascicular
  bifascicular bundle branch
  bifascicular heart
  bilateral bundle branch (BBBB)
  bundle branch (BBB)
  bundle branch heart
  complete AV (CAVB)
  complete congenital heart
  complete heart (CHB)
  conduction
  congenital complete heart
  congenital heart

block *(cont.)*
  congenital symptomatic AV
  deceleration-dependent
  divisional
  donor heart-lung
  entrance
  exit
  false bundle-branch
  familial heart
  fascicular
  first-degree AV
  first-degree heart
  fixed third-degree AV
  heart
  high-grade AV
  incomplete atrioventricular (IAVB)
  incomplete heart
  incomplete left bundle branch
    (ILBBB)
  incomplete right bundle branch
    (IRBBB)
  inflammatory heart
  infra-His
  intermittent third-degree AV
  interventricular
  intra-atrial
  intra-His
  intra-Hisian or intrahisian
  intranodal
  intravenous (IV)
  intraventricular conduction
  intraventricular heart
  ipsilateral bundle branch
  left anterior fascicular (LAFB)
  left anterior hemiblock
  left bundle branch (LBBB)
  left posterior fascicular (LPFB)
  Mobitz I or II second-degree AV
  Mobitz type I or II AV
  Mobitz type I on Wenckebach heart
  paroxysmal AV
  partial heart

block *(cont.)*
  peri-infarction (PIB)
  posterior fascicular
  pseudo-AV
  retrograde
  right bundle branch (RBBB)
  second-degree AV
  second-degree heart
  sinoatrial (SAB)
  sinoatrial exit
  sinus
  sinus exit
  sinus node exit
  supra-Hisian or suprahisian
  third-degree AV
  third-degree heart
  transient AV
  3:2 ("three to two") AV
  trifascicular
  2:1 ("two to one") AV
  unidirectional
  unifascicular
  VA (ventriculoatrial)
  ventricular
  vesicular
  Wenckebach AV
  Wilson
blockade
  adrenergic
  alpha-
  alpha-adrenergic
  beta-
  beta-adrenergic
  beta-adrenergic reception
  neuromuscular
blockage of bronchus
blockage of pulmonary artery
Block cardiac device
blocked APC (atrial premature
  contraction)
blocked artery
blocked bronchus

blocked pleurisy
blocker
　alpha-adrenergic
　alpha-adrenoreceptor
　beta-
　calcium channel
　calcium entry
　potassium channel
　sodium channel
　slow channel
blocking agent, beta-adrenoceptor
blocking of histamine receptors
Block right coronary guiding catheter
blood
　arterial
　artificial (100% O_2+fluorocarbons)
　autologous
　coagulability of
　cord
　defibrinated
　deoxygenated
　egress of
　expectoration of
　extravasated
　frank blood cardioplegia
　heparinized
　laky
　nonoxygenated
　normally oxygenated
　occult
　oxygenated
　peripheral
　shunted
　sludged
　unoxygenated
　venous
　whole
blood bank
blood-brain barrier
blood clot
blood-clotting mechanism
blood coagulability, increased

blood coagulation
blood coagulation factors (see *factors*)
blood-conservation techniques
blood count
　complete (CBC)
　differential white
　Schilling
blood dyscrasia
blood flow, antegrade
blood flow at capillary level
blood flow on Doppler echo-
　cardiogram
blood flow to tissue beyond obstruction
blood flow velocity
blood gas(es) (arterial) panel
　base excess
　bicarbonate
　HCO_3
　O_2 saturation (percent)
　$PaCO_2$
　PaO_2
　pCO_2
　pH
　pO_2
　venous
blood gases on oxygen
blood gases on room air
blood group
　ABO
　Auberger
　Cartwright
　Diego
　Dombrock
　Duffy
　high frequency
　I
　Kell
　Kidd
　Lewis
　low frequency
　Lutheran
　MNS

blood group *(cont.)*
  P
  Rh
blood leak into interstitial space
blood leak into intra-alveolar space
bloodless fluid
blood lipids
blood loss, nil
blood perfusion
blood perfusion monitor (BPM),
  Laserflo
blood plasma
blood plate thrombus
blood-pool imaging
blood-pool radionuclide angiography
blood-pool radionuclide echocardiography
blood pool, white-appearing
blood pressure (BP)
  arterial
  baseline
  baseline standing
  basic
  diastolic (DBP)
  high
  labile
  low
  maximum
  mean
  minimum
  orthostatic
  standing
  supine
  systolic (SBP)
  systolic/diastolic (SDBP)
blood pressure discrepancy in upper
  and lower extremities
blood pressure response
blood sample
blood serum
blood speckle
blood-streaked sputum

blood stream, bloodstream
blood substitute, oxygenated
  perfluorocarbon
blood supply, accessory
blood supply of thymus
blood test, cold agglutinins
blood-tinged expectoration
blood-tinged sputum
blood transfusion
  autogenous
  autologous
  homologous
  multiple
blood type
blood type, cross, and match
blood urea nitrogen (BUN)
blood vessel thermography
blood viscosity
blood volume
  central
  circulating
Bloodwell forceps
bloody exudate
bloody fluid
bloody nasal mucus
bloody pericardial fluid
bloody sputum
Bloom DTU 201 external stimulator
Bloom programmable stimulator
blooming, signal
blow-by, anesthesia
blowing murmur
blowing pansystolic murmur
blowing pneumothorax
blow-out, aortic stump
blue and white Tycron sutures
blue baby
blue bloater
blue finger syndrome
Blue FlexTip catheter
Blue Max balloon
Blue Max triple-lumen catheter

blue of Gregoire syndrome
blue phlebitis
blue sclerae
blue toe syndrome ("trash foot")
blue velvet syndrome
bluish coloration of sclerae
bluish nail lacunae
bluish skin color (cyanosis)
blunt border of lung
blunt chest trauma
blunt dissection
blunted chronotropic response
blunt forceps
blunt Hasson grasper
blunt injury
blunt thoracic trauma
blurring of aortic knob
blurring of costophrenic angle
  (on x-ray)
BML (billowing mitral leaflet)
B-mode (B-scan)
B-mode echocardiography
B-mode echography
B-mode, pseudocolor
body, bodies
  Amato
  aortic
  Arantius
  asbestos
  Aschoff
  bamboo
  Bracht-Wächter
  central fibrous
  coccoid x
  Deetjen
  ferruginous
  fibrin (of pleura)
  foreign
  gelatin compression
  Heinz
  Howell-Jolly
  Levinthal-Coles-Lillie (LCL)

body *(cont.)*
  Masson
  multilaminar
  Pappenheimer
  Reilly
  Zuckerkandl
body box/plethysmography
body contour orbit, body artifacts due
  to
body habitus
body of sternum
body surface area (BSA)
body surface potential mapping
Boeck sarcoid
Boettcher artery forceps
Bohr effect
bolster, Teflon felt
bolus, intravenous
bolus intravenous injection
bolus of medication
boluses of air
bone marrow embolism
bone wax
bony landmarks
Bookwalter retractor
booming diastolic rumble
BOOP (bronchiolitis obliterans
  organizing pneumonia)
booster phenomenon
boot-shaped heart
boot-strap two-vessel angioplasty
border, borders
  anterior
  cardiac
  ciliated
  inferior (of heart)
  lower sternal (LSB)
  mid-left sternal border
  sternocleidomastoid muscle
  upper sternal
borderline hypertension
borderline severe rejection

border of heart
  anterior
  inferior
  left
  posterior
  right
  superior
Borg scale (1-5) for programming
  pacers
Borg scale of perceived exertion
Borg scale of treadmill exertion
boring pain
Bornholm disease
Borrelia burgdorferi
Bosch ERG 500 ergometer
bottle nose forceps
bottle sound
bottle, suction
Bouillaud disease
Bouillaud sign
Bouillaud syndrome
bounding arterial pulse
bounding peripheral pulses
bounding water-hammer pulse
bouts of tachycardia
Bouchut respirations
Bouveret disease
Bouveret-Hoffmann syndrome
bovine allograft
bovine heterograft
bovine lavage extract surfactant
bovine pericardial bioprosthesis
bovine pericardial patch augmentation
  of aortic arch
bovine respirations
bovine tuberculosis (transmissible to
  humans)
bovine valve prosthesis
bovinum, cor
Bowditch effect
Bowditch staircase phenomenon

Bowditch, treppe (staircase)
  phenomenon of
bowing of mitral valve leaflet
Boyd formula
Boyd perforating vein
Bozzolo sign
BP (arterial blood pressure)
BPD (bronchopulmolnary dysplasia)
BPM or bpm (beats per minute)
BPP (biophysical profile)
BPV (balloon pulmonary valvuloplasty)
brachial approach
brachial artery
brachial artery compression
brachial artery cuff pressure
brachial artery pressure
brachial artery pulse pressure
brachial-basilar insufficiency
brachial bypass
brachial plexus
brachial plexus compression
brachial plexus injury
brachial pulse
brachioaxillary interposition graft
brachiocephalic (innominate) veins
brachiocephalic arteritis
brachiocephalic artery
brachiocephalic ischemia
brachiocephalic lymph nodes
brachiocephalic systolic murmur
brachiocephalic trunk
brachiocephalic vein
brachiocephalic vessels
brachiocrural symptoms
Bracht-Wächter bodies
Bradbury-Eggleston syndrome
Bradbury-Eggleston triad
bradyarrhythmia
  digitalis-induced
  vasovagal

bradyarrhythmic cardiac arrest
bradycardia
  Branham
  central
  essential
  fetal
  idioventricular
  intermittent junctional
  junctional
  nodal
  postinfective
  pulseless
  sinoatrial
  sinus (SB)
  symptomatic
  vagal
bradycardia pacing
bradycardia pacing zone
bradycardia-tachycardia syndrome
bradycardic agonal phase
bradydysrhythmia
bradykinin
bradypnea
bradypneic
bradysphygmia
bradytachycardia syndrome
bradytachydysrhythmia syndrome
braided lead
braided polyester sutures
braided suture
braided tape
brain abscess
brain anoxia
branch, branches (see also *artery*)
  acute marginal
  AV (atrioventricular) groove
  bifurcating
  bronchial
  caudal
  diagonal
  first diagonal
  first major diagonal

branch *(cont.)*
  first septal perforator
  inferior wall
  large obtuse marginal
  left bundle
  marginal
  midmarginal
  nonlingular
  obtuse marginal (OMB)
  posterior descending
  posterior intercostal
  posterior ventricular
  ramus
  ramus intermedius artery
  ramus medialis
  right bundle
  second diagonal
  septal
  septal perforating
  side
  subcostal
  superior phrenic
  ventricular
branching, mirror-image brachiocephalic
Branham bradycardia
Branham sign (arteriovenous fistula)
Branhamella catarrhalis
Brasdor method
brassy bruit
brassy cough
BRAT cell saver
Braunwald-Cutter ball prosthetic valve
Braunwald sign
brawny edema
brawny induration
bread-and-butter heart
bread-and-butter pericarditis
break, lead insulation
breakthrough vasodilatation
breast, pigeon
breast thrombophlebitis

breast tissue, attenuation by
breathhold, five-second
breathing
  amphoric
  apneustic
  assisted
  atactic
  Biot
  bronchial
  bronchovesicular
  cavernous
  Cheyne-Stokes
  cogwheel
  continuous positive pressure
    (CPPB)
  diaphragmatic
  frog
  glossopharyngeal
  intermittent positive pressure
    (IPPB)
  Kussmaul
  labored
  mouth
  periodic
  positive-negative pressure (PNPB)
  pursed-lip
  rapid shallow
  resistive (through fixed orifice)
  shallow
  sighing
  spontaneous
  stertorous
  stridulous
  tidal
  tubular
  vesicular
breathing apparatus
breathing pattern, tachypneic
breathing treatments via machine
breathlessness after activity
breathlessness at rest
breathlessness on waking

breathless when wheezing
breath pentane measurement
breath, shortness of
breath sounds (see also *sounds*)
  absent
  adventitious
  amphoric
  audible
  bronchial
  bronchovesicular
  cavernous
  coarse
  cogwheel
  decreased
  distant
  faint
  inspiratory-expiratory
  muffled
  normal
  reduced
  sibilant
  tubular
  vesicular
Brechenmacher fiber
Brechenmacher tract
Brecher and Cronkite technique for
  platelet counting
Brescio-Cimino AV (arteriovenous)
  fistula
Bretschneider-HTK cardioplegic
  solution
Brett syndrome
bridge, Wheatstone
bridging, muscular
brief anterior thrust
bright, highly mobile echoes
bright red flush
Brisbane method of aortic valve and
  ascending aorta replacement
brisk bifid arterial pulse
brisk drainage
Broadbent inverted sign

broadened P waves
broadened T wave
broad maxillary ridge
Brock cardiac dilator
Brock clamp
Brock commissurotomy knife
Brockenbrough-Braunwald sign
Brockenbrough cardiac device
Brockenbrough catheter, modified
    bipolar
Brockenbrough mapping catheter
Brockenbrough needle
Brockenbrough sign
Brockenbrough transseptal catheter
Brockenbrough transseptal method for
    commissurotomy
Brockenbrough transseptal needle
Brock middle lobe syndrome
Brock transventricular closed
    valvotomy
Brodie-Trendelenburg test for varicose
    veins
Brom repair of aortic stenosis
Brom repair of congenital supravalvu-
    lar aortic stenosis
bronchi (pl. of bronchus)
bronchial adenoma
bronchial annular cartilage
bronchial arteriography
bronchial artery
bronchial asthma
bronchial biopsy
bronchial branch
bronchial breath sounds
bronchial brushing
bronchial bud
bronchial calculus
bronchial caliber
bronchial carcinoma myasthenia
    syndrome
bronchial cartilage absence-bronchiec-
    tasis-bronchomalacia syndrome

bronchial cartilage, absent
bronchial collapse on forced expiration
bronchial collateral circulation
bronchial cyst
bronchial dehiscence
bronchial distortions
bronchial hyperreactivity to TDI
    (toluene diisocyanate)
bronchial hyperresponsiveness
    allergen-induced
    persistent
bronchial kinkings
bronchial lumen
bronchial mucosa
bronchial mucosal edema
bronchial murmur
bronchial obstruction
bronchial provocation
    HDM (house dust mites)
    methacholine
bronchial provocation testing
bronchial reactivity
bronchial respirations
bronchial secretions
bronchial septum
bronchial smooth muscle spasm
bronchial spasm
bronchial stenosis
bronchial stricture
bronchial suctioning
bronchial tree
bronchial type B disease
bronchial vessels
bronchial washings
bronchial washings cytology
bronchic cell
bronchiectasis
    acquired
    capillary
    congenital
    cylindrical
    cystic

bronchiectasis *(cont.)*
  dry
  follicular
  fusiform
  Polynesian
  postinfectious
  Pseudomonas
  recurrent
  saccular
  tuberculous
  varicose
bronchiectasis-ethmoid sinusitis
bronchiectasis-like quantities of
  purulent material
bronchiectasis-megaesophagus-
  osteopathy syndrome
bronchiectatic pattern
bronchi lobares
bronchiloquy
bronchiocele
bronchiolar carcinoma
bronchiolar edema
bronchiolar emphysema
bronchiolar epithelium
bronchiolar narrowing, irreversible
bronchiolar obstruction
bronchiolar passages, narrowing of
bronchiole, bronchioles
  alveolar
  lobular
  respiratory
  terminal
bronchiolectasis
bronchioli (pl. of bronchiolus)
bronchiolitis
  exudative
  proliferative
  vesicular
bronchiolitis exudativa
bronchiolitis fibrosa obliterans
bronchiolitis obliterans organizing
  pneumonia

bronchiolus (pl. bronchioli)
bronchiospasm
bronchiostenosis
bronchi principales dexter-sinister
bronchi segmentales
bronchismus
bronchitic
bronchitis
  acute
  acute infectious
  acute irritative
  acute laryngotracheal
  arachidic
  asthmatic
  bacterial
  capillary
  Castellani
  catarrhal
  cheesy
  chemical
  chronic
  chronic obstructive
  croupous
  dry
  emphysematous
  Enterobacter aerogenes
  ether
  exudative
  fetid
  fibrinous
  Haemophilus influenzae
  hemorrhagic
  infectious asthmatic
  infectious avian
  irritative
  laryngotracheal
  membranous
  mucopurulent
  necrotizing
  obstructive
  phthinoid
  plastic

bronchitis *(cont.)*
pneumococcal
productive
pseudomembranous
purulent
putrid
secondary
septic
staphylococcal
streptococcal
suffocative
vesicular
viral
bronchitis obliterans
bronchitis with bronchospasm
Bronchitrac L flexible suction catheter
bronchoadenitis
bronchoalveolar
bronchoalveolar cell carcinoma
bronchoalveolar lavage (BAL)
bronchoalveolar lavage fluid (BALF)
bronchoalveolitis
bronchoaspergillosis
bronchoblastomycosis
bronchoblennorrhea
bronchocandidiasis
Broncho-Cath double-lumen endo-
    tracheal tube
bronchocavernous
bronchocele
bronchocentric granulomatosis
bronchocentric inflammatory infiltrate
bronchoconstriction
    exercise-induced
    isocapnic hyperventilation-induced
bronchoconstrictor
bronchocutaneous fistula
bronchocutaneous fistulectomy
bronchodilatation or bronchodilation
bronchodilator
    inhaled
    long-acting

bronchodilator *(cont.)*
    nebulized
    parenteral
    short-acting
    weaned off
bronchodilator effect
bronchodilator therapy
bronchoegophony
bronchoesophageal fistulectomy
bronchoesophagoscopy
bronchofiberscope, -scopy
bronchogenic carcinoma
bronchogram, -graphy
    air
    tantalum
bronchographic
broncholith
broncholithiasis
bronchology
bronchomalacia
bronchomediastinal lymph trunk
bronchomotor effects
bronchomucotropic
bronchomycosis
bronchonocardiosis
bronchopathy
bronchophony
    pectoriloquous
    sniffling
    whispered
bronchoplasty, fiberoptic
bronchoplegia
bronchopleural fistula
bronchopleural fistula with empyema
bronchopleuromediastinal fistulectomy
bronchopleuropneumonia
bronchopneumonia (see *pneumonia*)
    bibasilar
    hemorrhagic
    hypostatic
    inhalation
    postoperative

bronchopneumonia *(cont.)*
  subacute
  tuberculous
  virus
bronchopneumonitis
bronchopneumopathy
bronchopulmonary allergy
bronchopulmonary aspergillosis,
  allergic
bronchopulmonary dysplasia (BPD)
bronchopulmonary lavage
bronchopulmonary lymph node
bronchopulmonary segment
bronchoradiography
bronchorrhagia
bronchorrhaphy
bronchorrhea
bronchoscope
  balloon-tipped, dual-channel
    fiberoptic
  directable tip of
  fiberoptic
  Jackson
  Jackson-Olympus
  Olympus BF1G10
  Olympus BF3C4
  Olympus BF4B2
  Olympus BFP-10
  rigid
  ultrathin
bronchoscopic shuttle technique
bronchoscopy
  fiberoptic
  flexible
  rigid
bronchoscopy lavage
bronchosinusitis
bronchospasm
  paradoxical
  uncontrolled
bronchospastic effects
bronchospirometry

bronchostaxis
bronchostenosis
bronchostomy
bronchotome
bronchotomy
bronchotracheal
bronchovesicular breath sounds
bronchovesicular breathing
bronchovisceral fistulectomy
bronchus (pl. bronchi)
  anterior
  anterior basal
  apical
  apicoposterior
  beaded
  cardiac
  contracted
  dilated
  edematous
  eparterial
  extrapulmonary
  granulomatous inflammation of
  hyparterial
  inflamed
  intermediate
  intrapulmonary
  lateral basal
  left main stem
  lingular
  lobar
  medial
  medial basal
  medium-sized
  normal-appearing
  posterior basal
  primary (right and left)
  right main stem
  secondary
  secretion-filled
  segmental
  stem
  subapical

bronchus *(cont.)*
   subsegmental
   superior
   tracheal
bronchus intermedius
Broviac atrial catheter
Brown Adson forceps
brown atrophy
Brown-Dodge method for angiography
brown induration of the lung
brown lung
brown pulmonary induration
Bruce protocol (exercise stress testing)
   modified
   standard
   treadmill exercise
brucellosis
Brugia malayi infection
bruit, bruits (see also *murmur*, *sound*)
   abdominal
   aneurysmal
   audible
   buzzing venous murmur
   carotid artery
   clashing noise
   clear ringing musical (brassy) note
   crackling pericardial
   crackling pleural
   creaking noise
   dull wooden nonmusical note
   epigastric
   false
   flank
   flapping rustle
   grating
   interscapulovertebral arterial
   palpable
   rasping
   rattling
   renal artery
   Roger
   rubbing sound

bruit *(cont.)*
   rustling murmur from pericardial
   seagull
   skodaic
   slowing sound
   splashing
   subclavian
   supraclavicular
   systolic
   to-and-fro
   Traube (gallop)
   Verstraeten
   waterwheel
bruit d'airain (brass)
bruit de bois (wood)
bruit de canon (cannon)
bruit de choc (shock, clash)
bruit de clapotement (rippling)
bruit de craquement (crackling)
bruit de cuir neuf (new leather)
bruit de diable (humming top)
bruit de drapeau (flag)
bruit de felé (cracked)
bruit de froissement (clashing)
bruit de frolement (rustling)
bruit de frottement (friction)
bruit de galop (gallop rhythm)
bruit de grelot (rattle)
bruit de lime (file)
bruit de moulin (mill)
bruit de parchemin (parchment)
bruit de piaulement (whining)
bruit de pot felé (cracked-pot sound)
bruit de rape (grater)
bruit de rappel (drum beating to arms)
bruit de Roger
bruit de scie (saw)
bruit de soufflet (bellows)
bruit de tabourka (drum)
bruit de tambour (drum)
bruit de triolet (a little trio)
bruit placentaire (placental)

bruit skodique
Brunschwig artery forceps
Brushfield spots
brushing, bronchial
BSA (body surface area)
BSA ejection fraction
bud, buds
   bronchial
   capillary
   vascular
bubbling cough
bubbling rales
bubbly lung syndrome
Buchbinder Omniflex catheter
Buchbinder Thruflex catheter
Buchbinder Thruflex Over-the-Wire
Buckberg cardioplegia
Buckberg solution
buckled innominate artery syndrome
buckling of mitral valve, midsystolic
Budd-Chiari syndrome
budgie (shell parakeet)-fancier's
   disease
Buerger-Gruetz disease
Buerger symptoms
Buerger thromboangiitis obliterans
   disease
buffer
buffy coat positive
buffy coat smear
bulb
   aortic
   carotid
   internal jugular
bulbar intracerebral hemorrhage
bulbar septum
bulb of heart
bulb of inferior jugular vein
bulb of superior jugular vein
bulbous-tip electrode
bulbus aortae
bulbus arteriosus

bulbus cordis
bulge
   bilateral anterior chest
   late systolic
   palpable presystolic
   parasternal
bulging precordium
bulging, suprasternal
bulla (pl. bullae), emphysematous
bulldog clamp
bulldog Hasson grasper
bull neck appearance
bullous emphysema
bullous lung disease
bull's eye images
bump, ductus
BUN (blood urea nitrogen)
bundle
   artery-vein-nerve
   AV (atrioventricular)
   Bachmann
   common
   fascicular
   Gierke respiratory
   His
   intercostal
   intercostal neuromuscular
   James
   Keith sinoatrial
   Kent
   Kent-His
   Mahaim
   main
   sinoatrial
   Thorel
   vascular
bundle branch block (BBB)
bundle branch heart block (on EKG)
bundle branch reentrant ventricular
   tachycardia
bundle branch reentry (BBR)
bundle of His ablation

bundle of Kent accessory bypass fibers
bundle of Stanley Kent
bur (see *burr*)
Burford-Finochietto rib spreader
Burford retractor
Burford rib spreader
Burghart symptoms
Burke syndrome
burning, substernal
Burns space
burr or bur
    atherectomy
    diamond-coated
    elliptical
    high-speed
    rotating
burst cycle length
burst
    multicapture
    respiratory
burst of arrhythmia
burst of ventricular ectopy
burst of ventricular tachycardia
burst pacing, adaptive
burying of P_2 sound
Buselmeier shunt
butterfly pattern of infiltrates
butterfly shadow (on x-ray)
butterfly, silicone
buttock claudication
button device for transcatheter
    occlusion of atrial septal defect
buttonhole opening
buttonhole stenosis
button of aorta
button, skin
button technique
buzzing murmur
BVAD (biventricular assist device),
    Thoratec
BVM (bag-valve-mask) resuscitating
    device

BVS (biventricular support system)
BV2 needle
bypass (see also *bypass graft*, *graft*)
    aorta-iliac-femoral
    aorta-renal
    aorta-subclavian-carotid
    aorta-subclavian-carotid-axillo-
        axillary
    aorta to first obtuse marginal
        branch
    aorta to LAD
    aorta to marginal branch
    aorta to posterior descending
    aortic-femoral
    aortic-superior mesenteric
    aortobifemoral
    aortocarotid
    aortoceliac
    aortocoronary
    aortocoronary-saphenous vein
    aortofemoral
    aortofemoral-thoracic
    aortoiliac
    aortoiliac-popliteal
    aortoiliofemoral
    aortopopliteal
    aortorenal
    apico-abdominal
    atrial-femoral
    atrial-femoral artery
    axillary
    axillary-brachial
    axillary-femoral
    axilloaxillary
    axillobifemoral
    axillofemoral
    axillopopliteal
    brachial
    cardiopulmonary (CPB)
    carotid-axillary
    carotid-carotid
    carotid-subclavian

bypass *(cont.)*
  common hepatic-common iliac-
    renal
  coronary
  coronary artery (CAB)
  cross femoral-femoral
  crossover
  distal arterial
  DTAF-F (descending thoracic
    aortofemoral-femoral)
  extra-anatomic
  extracranial-intracranial (EC-IC)
  fem-fem (femoral-femoral)
  fem-pop (femoral-popliteal)
  femoral-above-knee popliteal
  femoral crossover
  femoral to tibial
  femoral vein-femoral artery
  femoral-femoral
  femoral-popliteal
  femoral-tibial-peroneal
  femoral venoarterial
  femoroaxillary
  femorodistal
  femorofemoral
  femorofemoral crossover
  femorofemoropopliteal
  femoroperoneal
  femoropopliteal
  femoropopliteal saphenous vein
  femorotibial
  heart-lung
  hypothermic cardiopulmonary
  iliofemoral
  iliopopliteal
  in situ
  infracubital
  infrainguinal stenosis
  ipsilateral nonreversed greater
    saphenous vein
  left atrium to distal arterial aortic
  left heart

bypass *(cont.)*
  lesser saphenous vein in situ
  Litwak left atrial-aortic
  mammary-coronary artery
  marginal circumflex
  microscope-aided pedal
  nonreversed translocated vein
  normothermic cardiopulmonary
  obtuse marginal
  partial
  partial cardiopulmonary
  percutaneous femoral-femoral
    cardiopulmonary
  popliteal
  popliteal in situ
  popliteal to distal in situ
  pulsatile cardiopulmonary
  renal artery-reverse saphenous vein
  reversed
  right heart
  sequential in situ
  subclavian-carotid
  subclavian-subclavian
  superior mesenteric artery
  temporary aortic shunt
  tibial in situ
  total cardiopulmonary
  upper extremity in situ
bypass circuit
bypass graft
  aortobifemoral
  aortobiprofunda
  aortocoronary saphenous vein
  ascending aorta-abdominal aorta
  axillary-axillary
  axillary-femorofemoral
  axillobifemoral
  axillofemoral
  carotid-carotid venous
  femoral-femoral
  femoral-distal popliteal
  femoroperoneal

bypass graft *(cont.)*
  femorotibial
  hepatorenal
  hepatorenal saphenous vein
  iliac-renal
  ilioprofunda
  infrainguinal vein
  saphenous vein
  sequential
  splenorenal arterial
  supraceliac aorta-femoral artery
  supraceliac aortic
  supraceliac aortofemoral
  thoracic aorta-femoral artery

bypass tract
  atrio-Hisian or atriohisian
  AV (atrioventricular) nodal
  concealed
  fasiculoventricular bypass
  nodo-Hisian
  nodoventricular
  right ventricular
bypass-tract-mediated AV (atrioventricular) nodal reentrant
  tachycardia
Byrel SX pacemaker
Byrel-SX/Versatrax pacemaker
byssinosis

C, c

C (click)
C-A, CA (cardiac-apnea) monitor for
  newborns
C-A amplitude of mitral valve
CA (cardiac arrest)
CA (coronary artery)
CAB (coronary artery bypass)
"cabbage" (pronunciation of CABG)
CABG (coronary artery bypass graft)
cabinet respirator
cable
  alligator pacing
  fibrillator
  percutaneous
Cabot-Locke murmur
Cabrol I anastomosis
Cabrol I shunt
Cabrol I tube graft
Cabrol II coronary ostial revascular-
  ization
Cabrol II interposition coronary
  prosthetic graft
Cabrol II modification of Bentall
  procedure
CABS (coronary artery bypass
  surgery)
cachectic endocarditis

cachectic patient
cachexia, cardiac
CAD (coronary artery disease)
cadaverous
Cadence AICD (automatic implantable
  cardioverter-defibrillator)
Cadence biphasic ICD (implantable
  cardioverter-defibrillator)
Cadence ICD (implantable cardioverter-defibrillator)
cadence, rhythmic auscultatory
Cadence TVL nonthoracotomy lead
cadmium iodide detector
CADs (computer-assisted diagnostics)
CAEP (chronotropic assessment
  exercise protocol)
caerulea dolens, phlegmasia
caisson syndrome
calcareous deposits in pericardium
calcific aortic stenosis
calcific arteriosclerosis
calcific artery
calcification
  annular
  aortic
  aortic valve
  basketlike

75

calcification *(cont.)*
  coronary
  dystrophic
  eggshell
  idiopathic pleural
  intracardiac
  linear
  mitral annular
  mitral ring
  mitral valve
  Mönckeberg (Moenckeberg)
  subannular
  valve
  valvular
calcification of myocardium
calcification of pericardium
calcific constrictive pericarditis
calcific spur
calcified artery
calcified granulomatous disease
calcified irregular mass, polypoid
calcified pericardium
calcified plaque
calcified thrombus
calcified valvular leaflets
calcium antagonist
calcium channel antagonists
calcium channel blocker
calcium deposit
calcium entry blocker
calcium, intracardiac
calcium layering at aortic knob
calculus
  bronchial
  hemic
  lung
calf claudication
calf muscle tenderness
calf vein thrombus
caliber
  good
  excellent

caliber *(cont.)*
  internal
  luminal
  medium
  modest
  normal
  tracheal
  vessel
  wide
caliber of bronchus
caliber of vessel, borderline
caliber of vessel, suitable
California disease
caliper
callused elbows from repeated
  assumption of tripod position
Calman carotid artery clamp
Calman ring clamp
camera
  Anger-type scintillation
  gamma
  GE Starcam single-crystal
    tomographic
  multicrystal gamma
  scintillation
  Starcam
cameral fistula
CAMV (congenital anomaly of mitral
  valve)
Canadian Class system (I-IV) for
  severity of angina
Canadian Society of Cardiology
  criteria for effort angina
canal
  Arantius
  arterial
  atrioventricular (AV)
  common atrioventricular
  complex atrioventricular
  Cuvier
  Hunter
  perivascular

canal *(cont.)*
  persistent common atrioventricular
  pulmoaortic
  Sucquet-Hoyer
canalization
canalize
cancer embolus
candidal esophagitis
candidate for transplant
  excellent
  marginal
  suitable
candidemia, pulmonary artery catheter-related
candidiasis
cannabinosis
cannon a wave of jugular venous pulse
Cannon formula
cannon wave
cannula (pl. cannulae, cannulas)
  Bard
  aortic arch
  apex
  arterial
  atrial
  Bard arterial
  Bardic
  Cope needle introducer
  coronary artery
  coronary perfusion
  external jugular venous
  flexible suction
  femoral artery
  Gregg-type
  high-flow
  infusion
  inlet
  internal jugular venous
  intra-arterial
  introducer
  Litwak
  LV (left ventricular) apex

cannula *(cont.)*
  metallic tip
  nasal (for oxygen)
  outlet
  Pacifico venous
  perfusion
  peripheral arterial
  peripheral venous
  Polystan perfusion
  Portnoy ventricular
  Sarns aortic arch
  Sarns two-stage
  Sarns venous drainage
  single-bore
  Storz needle
  two-stage Sarns
  two-stage venous
  vena cava
  Venflon
  venous
  ventricular
  washout
  Webster infusion
cannulate, percutaneously
cannulated central vein
cannulation
  aortic
  arterial
  atrial
  bicaval
  direct caval
  left atrial
  ostial
  single-cannula atrial
  two-stage venous
  venoarterial
  venous
  venovenous
cannulization
  selective
  subselective
CaO_2 (arterial oxygen content)

cap
  hilar
  pleural
  pleural apical hematoma
  thin fibrous
capacious veins
capacitance
capacity
  cardiac functional
  closing (CC)
  decreased diffusing
  decreased exercise
  decreased ventilatory
  diffusing
  exercise
  exertional
  forced vital (FVC)
  functional residual (FRC)
  impaired exercise
  O_2 carrying
  reduced diffusing
  total lung (TLC)
  ventilatory
  vital
capacity for work, maximal
CAPD (continuous ambulatory
  peritoneal dialysis)
Capetown aortic prosthetic valve
capillary, capillaries
  arterial
  lymph
  Meigs
  permeability of
  venous
capillary bed
capillary blood sugar (CBS)
capillary blood volume
capillary bud
capillary congestion
capillary embolism
capillary endothelium
capillary filling, compensatory

capillary filtration coefficient (CFC)
capillary fragility test
capillary hemangioma ("strawberry
  mark")
capillary hemangiomas with (or without) extensive purpura
capillary hydrostatic pressure
capillary hyperpermeability
capillary leak (or leakage), generalized
capillary leak syndrome
capillary malformation (CM)
capillary pneumonia
capillary pressure
capillary pulsation
capillary refill
capillary resistance test
capillary stick
capillary stick on warmed heel
  of neonate
capillary walls
capillary wedge pressure, pulmonary
capillary-lymphatic malformation
  (CLM)
capillary-venous malformation (CVM)
Capiox-E bypass system oxygenator
Caplan syndrome
capnograph
capsular thrombosis
CapSure lead
Captopril-stimulated renal scan
capture
  atrial
  failure to
  lack of pacemaker
  1:1 retrograde
  pacemaker
  resistance
  retrograde atrial
  ventricular
capture threshold
Carabello sign
carbohydrate-inducible hyperlipemia

CarboMedics valve device
carbon dioxide (CO_2), extracorporeal
   removal of
carbon dioxide narcosis
carbon dioxide retention
carbon monoxide diffusion, decreased
carbon-11 palmitic acid radioactive
   tracer
carbonic acid deficit
Carbo-Seal cardiovascular composite
   graft
carboxyhemoglobin
carcinoid heart disease
carcinoid syndrome
carcinoid tricuspid valve disease
carcinoid tumor of bronchus
carcinoma
   adenosquamous
   alveolar
   alveolar cell
   bronchiolar
   bronchoalveolar cell
   bronchogenic
   cavitating
   clear cell
   endobronchial
   esophageal
   giant cell
   large cell
   non-small cell (of lung)
   oat cell
   small cell of the lung
   squamous cell
carcinoma en cuirasse
carcinomatosis, pulmonary
carcinosis, pulmonary
Cardarelli sign
cardiac action commences in sinus
   rhythm
cardiac action potentials
cardiac allograft
cardiac amyloidosis

Cardiac Angioplasty Analysis System
   (CAAS)
cardiac anomaly, Ebstein
cardiac apex
cardiac-apnea (CA) monitor for
   newborns
cardiac-arm syndrome
cardiac arrest (CA)
   asystolic
   bradyarrhythmic
   recurrent
   sudden
cardiac arrhythmia with Stokes-Adams
   attack
cardiac asthma
cardiac ballet
cardiac blood pool imaging
cardiac borders
cardiac bradyarrhythmia
cardiac branch
cardiac cachexia
cardiac catheter
cardiac catheterization
   retrograde
   transseptal
cardiac cirrhosis
cardiac compression
cardiac contractility, depressed
cardiac contractions
cardiac cycle
cardiac death
   recurrent, not-so-sudden
   sudden
cardiac decompensation
   end-stage
   fetal
cardiac decompression
cardiac decortication
cardiac denervation
cardiac device
   Baim-Turi
   Balloon-on-a-Wire

cardiac device *(cont.)*
  Block
  Brockenbrough
  Champ
  Cournand
  Durathane
  El Gamal
  Finesse
  Gensini
  Goetz
  Goodale-Lubin
  Hi-Per
  Ideal
  King
  Lehman
  Linx guide wire extension
  NBIH
  Nycore
  Positrol
  Presso
  Propel coating
  Probe
  Rashkind
  Super-9 guiding
  Symbion
  Tandem
  Thermetics
  Thoratec
  Veri-Flex
  Williams
  Wizard
  XT
  Zucker and Myler
cardiac dilatation
cardiac dullness during respiration
cardiac dynamics
cardiac dysrhythmia
cardiac ectopy
cardiac efficiency
cardiac enlargement
cardiac enzymes (see *isoenzymes*)
cardiac failure (see *heart failure*)

cardiac fibroma
cardiac fibrosarcoma
cardiac filling pressure
cardiac fossa
cardiac function
cardiac function tests (CFTs)
cardiac functional capacity
cardiac glycogenosis
cardiac glycosides
cardiac hamartoma
cardiac hemangioma
cardiac histiocyte
cardiac hypertrophy
cardiac hypokinesis
cardiac impression
cardiac index (CI) (pl. indices)
cardiac infarct
cardiac insufficiency
cardiac irritability
cardiac isoenzymes, serial
cardiac laminography
cardiac leads (see *lead*)
cardiaclike chest pain
cardiac-limb syndrome
cardiac lipoma
cardiac lung
cardiac lymphangioma
cardiac mapping
cardiac margins on x-ray
cardiac massage
cardiac monitor, MemoryTrace AT
cardiac murmur of unknown type
cardiac muscle fibers
cardiac myxoma
cardiac neurosis syndrome
cardiac node
cardiac notch
cardiac output (CO) (see also *output*)
  adequate
  augmented
  inadequate
  reduced

cardiac output *(cont.)*
  reduced systemic
  thermodilution
cardiac output measurement
  Fick oxygen method of
  indicator-dilution method of
  indocyanine green dye method of
  thermodilution method
cardiac overload (or overloading)
cardiac oxygenation
cardiac paraganglioma
cardiac perforation
cardiac plexus
cardiac psychosis
cardiac pumping ability
cardiac radiation syndrome
cardiac recovery
cardiac referred pain
cardiac reflexes
cardiac rehabilitation program
cardiac reserve
cardiac retraction clip
cardiac rhabdomyoma
cardiac rhabdomyosarcoma
cardiac rhythm
cardiac rhythm disturbance
cardiac risk assessment
cardiac risk factors
  age
  alcohol consumption
  alcoholism
  behavior
  blood pressure
  caffeine consumption
  cigarette smoking
  coffee drinking
  diabetes mellitus, type I
  diabetes mellitus, type II
  diet
  elevated cholesterol
  elevated blood lipids
  elevated triglycerides

cardiac risk factors *(cont.)*
  environment
  familial disposition
  family history
  gender (male more than female
    until menopause)
  genetic
  heredity
  high blood pressure (HBP)
  high plasma LDL (low-density
    lipoproteins)
  hypercalcemia
  hypercholesterolemia
  hypercoagulability
  hyperlipidemia
  hypertension
  hypertriglyceridemia
  hyperuricemia
  lack of exercise
  lipidemia
  low plasma HDL (high-density
    lipoproteins)
  menopause
  obesity
  oral contraceptive use
  personality type A
  physical inactivity
  race
  saturated fat consumption
  sedentary lifestyle
  smoking of cigarettes
  stress
  tobacco use
  type A personality
  vasectomy
  water hardness
cardiac rupture
cardiac sarcoma
cardiac series (x-rays)
cardiac shadow
cardiac shape
cardiac shunt

cardiac silhouette (on x-ray)
  borderline-enlarged
  enlarged
  large thymus shadow obscuring
cardiac sling
cardiac souffle
cardiac source
cardiac standstill
cardiac steady state
Cardiac Stimulator
cardiac syphilis
cardiac stroke volume
cardiac surgery intensive care unit
  (CSICU)
cardiac sympathectomy
cardiac sympathomimetic amines
cardiac syncope
cardiac tamponade, low-pressure
cardiac teratoma
cardiac thrombosis
cardiac thrust
cardiac tone
cardiac transplant donor (CTD)
cardiac transplant recipient (CTR)
cardiac trauma
cardiac troponin T test
cardiac tumor embolization
cardiacus, plexus
cardiac valvar operation
cardiac valve mucoid degeneration
cardiac valve prosthesis, Omniscience
  single leaflet
cardiac valves
cardiac vasculature
cardiac vein, great
cardiac waist
cardialgia
cardiasthma
cardiectasis
Cardifix EZ pacing lead
cardinal event
cardinal physical finding

cardinal signs of inflammation
cardinal symptom
cardioangiography
cardioangioscope
cardioarterial interval carcinoid
cardioauditory syndrome
Cardiobacterium hominis
cardiocele
cardiocentesis
cardiochalasia
cardiocirrhosis
cardiocutaneous syndrome
Cardio Data MK3 Holter scanner
cardiodefibrillator, Endotek
CardioDiary heart monitor
cardiodilator
cardiodiosis
cardiodynamics
cardiodynia
cardioesophageal
cardiofacial defect
cardiofacial syndrome
cardiogenesis
cardiogenic embolic stroke
cardiogenic embolism
cardiogenic pulmonary edema
cardiogenic shock, advanced
cardiogenic shock heart
cardiogram
  apex (ACG)
  electro-
  precordial
  ultrasonic (UCG)
  vector
cardiograph, -graphy
Cardio-Green dye
cardiohemic system
cardiohepatic
cardiohepatomegaly
cardioinhibitor
cardioinhibitory
cardioinhibitory carotid sinus syncope

cardioinhibitory carotid sinus
  syndrome
cardioinhibitory responses
cardioinhibitory/vasodepressor
cardiointegram (CIG)
cardiokinetic
cardiokymographic test
cardiokymography (CKG)
Cardiolite (^{99m}Tc sestamibi) scan
cardiologist
cardiology, invasive
cardiolysis
cardiomalacia
cardiomegaly
  alcoholic
  familial
  globular
  hypertensive
  iatrogenic
  idiopathic
  postoperative
cardiomotility
cardiomyoliposis
cardiomyopathic carnitine deficiency
cardiomyopathic lentiginosis
cardiomyopathy
  alcoholic
  alcoholic dilated
  amyloidotic
  apical hypertrophic (AHC)
  arrhythmogenic right ventricular
  beer-drinker's
  beriberi
  concentric hypertrophic
  congenital dilated
  congestive
  constrictive
  diabetic
  diffuse symmetric hypertrophic
  dilated (DCM)
  end-stage
  familial

cardiomyopathy *(cont.)*
  familial hypertrophic (FHC)
  Friedreich ataxic
  histiocytoid
  hypertrophic (HCM)
  hypertrophic obstructive (HOC
    or HOCM)
  idiopathic
  idiopathic dilated (IDC)
  idiopathic restrictive
  infantile histiocytoid
  infectious
  infiltrative
  ischemic
  ischemic congestive
  left ventricular
  metabolic
  mucopolysaccharidosis
  myotonia atrophica
  noncoronary
  nonischemic congestive
  nonobstructive
  obliterative
  obscure
  obstructive
  obstructive hypertrophic
  peripartum
  peripartum dilated
  postmyocarditis dilated
  postpartum
  primary
  restrictive (RCM)
  right ventricular
  right-sided
  secondary
  tachycardia-induced
  thyrotoxicotic
  toxic
  viral
cardiomyopathy with restrictive
  component
cardiomyoplasty

cardiomyotomy
cardionecrosis
cardionephric
cardioneural
cardio-omentopexy
Cardio-Pace Medical Durapulse
    pacemaker
cardiopathia nigra (Ayerza syndrome)
cardiopathic
cardiopathy
    hypertensive
    infarctoid
    obscure
cardiopathy nigra syndrome
cardiopericardiopexy
cardiopericarditis
cardiopexy, ligamentum teres
cardiophobia
cardiophrenia
cardiophrenic angle
cardiophrenic junction
cardioplasty
cardioplegia
    Buckberg
    cold
    cold blood
    cold blood hyperkalemic
    cold crystalloid
    cold potassium
    cold retrograde blood
    cold sanguineous
    continuous warm blood
    crystalloid potassium
    hyperkalemic
    nutrient
    potassium chloride
    St. Thomas Hospital
    warm continuous retrograde
cardioplegic arrest, hypothermic
cardioplegic needle
cardioplegic solution (see also
    cardioplegia)

cardioplegic solution *(cont.)*
    Bretschneider-HTK
    Buckberg
    hyperkalemic crystalloid
    infusion of
    leukocyte-depleted terminal blood
    retrograde
    St. Thomas
cardiopneumatic
Cardiopoint
cardioprotective
cardioptosis, Wenckebach
cardiopulmonary arrest
cardiopulmonary bilharziasis
cardiopulmonary bypass (CPB)
cardiopulmonary bypass time
cardiopulmonary deterioration
cardiopulmonary insufficiency
cardiopulmonary obesity
cardiopulmonary resuscitation (CPR)
cardiopulmonary schistosomiasis
cardiopulmonary support pump
    Bard
    percutaneous
cardiopulmonary support system (CPS)
cardiopulmonary support, temporary
    percutaneous
cardiopuncture
cardiopyloric
cardiorenal disease
cardiorespiratory distress
cardiorespiratory sign
cardiorrhaphy
cardiorrhexis (rupture of heart)
cardiosclerosis
cardioscope U system
cardioselective agent
cardioselective beta-blocker drug for
    hypertension and angina
cardiospasm
cardiosplenopexy
cardiotachometer, -metry

Cardio Tactilaze peripheral angio-
    plasty laser catheter
CardioTec or Cadiotec (^{99m}Tc tebor-
    oxime) scan
cardiotherapy
cardiothoracic index
cardiothoracic ratio (CTR)
cardiothoracic surgeon
cardiothyrotoxicosis
cardiotocograph, -graphy
cardiotomy
cardiotomy reservoir
cardiotonic drug
cardiotopometry
cardiotoxic
cardiotoxicity
    Adriamycin
    digitalis
    doxorubicin
cardiouremia
cardiovalvular
cardiovalvulitis
cardiovalvulotome
cardiovalvulotomy
cardiovascular accident (CVA)
cardiovascular anomalies
cardiovascular collagenosis
cardiovascular hemodynamics
cardiovascular radioisotope scan and
    function study
cardiovascular renal disease
cardiovascular resuscitation
cardiovascular shunt
cardiovascular silk suture
cardioversion
    DC (direct-current)
    electrical
    endocavitary
    pharmaceutical
    spontaneous
    synchronized DC
cardioversion zone

cardiovert, attempt to
cardioverted
cardioverter
cardioverter-defibrillator (see also
    pacemaker and *pulse generator*)
    automatic implantable (AICD)
    internal
    implantable
    implantable automatic atrial
    nonthoracotomy
    Res-Q AICD
cardioverter-defibrillator implantation
cardiovocal syndrome
carditis
    Lyme
    rheumatic
    streptococcal
    verrucous
Carey Coombs murmur
carina of trachea
carinatum, pectus
Carmalt forceps
C-arm digital fluoroscopy
Carmeda BioActive Surface
carnitine deficiency
carnitine deficiency syndrome
carotid arterial dissection
carotid arterial pulse, synchronous
carotid artery
    kinking
    redundant
carotid artery aneurysm
carotid artery bruit
carotid artery pulsations, transmitted
carotid artery-cavernous sinus fistula
carotid baroreceptor
carotid bifurcation
carotid bruit
carotid bulb
carotid-cavernous fistula
carotid duplex study
carotid ejection time

carotid endarterectomy
carotid glomectomy
carotid massage, chest pain relieved by
carotid occlusive disease
carotid phonoangiography
carotid pulse
carotid pulse collapse
carotid pulse peak
carotid pulse tracing
carotid pulse upstroke
carotid shudder
carotid sinus
carotid sinus hypersensitivity (CSH)
carotid sinus massage
carotid sinus reflex, hyperactive
carotid sinus syncope
carotid sinus syndrome
carotid string sign
carotid system, extracranial
carotid upstroke, brisk
carotid-carotid venous bypass graft
carotid-subclavian bypass
carotids, equal
carotidynia
Carpenter syndrome
Carpentier annuloplasty ring prosthesis
Carpentier-Edwards aortic valve
Carpentier-Edwards bioprosthetic
    valve
Carpentier-Edwards glutaraldehyde-
    preserved porcine xenograft bio-
    prosthesis
Carpentier-Edwards mitral annulo-
    plasty valve
Carpentier-Edwards pericardial valve
Carpentier-Edwards Porcine
    SupraAnnular valve (SAV)
Carpentier method
Carpentier ring
Carpentier technique
Carpentier tricuspid valvuloplasty
CAR (carotid arterial) pulse

Carrel button
Carrel patch
Carrel technique
Carrel, triangulation of
Carter equation
cartilage
    absent bronchial
    aortic
    bronchial annular
    costal
    costal interarticular
    cricoid
    hyaline
    laryngeal
    main stem bronchial
    pulmonary
    sternal
    thyroid
    tracheal
    xiphoid
Carvallo sign in tricuspid regurgitation
CAS (coronary artery spasm)
cascade
    arachidonic acid
    coagulation
cascade of abdomen
caseating tuberculosis with cavity
    formation
CASE computerized exercise EKG
    system
caseous necrosis
CASS (Coronary Artery Surgery
    Study)
CASS scoring of left ventricular
    function
Castaneda anastomosis clamp
Castaneda vascular clamp
Castellani bronchitis
Castellani disease
Castellino sign
Castillo catheter
Castroviejo needle holder

cat-eye syndrome (or cat's eye)
CAT (computed axial tomography)
catacrotic
catacrotism
catadicrotism
catadicrotic pulse
catatricrotism
catarrhal croup
catarrhal laryngitis
catarrhal tracheitis
catastrophe, vascular
catch
catching feeling
catechol excess
catecholamines, circulating
catgut absorbable suture material
cath (catheterization)
cathed or cath'd (catheterized)
catheter
  ACE
  Achiever balloon dilatation
  ACS (Advanced Catheter or
    Cardiac Systems)
  ACS angioplasty
  ACS balloon
  ACS JL4 (Judkins left 4 French)
  ACS mini
  ACS RX coronary dilatation
  AL-1
  AL II guiding
  Alzate
  Amplatz cardiac
  Amplatz femoral
  Amplatz right coronary
  Angio-Kit
  Angiocath PRN flexible
  angiographic balloon occlusion
  Angiomedics
  angiopigtail
  angioplasty balloon
  angled balloon
  angulated

catheter *(cont.)*
  Anthron heparinized antithrombo-
    genic
  aortogram
  AR-2 diagnostic guiding
  Arani double loop guiding
  Arrow-Berman balloon
  ArrowGard Blue Line
  ArrowGard central venous
  Arrow-Howes multilumen
  Arrow pulmonary artery
  Arrow Twin Cath
  Arrow Twin Cath multilumen
    peripheral
  arterial embolectomy
  atherectomy
  atherectomy, peripheral
  AtheroCath
  Atlas LP PTCA balloon dilatation
  Atlas ULP balloon dilatation
  Atri-pace I bipolar-flared pacing
  Auth atherectomy
  AV-Paceport thermodilution
  Axiom DG balloon angioplasty
  bail-out
  Baim pacing
  Baim-Turi monitor/pacing
  balloon biliary
  balloon dilatation
  balloon dilating
  balloon embolectomy
  balloon flotation
  balloon septostomy
  balloon-flotation pacing
  balloon-tipped angiographic
  balloon-tipped end-hole
  balloon-tipped flow-directed
    pulmonary artery
  ball-wedge
  Bard guiding
  Bardic cutdown
  Baxter

catheter *(cont.)*
　Berman angiographic
　Bernstein
　bicoudate
　bifoil balloon
　bipolar pacing electrode
　bipolar temporary pacemaker
　Block right coronary guiding
　Blue FlexTip
　Blue Max triple-lumen
　Brockenbrough
　Brockenbrough mapping
　Brockenbrough modified bipolar
　Brockenbrough transseptal
　bronchial
　Bronchitrac L
　bronchospirometric
　Broviac
　Broviac atrial
　Buchbinder Omniflex
　Buchbinder Thruflex
　Buerhenne steerable
　Camino microventricular bolt
　cardiac
　Cardiomarker
　Cardio Tactilaze peripheral
　　angioplasty laser
　Castillo
　Cath-Finder
　central venous (CVC)
　Chemo-Port
　Cloverleaf
　coaxial
　Cobra
　Cobra over-the-wire balloon
　cobra-shaped
　coil-tipped
　Comfort Cath I or II
　conductance
　Cook arterial
　Cook pigtail
　Cook TPN

catheter *(cont.)*
　Cordis Brite Tip guiding
　Cordis Ducor I (or II, III) coronary
　Cordis Ducor pigtail
　Cordis high-flow pigtail
　Cordis Son-II
　coronary dilatation
　coronary guiding
　coronary sinus thermodilution
　corset balloon
　coudé
　Cournand cardiac
　CR Bard
　Critikon
　cryoablation
　cutdown
　CVP (central venous pressure)
　Dacron
　Datascope DL-II percutaneous
　　translucent balloon
　decapolar
　deflectable quadripolar
　diagnostic
　Diasonics
　dilatation balloon
　dilating
　DLP cardioplegic
　Doppler coronary
　Dorros brachial internal mammary
　　guiding
　Dorros infusion/probing
　Dotter
　Dotter caged balloon
　Dotter coaxial
　Double J indwelling
　Double J ureteral
　double-lumen
　Ducor balloon
　DVI Simpson atherocath
　EAC (expandable access catheter)
　EchoMark
　EchoMark angiographic

catheter *(cont.)*
Edwards diagnostic
Elecath thermodilution
electrode
11 French JCL 3.5 guiding
El Gamal coronary bypass
Elite
embolectomy
end-hole
Endosound endoscopic ultrasound
Endotak C lead
enhanced torque 8F (8 French)
  guiding
Eppendorf
Erythroflex
Erythroflex hydromer-coated
  central venous
expandable access (EAC)
Express
Express PTCA
extraction
extrusion balloon
FAST (flow-assisted, short-term)
  balloon
femoral guiding
Finesse large-lumen guiding
Flexguard Tip
flotation
flow-directed
flow-oximetry
fluid-filled
Fogarty adherent clot
Fogarty arterial embolectomy
Fogarty balloon
Fogarty balloon biliary
Fogarty embolectomy
Fogarty graft thrombectomy
Fogarty occlusion
Fogarty venous thrombectomy
Fogarty-Chin extrusion balloon
Force balloon dilatation
French

catheter *(cont.)*
French 5 (5 French) angiographic
French MBIH
FR4 guiding
Ganz-Edwards coronary infusion
Gensini coronary
Gentle-Flo suction
Goodale-Lubin cardiac
Gorlin pacing
Gould PentaCath 5-lumen thermo-
  dilution
graft-seeking
Grollman
Grollman pigtail
Groshong
Groshong double-lumen
Gruentzig (Grüntzig)
Grüntzig arterial balloon
Grüntzig Dilaca
guiding
Halo
Hanafee
Hartzler ACX-II or RX-014 balloon
Hartzler LPS dilatation
Hartzler Micro II
Hartzler Micro XT dilatation
headhunter visceral angiography
helical-tip Halo
helium-filled balloon
hexapolar
Hickman indwelling right atrial
Hidalgo
Hieshima coaxial
high-fidelity
high-fidelity microtipped
high-flow
high-speed rotation dynamic
  angioplasty
hot-tip
HydraCross TLC PTCA
IAB (intra-aortic balloon)
Illumen-8 guiding

catheter *(cont.)*
ILUS (intraluminal ultrasound)
indwelling
Infiniti
Inoue balloon
intra-aortic balloon
intra-aortic balloon double-lumen
Intracath
intracoronary guiding
intracoronary perfusion
intravascular ultrasound
intravenous pacing
intrepid PTCA angioplasty
ITC balloon
Jackman orthogonal
Jelco intravenous
JL4 (Judkins left 4 cm curve)
JL5 (Judkins left 5 cm curve)
JR4 (Judkins right 4 cm)
Judkins left 4 cm (JL4)
Judkins left coronary
Judkins right 4 cm (JR4)
Judkins right coronary
Judkins USCI
KDF-2.3
Kensey
Kensey atherectomy
Kifa
King multipurpose coronary graft
Kinsey atherectomy
Kontron balloon
large-bore
large-lumen
laser
left coronary
left heart
left Judkins
left ventricular sump
Lehman
Lehman ventriculography
Lo-Profile balloon
Lo-Profile II balloon

catheter *(cont.)*
Lo-Profile steerable dilatation
Longdwel Teflon
low-speed rotation angioplasty
LPS
Lumaguide
Mallinckrodt angiographic
manometer-tipped cardiac
Mansfield
Mansfield Atri-Pace 1
Mansfield orthogonal electrode
Mansfield Scientific dilatation
   balloon
Marathon guiding
Max Force
McGoon coronary perfusion
McIntosh double-lumen
Medi-Tech balloon
Medtronic balloon
Micro-Guide
micromanometer-tip
midstream aortogram
Mikro-tip micromanometer-tipped
Millar
Millar micromanometer
Millar MPC-500
Millar pigtail angiographic
Miller septostomy
Mini-Profile dilatation
Mirage over-the-wire balloon
Mitsubishi angioscopic
Molina needle
Monorail angioplasty
Monorail balloon
MPF
Mullins transseptal
multi-electrode impedance
Multi-Med triple-lumen infusion
multifiber
multilumen
multipolar impedance
multipurpose

catheter *(cont.)*
MVP
Mylar
NBIH
NIH (National Institutes of Health)
NIH cardiomarker
NIH left ventriculography
9 Fr JL 4 guiding (9 French Judkins
   left 4 guiding)
nontraumatizing
NoProfile balloon
Nycore
Nycore angiography
octapolar
Omniflex balloon
one-hole angiographic
Optiscope
over-the-wire balloon
oximetric
PA Watch position-monitoring
Paceport
Pacewedge dual-pressure bipolar
   pacing
pacing
Pathfinder
PE Plus II balloon dilatation
Percor DL balloon
Percor DL-II balloon
Percor-Stat-DL
percutaneous
perfusion
peripherally inserted central (PICC)
pervenous
Phantom V Plus
PIBC (percutaneous intra-aortic
   balloon counterpulsation)
pigtail
polyethylene
Polystan venous return
Positrol II
preformed
preshaped

catheter *(cont.)*
probing
Profile Plus dilatation
Proflex 5 dilatation
Pro-Flo
Pruitt-Inahara balloon-tipped
   perfusion
PTCA (percutaneous transluminal
   coronary angioplasty)
pulmonary artery
pulmonary flotation
pulmonary triple-lumen
quadripolar electrode
quadripolar steerable electrode
Quanticor
Quinton
Raaf Cath vascular
radial artery
Rashkind balloon
Rashkind septostomy balloon
recessed balloon septostomy
RediFurl TaperSeal IAB
Rentrop infusion
retroperfusion
RF (radiofrequency-generated
   thermal) balloon
right coronary
right heart
right Judkins
Robinson
Rodriguez
Rodriguez-Alvarez
Royal Flush angiographic flush
Rumel
Sarns wire-reinforced
Schneider
Schneider-Shiley
Schoonmaker femoral
Schoonmaker multipurpose
Schwarten balloon
Schwarten balloon dilatation
Sci-Med SSC "Skinny"

catheter *(cont.)*
  sensing
  serrated
  shaver
  Sheldon
  Shiley guiding
  Shiley-Ionescu
  Skinny
  SHJR4s (side-hole Judkins right,
    curve 4, short)
  side-hole
  sidewinder
  Silastic
  Silicore
  Simmons-type (sidewinder)
  Simplus PE/t dilatation
  Simpson peripheral AtheroCath
  Simpson Ultra Lo-Profile II balloon
  Simpson-Robert
  single-stage
  sliding rail
  Smec balloon
  snare
  Softip arteriography
  Softip diagnostic
  Softouch guiding
  Sones cardiac
  Sones Cardio-Marker
  Sones Hi-Flow
  Sones Positrol
  Stack perfusion coronary dilatation
  standard Lehman
  steerable electrode
  Steerocath
  Stertzer brachial guiding
  Stertzer guiding
  stimulating
  straight flush percutaneous
  SULP II
  sump
  Swan-Ganz balloon-flotation
    pulmonary artery

catheter *(cont.)*
  Swan-Ganz flow-directed
  Swan-Ganz Guidewire TD
  Swan-Ganz Pacing TD
  Swan-Ganz thermodilution
  TAC atherectomy
  Teflon
  temporary pacing
  Tennis Racquet angiographic
  tetrapolar esophageal
  thermistor
  thermodilution balloon
  thermodilution pacing
  thermodilution Swan-Ganz
  thoracic
  thrombectomy
  Thruflex PTCA balloon
  toposcopic
  Torcon NB selective angiographic
  Tracker
  transcutaneous extraction
  transducer-tipped
  transluminal extraction (TEC)
  transseptal
  transvenous pacemaker
  trefoil balloon
  Triguide
  triple thermistor coronary sinus
  triple-lumen central venous
  tripolar
  tripolar electrode
  Tygon
  ULP (ultra-low profile)
  ultra-low profile fixed-wire balloon
    dilatation
  UMI
  USCI Bard
  USCI guiding
  USCI Mini-Profile balloon
    dilatation
  valvuloplasty balloon
  Van Andel

catheter *(cont.)*
  Van Tassel pigtail
  Variflex
  venous
  venous thrombectomy
  venting
  ventriculography
  VIPER PTA
  Vitalcor venous
  Voda
  Webster coronary sinus
  Webster orthogonal electrode
  Wexler
  Williams L-R guiding
  Wilton-Webster coronary sinus
  Zucker
cathéter `a demeure (indwelling)
catheter advanced under fluoroscopic
  guidance
catheter artifact
catheter balloon valvuloplasty
catheter coated with cefazolin
catheter damping
catheter deployment
catheter electrode
catheter embraced by plaque
catheter exchanged over a guide wire
catheter impact artifact
catheter inched up the artery
catheter-induced bacteremia
catheter-induced coronary artery spasm
catheter, introduction of
catheterization
  antegrade transseptal left heart
  cardiac
  central venous (CVC)
  Fogarty balloon
  left heart
  Mullins modification of transseptal
  PTCA (percutaneous transluminal
    coronary angioplasty)

catheterization *(cont.)*
  retrograde
  retrograde arterial
  retrograde left heart
  right heart
  selective cardiac
  simultaneous right and left heart
  subclavian vein
  transseptal cardiac
  transseptal heart
  transseptal left heart
catheterizing
catheter kinking
catheter mapping
catheter migration
catheter passage, tortuosity precluding
catheter sheath
catheter-skin interface
catheter tip hockey-stick appearance
catheter tip motion artifact
catheter-tipped manometer
catheter-tissue contact
catheter whip artifact
catheter with preformed curves
cathodal lead
cathodal patch electrode, posterior
cathode
  defibrillation
  epicardial patch
caudad
caudal branch
caudal collaterals
caudal view
causative organism
causative virus
cautery
cautious dissection
cava, juxtarenal
caval-atrial (or cavoatrial) junction
caval-pulmonary artery anastomosis
caval snare

caval tourniquet
CAVB (complete atrioventricular
   block)
cavernous angiosarcoma
cavernous breath sounds
cavernous breathing
cavernous hemangioma
Caves-Schulz bioptome
cavitary lung mass
cavitary mass
cavitary tuberculosis
cavitating carcinoma
cavitation
cavity
   coexistent
   pericardial
   pulmonary
   thoracic
cavity in the lung
cavoatrial (caval-atrial) junction
cavogram
cavopulmonary anastomosis,
   bidirectional
cavopulmonary connection
Cayler syndrome
CBC (complete blood cell count)
   hematocrit
   hemoglobin
   MCH (mean corpuscular
      hemoglobin)
   MCHC (mean corpuscular
      hemoglobin concentration)
   MCV (mean corpuscular volume)
   RBC (red blood cell) count
   WBC (white blood cell) count
CBC with diff (differential)
CBC with WBC and differential
CBS (capillary blood sugar)
CBV (catheter balloon valvuloplasty)
CC (closing capacity)
CCA (common carotid artery)
C-C (convexo-concave) heart valve

cc/min. (cubic centimeters per minute)
C, C, or E (clubbing, cyanosis, or
   edema)
CCU (coronary care unit) protocol
CCU (critical care unit) protocol
CD (conduction defect)
CDI blood gas-monitoring system
C_{dyn} (dynamic lung compliance)
C-E amplitude of mitral valve
CECG (continuous electrocardio-
   graphic monitoring)
Cedars-Sinai classification of pump
   failure
Ceelen-Gellerstedt syndrome
cefazolin, catheter coated with
Cegka sign
celer, pulsus (quick pulse)
C-11 (^{11}C) (carbon-11)
C-11 acetate imaging
C-11 hydroxylase deficiency
C-11 palmitate uptake on PET scan
celiac angiography
celiac artery
celiac artery compression syndrome
celiac axis syndrome
cell, cells
   adventitial
   air
   alveolar (type I or II)
   Anichkov (or Anitschkow)
   APUD (amine precursor uptake and
      decarboxylation)
   Aschoff
   automatic
   basket
   Beale ganglion
   bend
   blood
   bronchic
   caterpillar
   chicken-wire myocardial
   Clara

cell *(cont.)*
  dust
  endothelioid
  epithelioid
  foamy myocardial
  goblet
  heart-disease
  heart-failure
  heart-lesion
  Marchand
  mast
  mononuclear
  multinucleate giant
  myocardial
  oat
  oat-shaped
  P
  pacemaker
  packed red blood
  perithelial
  perivascular
  plasma
  pleomorphic mononuclear
  pulmonary capillary endothelial
  pulmonary epithelial
  Purkinje
  spider
  strap
  T
  tennis racquet
  transitional
  virus-infected
Cellano phenotype
cell count
cell necrosis, myocardial
cellophane rales
Cell-Saver autotransfusor
cell saver, BRAT
Cell Saver Haemolite
Cell Saver Haemonetics Autotransfusion System
celltrifuge

cellular debris
cellular hypo-osmolality
cellular infiltrates
cellular infiltration
cellulitis
cellulitis-phlebitis
cell washings for cytologic study
Cenflex central monitoring system
central alpha-agonists
central aortic pressure
central aortic pulse pressure
central aortopulmonary shunting
central apnea
central arterial return
central blood volume
central cyanosis
central fibrous body
central hilar structures
central hypoventilation
central intra-aortic pressure curve
central jet
central splanchnic venous thrombosis
  (CSVT)
central vein, cannulated
central venous line
central venous pressure (CVP)
central venous pressure elevation
centriacinar emphysema
centrifugal mechanical assist (CMA)
centrilobular emphysema
cephalad
cephalic vein, cutdown over
cephalization of pulmonary flow
  pattern
cerebellar intracerebral hemorrhage
cerebral aneurysm
cerebral anoxia
cerebral arteries
cerebral arteriovenous fistula
cerebral arteritis
cerebral blood flow, decreased
cerebral carotid sinus syncope

cerebral embolism
cerebral hypoperfusion, global
cerebral hypoxia
cerebral infarction
cerebral intracerebral hemorrhage
cerebral ischemia
cerebral perfusion pressure
cerebral thrombosis
cerebromeningeal intracerebral
  hemorrhage
cerebrovascular accident (CVA)
  (stroke)
ceroid lipofuscinosis
cervical aorta syndrome
cervical extension incision
cervical pleura
cervical radiculitis
cervical vein pulsation
cervical venous hum
cervicocephalic arterial dissection
cesium chloride
cessation of normal cardiac
  contractions
cessation of smoking
cestodic tuberculosis
CFC (capillary filtration coefficient)
CFR (coronary flow reserve)
CFTs (cardiac function tests)
CGR biplane angiographic system
Chagas disease
chain reaction, polymerase (PCR)
chain, sympathetic
challenge
  exercise
  fluid
  HDM (house dust mites)
  histamine
  hypertonic saline
  inhalation aspirin
  methacholine chloride
  methacholine inhalation
  nasal antigen

chamber
  cardiac
  false aneurysmal
  hyperbaric
  infundibular
  left atrial
  left ventricular
  reduced compliance of
  right atrial
  right ventricular
  rudimentary outlet
chamber compression
chamber dilatation
chamber of heart
chamber size
chamber stiffness
Champ cardiac device
Chandler V-pacing probe
Chandra-Khetarpal syndrome
change, changes
  behavioral
  diagnostic ST segment
  EKG
  E to A
  hyaline
  ischemic
  nonspecific
  pulmonary parenchymal
  serial
  ST and T wave
  ST-T wave
  T wave
  transient repolarization
changes in sensorium
channel
  aberrant vascular
  blood
  calcium
  central
  false
  fast sodium
  slow calcium

channel *(cont.)*
   sodium
   thoroughfare
chaotic atrial tachycardia
character of pulse
characteristic findings
characteristic symptoms
Charcot-Bouchard aneurysm
Charcot-Leyden crystals
Charcot sign
Charcot-Weiss-Baker syndrome
Chardack-Greatbatch Implantable
   Cardiac Pulse Generator
Chardack-Greatbatch pacemaker
CHARGE (colobomas, choanal
   atresia, mental and growth
   deficiency, genital and ear
   anomalies) syndrome
charring
CHB (complete heart block)
CHD (congenital heart disease)
Check-Flo introducer
check-valve sheath
cheese handler's disease
cheese washer's disease
chemical ablation therapy for
   arrhythmia
chemical bronchitis
chemical derangement
chemical pneumonitis
chemical pulmonary edema
chemistry profile
chemoembolization
chemohormonal therapy
Chemo-Port perivena catheter system
chemotherapy, adjuvant
chest
   alar (flat)
   barrel-shaped
   blast
   cobbler's
   cylindrical

chest *(cont.)*
   flail
   flat
   foveated
   funnel
   globular
   hollow
   keeled
   paralytic
   phthinoid (flat)
   pigeon
   pounding
   pterygoid (flat)
   splinting of the
   symmetrical
   tetrahedron
chest cage abnormal
chest discomfort
chest excursion
   limited respiratory
   poor
chest heaviness
chest immobilization
chest lead
chest pain (see also *angina*)
   cardiaclike
   concomitant
   crushing
   evanescent
   ill-defined
   noncardiac
   pleuritic
   precordial
   substernal
chest pain relieved by carotid massage
chest PT (physiotherapy)
chest rawness
chest reexploration for bleeding
chest retraction on inspiration
chest thoracostomy site infection
chest tightness, waking with
chest tube (see *tube*)

chest tube, atelectasis following
  removal of
chest tube breakage upon removal
chest wall
  anterior
  lower
  upper
chest wall compliance
chest wall flattening
chest wall pain
chest wall paradoxical motion
chest wall phlebitis
chest wall tenderness
chest wall retractions
chest x-ray (CXR), baseline
Cheyne-Stokes breathing
Cheyne-Stokes respiration
CHF (congestive heart failure)
CH50 or CH_{50} (total hemolytic
  complement)
Chiari-Budd syndrome
Chiari syndrome
chicken fat clot
chicken-wire myocardial cell
childhood asthma
childhood tuberculosis
chill, chills
  brass
  brazier
  creeping
  fever and
  periodic
  shaking
  spelter
  teeth-chattering
  zinc
Chlamydia psittaci
chloral hydrate
chloride, chlorides
chlorotic phlebitis
chlorpromazine
choking

cholesterol
  "bad"
  "good"
  serum
  total plasma
cholesterol-carrying lipoproteins
cholesterol cleft
cholesterol crystal embolization,
  atheromatous
cholesterol debris
cholesterol effusion
cholesterol embolism
cholesterol embolization
  diffuse
  disseminated
cholesterol embolization syndrome
  peripheral
  renal
  visceral
cholesterol microembolization in toes
cholesterol pericarditis syndrome
cholesterol pleurisy
chondromatous hamartoma
chondrosternal junction
chordae (pl. of chorda)
  basal
  cleft
  commissural
  elongation of
  first order
  redundant
  ruptured
  second order
  shortening of
  strut
  third order
chordae tendineae cordis
  redundant
  ruptured
chordae tendineae rupture
chordal insertion
chordal length

chordal rupture
chorditis, fibrinous
chorditis nodosa
chorditis tuberosa
chorea
    cordis
    rheumatic
    Sydenham
choreiform movements, postoperative
choreoathetosis, postoperative
Chorus dual-chamber pacemaker
Chorus II dual-chamber pacemaker
Chorus RM rate-responsive dual-
    chamber pacemaker
Christmas blood coagulation factor
Christmas coagulation factor IX
Christmas disease (hemophilia B)
chromatography, gas
chromic catgut sutures
chromic suture
chronic airways obstruction
chronic allergic rhinitis
chronic arterial occlusive disease of
    extremities
chronic asthmatic diathesis
chronic atrial fibrillation with slow
    ventricular response
chronic bronchitis
chronic constrictive pericarditis
chronic discoloration of skin
chronic effusive pericarditis
chronic emphysema
chronic emphysematous mountain
    sickness
chronic eosinophilic pneumonia
chronic erythemic mountain sickness
chronic heart failure
chronic hemodynamic overload
chronic humoral rejection
chronic hypertensive disease
chronic hypertrophic emphysema
chronic hypertrophic myocarditis

chronic hyperventilation syndrome
chronic hypoxia
chronic indolent bacterial infection
chronic interstitial myocarditis
chronic intractable cough
chronic lead placement
chronic lung embolization by blood-
    borne eggs
chronic mountain sickness
    emphysematous-type
    erythremic-type
chronic nasopharyngitis
chronic necrotizing infection of
    bronchi
chronic obstructive bronchitis
chronic obstructive emphysema
chronic obstructive lung disease
    (COLD)
chronic obstructive pulmonary disease
    (COPD)
chronic parenchymal hemorrhage
chronic passive congestion of the lung
chronic pericarditis
chronic pernicious myocarditis
chronic pleurisy
chronic pneumonitis
chronic post-rheumatic fever arthritis
chronic pulmonary disease
chronic rejection of transplanted lung
chronic renal failure
chronic respiratory decompensation
chronic rheumatic heart disease
    (CRHD)
chronic rheumatic mediastinoperi-
    carditis
chronic rheumatic myopericarditis
chronic salicylate ingestion
chronic venous insufficiency
chronic vessel closure
Chronocor IV external pacemaker
chronotropic assessment exercise
    protocol (CAEP)

chronotropic effect
chronotropic incompetence
chronotropic response, blunted
chronotropic therapy
chunky sputum
Churchill-Cope reflex
Church scissors
Churg-Strauss syndrome
chyle
    effused
    pericardial
chyliform pleurisy
chylocele, nonfilarial
chyloid pleurisy
chylomicron
chylomicronemia, familial
chylopericardium
chylothorax (pl. chylothoraces)
chylous ascites
chylous pleurisy
CI (cardiac index)
Cibatome
CIE (counterimmunoelectrophoresis)
    of sputum
CIG (cardiointegram)
cigarette abuse
cigarette smoking, pack-years of
cilia
    dyskinetic
    immotile
ciliated border
cinchonism
cine CT (computed tomography)
    scanner
cine magnetic resonance, tagging
cine view in MUGA (cinematograph in
    multiple gated acquisition) scan
cineangiocardiography
cineangiogram, cineangiography
    biplane
    coronary
    left anterior oblique (LAO)

cineangiogram *(cont.)*
    left posterior oblique (LPO)
    left ventricular (LV)
    radionuclide
    right anterior oblique (RAO)
    right posterior oblique (RPO)
    selective coronary
    Sones technique for
    ventricular
cinecardioangiography
cinefluorography
cineloop
cineradiographic views
cineradiography
circ, CF, CX (circumflex artery)
Circadia dual-chamber rate-adaptive
    pacemaker
circadian event recorder
circadian periodicity
circadian rhythm of plasma aldosterone
circle of Vieussens
circle of Willis
circuit
    arrhythmia
    bypass
    macroreentrant
    microreentrant
    reentry
    shunting
circular aortotomy
circular cherry-red lesion
circular muscles
circular plane
circular shape factor
circular syncytium
circulating aldosterone level
circulating blood
circulating blood cells
circulating blood volume
circulating catecholamines
circulating fibrinogen pool
circulating lymphocytes

circulating renin
circulating water blanket
circulation
  abundant collateral
  adequate collateral
  allantoic
  arrested
  assisted
  balanced coronary
  bronchial collateral
  codominant
  codominant coronary
  collateral
  compensatory
  derivative
  extracorporeal
  fetal
  greater
  intervillous
  left circumflex-dominant
  left-dominant coronary
  lesser
  parasitic
  peripheral
  persistent fetal
  placental
  poor collateral
  portal
  precarious
  pulmonary
  pulmonary arterial
  reduced
  right-dominant coronary
  systemic
  thebesian
circulation time
circulatory abnormalities, occult
circulatory arrest
  profound hypothermic (PHCA)
  profoundly hypothermic total
circulatory assist devices
circulatory collapse

circulatory compromise
circulatory disturbances
circulatory embarrassment
circulatory failure
circulatory hyperkinetic syndrome
circulatory impairment
circulatory shock
circulatory stasis
circulatory support device, Elecath
circulatory support, mechanical
circumferential echodense layer
circumferential suture
circumflex (circ, CF, CX)
circumflex artery
circumflex branches
circumflex coronary artery
circumflex coronary system
circumflex groove artery
circumflex system
circumflex vessels
circumoral flush
circumoral pallor
circumscribed edema
circumscribed pleurisy
circumscript aneurysm
circumscript lesion
circus movement
circus-movement tachycardia (CMT)
cirrhosis
  cardiac
  congestive
  liver
  lung
  pulmonary
  vascular
cirsenchysis
cirsocele
cirsodesis
cirsoid aneurysm
cirsotome
cirsotomy
Citrobacter

CK (creatine kinase)
CK/AST ratio
CK isoenzymes (see *isoenzymes*)
   cardiac
CK-MB fraction (CK$_2$)
CKG (cardiokymography)
CL (cycle length)
clamminess
clammy skin
clamp or clip
   Adams-DeWeese vena caval clip
   Alfred M. Large vena cava
   Allis
   Allis-Adair
   anastomosis
   angled peripheral vascular
   aortic
   aortic aneurysm
   aortic occlusion
   appendage
   atraumatic vascular
   Atrauclip hemostatic
   Bahnson aortic
   Bailey aortic
   Beck
   Beck aortic
   Beck miniature aortic
   Beck-Potts
   Beck vascular
   Berman aortic
   Blalock-Niedner
   Blalock pulmonary
   Brock
   bulldog
   Calman carotid artery
   Calman ring
   Castaneda
   Castaneda anastomosis
   Castaneda vascular
   celiac
   coarctation

clamp *(cont.)*
   Cooley
   Cooley anastomosis
   Cooley aortic
   Cooley-Beck
   Cooley coarctation
   Cooley-Derra anastomosis
   Cooley iliac
   Cooley partial occlusion
   Cooley patent ductus
   Cooley pediatric
   Cooley renal
   Cooley-Satinsky
   Cooley vascular
   Cooley vena cava catheter
   Crafoord aortic
   Crafoord coarctation
   Crile
   curved
   curved Cooley
   Davidson vessel
   Davis aneurysm
   DeBakey aortic aneurysm
   DeBakey arterial
   DeBakey-Bahnson vascular
   DeBakey-Bainbridge
   DeBakey-Beck
   DeBakey bulldog
   DeBakey coarctation
   DeBakey cross-action bulldog
   DeBakey-Derra anastomosis
   DeBakey-Harken
   DeBakey-Howard
   DeBakey-Kay
   DeBakey patent ductus
   DeBakey pediatric
   DeBakey peripheral vascular
     bulldog
   DeBakey-Reynolds anastomosis
   DeBakey ring-handled bulldog
   DeBakey-Semb

clamp *(cont.)*
  DeBakey tangential occlusion
  DeBakey vascular
  DeMartel vascular
  Demos tibial artery
  DeWeese vena cava
  double-occluding
  exclusion
  Fogarty
  Fogarty Hydrogrip
  Fogarty-Chin
  Garcia aorta clamp
  Gerbode patent ductus
  Glover coarctation
  Glover patent ductus
  Glover vascular
  Goldblatt
  Grant aneurysm
  Gregory baby profunda clamp
  Gregory carotid bulldog
  Gregory external
  Gross coarctation occlusion
  Grover
  Gutgeman
  Harken auricle
  Heifitz
  hemostatic
  Hendrin ductus
  Henley vascular
  Hopkins aortic
  Hufnagel aortic
  Humphries aortic
  Jacobson-Potts
  Jahnke anastomosis
  Javid carotid artery
  Johns Hopkins coarctation
  Jones thoracic
  Kapp-Beck
  Kapp-Beck-Thomson
  Kartchner carotid artery
  Kay aorta
  Kay-Lambert

clamp *(cont.)*
  Kindt carotid artery
  Lambert aortic
  Lambert-Kay aorta
  Lambert-Kay vascular
  Lee microvascular
  Leland-Jones vascular
  Liddle aorta
  long Péan
  Mason vascular
  Mattox aorta
  metal
  metallic
  Michel aortic
  microvascular
  Mixter
  Mixter right-angle
  Morris aorta
  mosquito
  Muller pediatric
  Niedner anastomosis
  noncrushing vascular
  Noon AV fistula
  O'Neill
  occluding
  Omed bulldog vascular
  partial occlusion
  partially occluding vascular
  patent ductus
  Péan
  pediatric bulldog
  pediatric vascular
  Poppen-Blalock-Salibi
  Potts aortic
  Potts coarctation
  Potts-Nieder
  Potts patent ductus
  Potts-Satinsky
  Potts-Smith aortic occlusion
  Raney
  Reinhoff
  Reynolds vascular

clamp *(cont.)*
  right-angle
  Rumel myocardial
  Rumel thoracic
  Salibi carotid artery
  Sarot bronchus
  Satinsky aortic
  Satinsky vascular
  Satinsky vena cava
  Schnidt (*not* Schmidt)
  Schumaker aortic
  Schwartz
  Sehrt
  Selman
  Selverstone carotid
  side-biting
  sponge
  spoon
  stainless steel
  Stille-Crawford
  straight
  Subramanian
  Sugita right-angle aneurysm
  Swan aortic
  Thompson carotid artery
  tissue occlusion
  tube-occluding
  tubing
  vascular
  Vorse-Webster
  Wangensteen anastomosis
  Wangensteen patent ductus
  Weber aortic
  Weck
  Wister vascular
  Wylie carotid artery
  Yasargil carotid
clamp-and-sew technique
clamping, prolonged aortic
Clamshell Occluder
clapping
Clara cells

Clarke-Hadefield syndrome
Clark oxygen electrode
classic interstitial pneumonia
classical angina
classical hemophilia
classical triad of symptoms
classification (see also *index*)
  AHA (American Heart Association)
  AHA stenosis
  ASA (American Society of
    Anesthesia) risk
  Canadian system (I-IV) for severity
    of angina
  Cedars-Sinai pump failure
  Croften (for pulmonary eosino-
    philia)
  DeBakey (type I, II, III) (of aortic
    dissection)
  Dexter-Grossman mitral
    regurgitation
  Dubin and Amelar varicocele
  Fredrickson and Lees hyperlipo-
    proteinemia (type I-V)
  Fredrickson hyperlipoproteinemia
  Goldman
  Heath-Edwards
  Keith-Wagener-Barker (arteriolo-
    sclerosis, group 1-4)
  Killip heart disease
  Killip-Kimball heart failure
  Killip pump failure
  Lev complete AV (atrioventricular)
    block
  Levine-Harvey heart murmur
  Liebow and Carrington (for
    pulmonary eosinophilia)
  Lown ventricular arrhythmia
  Lown ventricular premature beat
  Minnesota EKG
  Mobitz atrioventricular block
  NYHA (New York Heart
    Association)

classification *(cont.)*
  NYHA angina (I-IV or A-D)
  NYHA congestive heart failure
  NYHA heart block, I-IV
  Pulec and Freedman (of congenital
    aural atresia)
  Stanford (type A, B, etc.) (of aortic
    dissection
  TIMI (thrombolysis in myocardial
    infarction) (II, IIA, etc.)
  Vaughn Williams antiarrhythmic
    drugs
classification of aortic dissection
classification of cardiomyopathy
Classix pacemaker
claudicant
claudication
  buttock
  calf
  hip
  intermittent
  intermittent venous
  leg
  lifestyle-limiting
  lower extremity
  nonlifestyle-limiting
  one-block
  one-flight
  progressive
  thigh
  three-block
  two-block
  two-flights-of-stairs
  venous
claustrophobic anxiety
claw grasper
Claybrook sign
clear airway
clear cell carcinoma of kidney
clear viscous sputum
clear zone
cleavage plane, subintimal

cleaving, plaque
cleft
  cholesterol
  horizontal chin
  Sondergaard
cleft chordae
cleft mitral valve
Clerc-Levy-Cristeco (CLC) syndrome
click
  aortic
  aortic ejection (AEC)
  aortic opening (AOC)
  apical midsystolic
  ejection (EC)
  fixed aortic ejection
  late systolic
  loud
  low-intensity systolic
  midsystolic
  mitral
  nonejection (NEC)
  nonejection systolic (NESC)
  palpable ejection
  pulmonary ejection (PEC)
  systolic (SC)
  systolic ejection
  systolic nonejection
  valvular
click louder when patient sits up
click murmur
click of maximal intensity when patient
    stands
clinical diagnosis
clinical picture
clinical remission
clinical sequelae
clinically significant
clinometry
clip (see *clamp*)
Clip On torquer
clipping, aneurysm
CLO (congenital lobar overinflation)

clockwise rotation of electrical axis on EKG
clockwise torque, constant (of electrode tip)
cloning
Clonorchis sinensis infection
closed lung biopsy
closed pleural biopsy
closed transventricular aortic valvotomy
closed tube thoracotomy
closing capacity (CC)
closing volume (CV)
clostridial infection
closure
  abrupt
  abrupt vessel
  acute vessel
  chronic vessel
  delayed sternal
  double umbrella
  ductus arteriosus
  impending
  patch
  patent ductus arteriosus
  patent ductus arteriosus (by double umbrella device)
  primary
  pulmonary valve
  secondary
  staged
  subcuticular
  subcuticular skin
  threatened vessel, post-PTCA
  tricuspid valve
  valve
  vein patch
closure of defect, spontaneous
closure of native aortic valve
clot
  agonal (or agony)
  antemortem

clot *(cont.)*
  autologous
  blood
  chicken fat
  currant jelly
  distal
  fibrin
  heart
  internal
  laminated
  marantic
  passive
  plastic
  postmortem
  proximal
  preformed
  stratified
  washed
  white
clot-dissolving mechanism
clot-dissolving treatment of coronary thrombosis
clot formation
clot lysis
clots and debris
clotting process
clotting time of whole blood
clouded consciousness
clouding of consciousness
cloudy swelling of the heart
Cloverleaf catheter
cloverleaf-shaped lumen
CLC (Clerc-Levy-Cristeco) syndrome
clubbing and cyanosis
clubbing, cyanosis, or edema (C, C, or E)
clubbing
  digital
  finger
clubbing of fingernails
clubbing of fingers and toes
clubbing of fingertips

clubbing of nail beds
clumps of sickled red cells
CM (continuous murmur)
CMA (centrifugal mechanical assist)
CM5 lead
CMR (congenital mitral regurgitation)
CMT (circus-movement tachycardia)
CNT (continuous nebulization therapy)
CO (cardiac output) (L/min)
coagulability of the blood
coagulable
coagulase-negative staphylococci
coagulase-positive *Staphylococcus aureus*
coagulation
    bipolar
    disseminated (or diffuse) intra-
        vascular (DIC)
    electric
coagulation cascade
coagulation factors of blood
    I: fibrinogen
    II: prothrombin
    III: thromboplastin
    IV: calcium ions
    V: proaccelerin (or AcG,
        accelerator globulin)
    VI: no factor VI
    VII: proconvertin (or SPCA, serum
        prothrombin conversion
        accelerator)
    VIII: antihemophilic (AHF)
        (von Willebrand)
    IX: plasma thromboplastin
        component (PTC) (Christmas)
    X: Stuart (or Stuart-Prower)
    XI: plasma thromboplastin
        antecedent (PTA)
    XII: Hageman
    XIII: fibrin stabilizing (FSF)
coagulation inhibitors

coagulation monitor, Biotrack
coagulator
    Biceps bipolar
    Concept bipolar
coagulopathic
coagulopathy
    consumption
    disseminated intravascular
coal miner's lung
coal worker's lung
coal worker's pneumoconiosis
Coanda effect
coaptation of valve leaflets
coaptation point
coapted leaflets
coarctation
    aortic
    atypical
    atypical subisthmic
    congenital isthmic
    isthmic
    juxtaductal
    preductal
    reversed
coarctation of aorta
    adult-type
    infantile-type
    juxtaductal
    postductal
    preductal
    reversed
coarctation repair
coarctectomy
coarcted aorta
coarcted segment
CoA reductase
coarse appearance
coarse bronchovascular markings
coarse crackles
coarse friction rub
coarse nodularity

coarse rales
coarse rhonchi
coarse sibilant expiratory rhonchi
coarse streaking
coated with cefazolin, catheter
coaxial catheter
coaxial catheter tip position
coaxial steering
cobbler chest syndrome
Cobe-Stockert heart-lung machine
Cobra catheter (mfg. by Sci-Med)
cobra-head appearance
cobra-head effect
Cobra over-the-wire balloon catheter
cobra venom factor (for myocardial
    ischemia)
cocaine-induced arrhythmias
cocaine-induced myocardial infarcts
cocaine-related cardiac death
cocaine-related fatal arrhythmias
cocaine-related fatal myocardial
    infarcts
cocci, gram-negative
Coccidioides immitis
coccidioidin test
coccidioidoma
coccidioidomycosis
    asymptomatic
    desert
    disseminated
    latent
    Posadas-Wernicke
    primary
    progressive
    San Joaquin Valley
    secondary
    valley
coccidioidal granuloma
coccidioidosis
coccidiosis
coccoid x bodies
Cockayne syndrome

cocktail, renal
Code Blue
codominant circulation
codominant coronary circulation
codominant system
codominant vessel
CO_2 electrode
CO_2 production
coeur en sabot (on x-ray)
coexistent cavity
coexisting disease
coffee worker's lung
cognitive dysfunction
cognitive symptoms
cogwheel breathing
coil
    defibrillation
    Gianturco
    Gianturco occlusion
    Gianturco wool-tufted wire
    proximal
    right ventricular
    surface
coil closure of coronary artery fistula
coil embolization (therapeutic)
coil embolization of fistula to
    pulmonary artery
coil embolization of unwanted vessel
coil soaked in thrombin
coil-tipped catheter
coil-to-vessel diameter
coin lesion (on x-ray)
coin sound
CO_2 laser
COLD (chronic obstructive lung
    disease)
cold agglutinin titer
cold agglutinins
cold blood cardioplegia
cold blood hyperkalemic cardioplegic
    solution
cold cardioplegia

cold cardioplegia arrest
cold cardioplegic solution
cold crystalloid cardioplegia
cold exposure
cold extremities
cold lactated Ringer's solution
cold potassium cardioplegia
cold potassium solution-induced
   cardiac arrest
cold pressor stimulation
cold pressor test (Hines and Brown
   test)
cold retrograde blood cardioplegia
cold spot myocardial imaging (thallium
   imaging, thallium scintigraphy)
cold stimulation test for Raynaud's
   syndrome
cold-induced angina
coldness of lower extremities
Cole-Cecil murmur
Colinet-Caplan syndrome
collagen degeneration
collagen hemostat
collagen-impregnated knitted Dacron
   velour graft
collagenosis, cardiac
collagenous deposits in alveolar septa
collagenous fibers
collagenous pneumoconiosis
collagen tissue proliferation
collagen vascular disease
collagen vascular screen (test)
collapse
   airway
   alveolar
   carotid pulse
   circulatory
   complete lung
   left lower lobe
   massive lung
   partial lung
collapsed lung field

collapsed portion of lung
collapse of alveoli
collapse of jugular venous pressure
collapse of venous pulse, diastolic
collapsing pulse
collar incision
collar prosthesis
collateral, collaterals
   antegrade
   aortopulmonary
   arcade of
   bridging
   caudal
   filled by
   filling via
   gives
   left to right
   persistent congenital stenosed
   receives
   retrograde
   right to left
   septal
collateral blood flow
collateral blood supply
collateral branch
collateral circulation
   abundant
   adequate
   bronchial
collateral hyperemia
collateralization, distal
collateralization of the airways
collateral supply
collateral system
collateral vessel filling
collateral vessels
collecting system, engorged
collection, loculated
collection of fluid in pleural cavity
collector, Lukens
Collins bicycle ergometer
Collins cycle ergometer

colloid osmotic pressure
colloid solution
colloids
Collostat hemostatic sponge
color
  blue bloater
  bluish skin
  beefy red
  dusky skin
  pink puffer
color Doppler recording
color-duplex interrogation
color flow Doppler real-time imaging
  of blood flow
color-flow duplex scan
color flow mapping
columnae carneae (trabeculae carneae)
columnar epithelium, pseudostratified
combination flow and pressure loads
combined hyperlipidemia
Comfeel Ulcus dressing
comma sign in truncus arteriosus
Command PS pacemaker
commence
commissural attachments
commissural chordae
commissural fusion
commissural incision
commissural leaflets
commissural neuron
commissural plication
commissural point
commissure
  anterior
  anteroseptal
  fused
  scalloped
  valve
  vestigial
commissurotomy
  Brockenbrough transseptal
  closed

commissurotomy *(cont.)*
  closed mitral
  mitral valve
  open mitral
  percutaneous catheter
  percutaneous transatrial mitral
  percutaneous transvenous mitral
    (PTMC)
  pulmonary valve
committed defibrillation shocks
committed shock
commode, bedside
common carotid artery
common faint
common femoral artery
common hepatic-common iliac-renal
  bypass
common iliac arteries
common pulmonary vein stenosis
Commucor A+V Patient Monitor
commune, ostium atrioventriculare
communicating vein incompetence
communicating veins
communication, interatrial
communicative disease
communicators, stripping of multiple
community-acquired pneumonia
comorbid condition
comp (comparison)
compartment
  anterior mediastinal
  superficial posterior
compartment syndrome
compensated congestive heart failure
compensating emphysema
compensatory enlargement
compensatory hypertrophy
compensatory mechanism
compensatory pause
compensatory polycythemia
competent valve
complaints, constitutional

complement activation
complementary increase in respiratory
    frequency
complement levels
complete atrioventricular block
complete atrioventricular dissociation
complete atrioventricular heart block
complete congenital heart block
complete graft preservation
complete heart block
complete lung collapse
complete occlusion of graft
complete stent expansion
complete transposition of the great
    arteries
complex
    aberrant QRS
    anisoylated plasminogen
        streptokinase activator
    anomalous
    aortic tract
    atrial
    atrial arrhythmias
    atrial premature (APC)
    AV (atrioventricular) junctional
        escape
    AV (atrioventricular) junctional
        premature
    biphasic EKG
    diphasic EKG
    Eisenmenger
    frequent spontaneous premature
    fusion QRS
    Ghon
    interpolated ventricular junctional
        premature
    Lutembacher
    monophasic contour of QRS
    multiform premature ventricular
    Mycobacterium avium (MAC)
    narrow QRS
    normal-voltage QRS

complex *(cont.)*
    parasystolic ventricular
    plasminogen streptokinase activator
    preexcited QRS
    premature atrial (PAC)
    premature AV (atrioventricular)
        junctional
    premature ventricular
    QRS
    QRST
    QS
    RS
    rS
    slurring of QRS
    Steidele
    symptom
    triphasic contour of QRS
    ventricular
    ventricular escape
    ventricular premature (VPC)
    wide QRS
    widening of QRS
complex cardiovascular defects
complex lesion
complex ventricular ectopic activity
compliance
    atrial
    chest wall
    decreased dynamic
    decreased lung
    decreased pulmonary vascular
    dynamic
    dynamic lung (C_{dyn})
    excellent
    good
    lung
    patient
    poor
    reduced pulmonary
    regional
    static lung (C_{STAT})
    ventricular

complicated hypertension
complicated silicosis
complicating meningitis
complications
  adverse
  perioperative
component
  actuator
  aortic
  first
  loud pulmonic
  markedly accentuated pulmonic
  pulmonic
  second
composite aortic valve
composite aortic valve replacement
composite graft
composite valve graft (CVG)
composite valve graft replacement
composite vein graft
compound
  artificial lung-expanding (ALEC)
  heparinoid
compressed Ivalon patch graft
compressible grape-like clusters of
  large venous spaces
compression
  brachial artery
  brachial plexus
  cardiac
  extrinsic
  iliocaval
  instrumental
  manual
  plaque
  pneumatic
  posterior fossa
  thermal
compression/atelectasis
compression cough
Compression Device, Kendall
  Sequential

compression garment, pneumatic foot
compression of tissues with pressure
  effects
compression stockings, Sigvaris
compression ultrasonography
compressor Deschamps
compromise
  circulatory
  respiratory
  systemic circulatory
  vascular
compromised flow
compromised respiratory status
compromised ventricular function
compromising flow
Compuscan Hittman computerized
  electrocardioscanner
computed ejection fraction
computed tomography (CT) scan
conal papillary muscle
conal portion of right ventricle
conal septum
Concato disease
concealed accessory pathway
concealed atrioventricular pathways
concealed bypass tracts
concealed conduction
concealed entrainment
concealed retrograde conduction
concentration
  albumin
  fibronectin
  histamine
  magnesium plasma
  neutrophil
  plasma
  potassium
  serum myoglobin (Mb)
  serum potassium
  24-hour urine creatinine
  24-hour urine potassium
  24-hour urine sodium

concentric atherosclerotic plaque
concentric hypertrophy
concentric left ventricular hypertrophy
concentric lesion
concentric plaque in arterial walls
concentric tear
Concept bipolar coagulator
concomitant antiarrhythmic therapy
concomitant arch repair
concomitant chest pain
concomitant condition
concomitant coronary artery bypass
concomitant defect
concomitant disease
concomitant findings
concomitant infarction
concomitant symptoms
concomitant therapy
concomitant tracheal injury
concordance, atrioventricular
concordant arterial connection
concordant atrioventricular connection
concretio cordis (dense pericardial
　　calcification)
concretio pericardii
concurrent infection
condition
　　comorbid
　　concomitant
　　improving
　　inherently unstable
　　precarious
conductance and resistance
conduction
　　aberrant
　　accelerated AV (atrioventricular)
　　　　node
　　accelerated atrioventricular
　　accessory atrioventricular
　　anomalous
　　antegrade
　　anterograde

conduction *(cont.)*
　　atrioventricular node
　　AV (atrioventricular) nodal
　　concealed
　　concealed retrograde
　　decremental
　　delayed
　　fast-pathway
　　infranodal
　　intra-atrial
　　intraventricular
　　preexcitation
　　preexcitation atrioventricular
　　reciprocating
　　retrograde
　　retrograde VA (ventriculoatrial)
　　slow-pathway
　　supernormal
　　ventriculoatrial (VA)
conduction abnormality
conduction block
conduction defect, intraventricular
conduction delay
conduction disturbance
conduction interval
conduction interval, intraatrial
conduction ratio (number of P waves to
　　number of QRS)
conduction system of heart
conduction time, sinoatrial (SACT)
conductive system of heart
conduit (see also *graft*)
　　afferent
　　apical aortic valved
　　apico-aortic (abdominal)
　　apico-aortic valved
　　efferent
　　valved
conduit graft
conduit valve
cone nose forceps
cone of apical tissue

confabulation
confidence interval
configuration
  bidirectional lead
  fishmouth (of mitral valve)
  inverted Y
  scalloped luminal
  spike-and-dome
  spike-dome
  thoracic cage
  undirectional lead
confluent consolidation
confluent fibrosis
confusion following open heart surgery
congenita
  myotonia
  paramyotonia
congenital absence of venous valves as
  cause of leg ulcers
congenital adrenal hyperplasia
congenital anemia of newborn
congenital aneurysm
congenital angiodysplasias of
  extremities
congenital anomaly of tricuspid valve
congenital aortic regurgitation
congenital aortic sinus aneurysm
congenital aortic stenosis
congenital arteriovenous fistula
congenital bicuspid aortic valve
congenital bleeding diathesis
congenital bronchiectasis
congenital cardiac anomaly
congenital cardiac defects
congenital cardiac malformation
congenital central hypoventilation
  syndrome
congenital cerebral aneurysm
congenital dilated cardiomyopathy
congenital fetal arrhythmia
congenital heart block
congenital heart disease, cyanotic

congenital heart failure
congenital heart murmur
congenital hypoplastic anemia
congenital interruption of aortic arch
congenital isolated hypoplasia
congenital isthmic coarctation
congenital lobar emphysema
congenital lobar overinflation (CLO)
congenitally absent pericardium
congenital mitral regurgitation
congenital mitral stenosis
congenital mitral valve disease
congenital pericardial absence
congenital pneumothorax
congenital polyvalvular dysplasia
congenital pulmonary fistula
congenital regurgitation
congenital rings of aortic arch
congenital rubella pneumonitis
congenital segmental renal hyperplasia
congenital stenosis of pulmonary vein
congenital subaortic stenosis
congenital subpulmonic obstruction
congenital subvalvular aortic stenosis
congenital supravalvular aortic
  stenosis, Brom repair of
congenital transposition, corrected
congenital valvular aortic stenosis
congenital vascular malformation
  (CVM)
congenital vascular-bone syndrome
  (CVBS)
congenital ventricular tachycardia
congestion
  active
  asymmetric pulmonary
  capillary
  chronic passive
  hepatic
  ʼ hypostatic
  passive vascular
  pulmonary

congestion *(cont.)*
  pulmonary venous
  symmetric pulmonary
  vascular
  venous
congestion stage
congestive atelectasis
congestive cardiomyopathy
congestive cirrhosis
congestive heart failure
conical heart
conjoined leaflet
conjunctive treatment
connection
  anomalous pulmonary venous
  cavopulmonary
  concordant arterial
  concordant atrioventricular
  discordant arterial
  discordant atrioventricular
  discordant ventriculoarterial
  partial anomalous pulmonary
    venous
  slip-in
  total anomalous pulmonary venous
    (TAPVC)
connective tissue proliferation
connective tissue septa
connector, three-way stopcock
Connolly eversion endarterectomy
Conn syndrome
conotruncal anomaly, congenital
conoventricular defect
Conradi-Hünermann syndrome
consciousness
  altered
  clouded
  diminished
  impaired
  near-loss of
  transient decrease
  transient loss of

consent, written informed
consequences, lethal
consolidated infiltrate
consolidated lung
consolidation
  alveolar
  confluent
  dense
  exudative
  lobar
  lung
  lung parenchyma
  patchy
  pulmonary
consolidation of alveoli
consolidation of lung
consolidative change
consolidative changes on chest x-ray
consolidative pneumonia
consolidative pneumonia due to
  Pneumococcus
conspicuous feature
constant clockwise torque of electrode
  tip
constant rate atrial pacing
constant tilt wave
constellation of findings
constellation of symptoms
constituent, plaque
constitutional complaints
constitutional disturbance
constitutional symptoms
constriction
  airway
  occult pericardial
  tangential
constriction of coronary arteries by
  cocaine
constriction of ductus arteriosus
constriction of peripheral arterioles
constrictive cardiomyopathy
constrictive lesion

constrictive pericardial disease
constrictive pericarditis
  advanced tuberculous
  effusive
construction of intra-atrial baffle
construction, venous valve
consumption
  myocardial oxygen (MVO$_2$)
  oxygen
  ventilatory oxygen (VO$_2$)
consumption coagulopathy
contact, stent-vessel wall
contagious disease
contained aneurysmal rupture
container, evacuator
contiguous segment
continuity equation
continuous ambulatory peritoneal
  dialysis (CAPD)
continuous electrocardiogram
continuous lateral rotation therapy
continuous mammary souffle
continuous mechanical ventilation
continuous monitoring of myocardial
  ischemia
continuous murmur (CM)
continuous positive airway pressure
  (CPAP)
continuous positive pressure ventilation
  (CPPV)
continuous rapid atrial pacing
continuous sampling of cardiac
  electrical activity
continuous sutures
continuous warm blood cardioplegia
continuous wave ablation
continuous wave Doppler recording
continuous wave Doppler ultrasonography
continuous wave laser system

contour
  aortic knob
  irregular hazy luminal
  precordial impulse contour
  S
contoured lead
contractile dysfunction
contractile force
contractile function, depressed right
  ventricular
contractile pattern
contractile performance, depressed
  myocardial
contractile reserve
contractile work index
contractility
  cardiac
  depressed
  depressed cardiac
  deranged left ventricular
  myocardial
contractility effect
contractility index
contracting factor, endothelium-
  derived
contraction
  atrial premature (APC)
  atrioventricular junctional
    premature
  automatic ventricular
  cardiac
  escaped ventricular
  force of
  isometric heart
  isotonic heart
  isovolumic (IVC)
  left atrial
  left ventricular
  myocardial
  nodal

contraction *(cont.)*
  nodal premature
  period of isovolumic
  premature atrial (PAC)
  premature junctional (PJC)
  premature nodal (PNC)
  premature ventricular (PVC)
  right atrial
  right ventricular
  R-on-T ventricular premature
  spastic
  supraventricular premature (SVPC)
  ventricular premature (VPC)
  ventricular segmental
contraction stress test (CST)
contraction time, isovolumic
contractor
  Bailey-Gibbon rib
  Bailey rib
  rib
contracture, myocardial
contraindicated drugs
contraindication to surgery
contralateral hemiparesis
contralateral pneumonectomy
contralateral vessel
contrast
  spontaneous echo
  tissue
contrast agent (see *contrast medium*)
contrast echo agents
contrast echocardiography
contrast laryngogram
contrast material (see *contrast medium*)
contrast medium (pl. media) (see also
  dye)
  Adenoscan
  Amipaque
  Angio-Conray
  Angiocontrast
  Angiovist

contrast medium *(cont.)*
  carbonated saline solution
  carbon-11 (^{11}C)
  ^{11}C palmitic acid radioactive
  ^{11}C-labeled fatty acids
  Cardio-Green (indocyanine green)
  Cardiolite (technetium Tc 99m
    sestamibi) (^{99m}Tc)
  CardioTec or Cardiotec (technetium
    Tc 99m teboroxime) (^{99m}Tc)
  CentoRx (monoclonal antibody 7E3)
  Conray
  degassed tap water
  dextrose 5% in water
  diatrizoate meglumine
  diatrizoate sodium
  Diatrizoate-60
  FDG (fluorodeoxyglucose)
  gadolinium-diethylenetriamine-
    pentaacetic acid
  gallium-68 (^{68}gallium)
  gold-195m
  hand-agitated
  Hexabrix
  high osmolar
  hydrogen peroxide
  Hypaque-76
  Hypaque Meglumine
  Hypaque Sodium
  indium 111 (^{111}In)
  ^{111}In imciromab pentetate
  ^{111}In-labeled antimyosin
  ^{111}In murine monoclonal antibody
    Fab to myosin
  ^{111}In pentetreotide
  ^{111}In radioisotope
  indocyanine green
  iodine 123, 125, or 131
    (^{123}I, ^{125}I, ^{131}I)
  ^{123}I heptadecanoic acid radioisotope
  ^{123}I pentylpentadecanoic acid
    (IPPA) radioisotope

contrast medium *(cont.)*
125I radioisotope
131I radioisotope
indocyanine green
iohexol
ionic
iopamidol
Iopamiron 310; 370
iothalamate meglumine
iothalamate sodium
iothalmic acid
ioversol
ioxaglate meglumine
Isopaque
Isovue-300; -370, Isovue-M 300
low osmolar
Magnevist
mannitol and saline 1:1 solution
MD-60; MD-76
meglumine
metaiodobenzulguanidine
metrizamide
metrizoic acid
Myoscint (indium 111 [111In]
  murine monoclonal antibody Fab
  to myosin; imciromab pentetate)
Myoview
nonionic
Omnipaque
OncoTrac (monoclonal antibodies)
Optiray
oxygen-15
31P
polygelin colloid
potassium-43 (43K)
Renografin-60
Renografin-76
Renovist
Renovist II
rubidium chloride (82Rb)
rubidium-82 radioisotope (82Rb)
sestamibi, technetium Tc 99m

contrast medium *(cont.)*
SHU-454
sodium bicarbonate solution
sodium chloride 0.9%
sonicated meglumine sodium
sonicated Renografin-76
sorbitol 70%
teboroxime, technetium Tc 99m
TechneScan Q-12
technetated (99mTc) aggregated
  albumin, human
technetium bound to DTPA
technetium bound to serum albumin
technetium bound to sulfur colloid
technetium-99m-labeled fibrinogen
technetium-99m-labeled red blood
  cells
technetium-99m pyrophosphate
technetium-99m sodium
  pertechnetate
technetium Tc 99m
technetium Tc 99m albumin
  aggregated
technetium Tc 99m biciromab
technetium Tc 99m DTPA
technetium Tc 99m furifosmin
technetium Tc 99m pentetate
technetium Tc 99m sestamibi
technetium Tc 99m teboroxime
technetium-99m-tin-pyrophosphate
thallium-201 (201Tl)
thallous chloride
Thorotrast
Ultravist
Urografin-76
Vascoray
ZK44012
contrast venography
control
C-arm
diluent
fluoroscopic

control *(cont.)*
  fluoroscopy
  histamine
  radiographic
  roentgenographic
controlled aortic root reperfusion
controlled ventilation
controlled ventricular response
control of hypertension
ControlWire guide wire
contusion
  myocardial
  pulmonary
conus arteriosus
conus artery
conus branch ostia
conus ligament
conus septum
convalesce
convalescence, uncomplicated
convalescent
conventional pulse sequence
convergence zone
conversion
  spontaneous
  successful
converting-enzyme inhibitors
convexo-concave disk prosthetic valve
convulsivum, asthma
Cook arterial catheter
Cook deflector
Cook introducer
Cook pacemaker
Cook yellow pigtail catheter
Cooley anastomosis clamp
Cooley anemia
Cooley aortic clamp
Cooley atrial retractor
Cooley-Baumgarten aortic forceps
Cooley-Beck clamp
Cooley clamp
Cooley coarctation clamp

Cooley-Cutter disk prosthetic valve
Cooley-Cutter valve prosthesis
Cooley-Derra anastomosis clamp
Cooley Dacron prosthesis
Cooley iliac clamp
Cooley intrapericardial anastomosis
Cooley modification of Waterston
  anastomosis
Cooley partial occlusion clamp
Cooley patent ductus clamp
Cooley pediatric clamp
Cooley renal clamp
Cooley retractor
Cooley-Satinsky clamp
Cooley trait
Cooley valve dilator
Cooley vascular clamp
Cooley vascular forceps
Cooley vena cava catheter clamp
Cooley woven Dacron graft
cooling
  core
  external cardiac
cooling blanket
Coombs murmur
Coombs test
  direct
  indirect
Cooper ligament
"coo sur coo" (coup sur coup)
COPD (chronic obstructive pulmonary
  disease), emphysematous
Cope biopsy needle
Cope needle introducer cannula
copious amounts of blood
copious sputum production
copious watery rhinorrhea
copper deficiency
copper wire effect
copper wiring (on eye exam)
cor (heart)
cor adiposum

coral reef atheroma
coral reef plaque
cor arteriosum
Coratomic prosthetic valve
cor biloculare
cor bovinum ("ox heart")
cord, cords
  fibrous
  rope-like (in thrombophlebitis)
  vocal
cordate
cor dextrum
cordis
  annuli
  atrium
  bulbus
  concretio (dense pericardial
    calcification)
  crux
  ectopia
  fibrosis
  morbus
Cordis Atricor pacemaker
Cordis Bioptone sheath
Cordis Brite Tip guiding catheter
Cordis dilator
Cordis Ducor brachial I (II, III)
  coronary catheter
Cordis-Ducor-Judkins catheter
Cordis Ducor pigtail catheter
Cordis electrode
Cordis fixed-rate pacemaker
Cordis Gemini pacemaker
Cordis high flow pigtail catheter
Cordis lead conversion kit
Cordis Multicor II pacemaker
Cordis pacing lead
Cordis Sequicor II pacemaker
Cordis sheath
Cordis Son-II catheter
Cordis tantalum stent
Cordis Ventricor pacemaker

cordlike mass
cordlike vein
corduroy arteries
core cooling
cor en cuirasse
core of atheroma
core temperature
CO_2 retention
cor hirsutum
cork handler's disease
cork handler's lung
cork worker's syndrome
Cormed pump
cor mobile
corneal arcus
corneal flattening
Cornelia de Lange syndrome
Cornell protocol (exercise stress
  testing)
Corometrics-Aloka echocardiograph
  machine
coronal image
coronal section
coronaropathy
coronary angiogram, -graphy
coronary angioplasty
coronary arterial thrombosis
coronary arteriography
coronary arteriosclerosis
coronary arteriosystemic fistula
coronary arteriovenous fistula
coronary arteritis
coronary artery
  anomalous pulmonary origin
  circumflex
  dominant left
  dominant right
  eccentric
  intramural
  left anterior descending
  ramus medialis
coronary artery bypass, concomitant

coronary artery bypass graft (CABG)
coronary artery cameral fistula
coronary artery disease (CAD)
coronary artery disease, post-transplant
coronary artery dominance
coronary artery embolus
coronary artery lesion
coronary artery malformation
coronary artery origin from pulmonary
   artery
coronary artery ostia
coronary artery patency
coronary (artery) perfusion pressure
   (CPP)
coronary artery spasm, catheter-
   induced
coronary artery steal syndrome
coronary artery thrombosis
coronary artery tree
coronary atherosclerosis
coronary balloon angioplasty
coronary blood flow, regional
coronary bypass
coronary bypass graft patency
coronary-cameral fistula
coronary care unit (CCU)
coronary cusp
coronary disease, three-vessel
coronary fistula
coronary flow reserve (CFR)
coronary groove
coronary heart disease (CHD)
coronary hyperemia
coronary ischemia
coronary nodal rhythm
coronary occlusion
coronary ostia
coronary ostial reimplantation
coronary ostial revascularization,
   Cabrol II
coronary ostium
coronary perfusion

coronary reocclusion, postthrombolytic
coronary reperfusion
coronary sclerosis
coronary sinus (CS)
coronary sinus lead
coronary sinus of Valsalva
coronary sinus orifice
coronary sinus os
coronary sinus ostium
coronary sinus retroperfusion
coronary sinus rhythm (CSR)
coronary sinus, roof of
coronary spasm
coronary steal phenomenon
coronary steal syndrome
coronary system
   dominant left
   dominant right
coronary thrombolysis, intravenous
coronary thrombosis
coronary tree
coronary vascular resistance
coronary vasomotion
coronary vasomotion disorder
coronary vessel aneurysm
COROSKOP C cardiac imaging
   system
cor pendulum
corporis diffusum universale,
   angiokeratoma
cor pulmonale (c. pulmonale)
corpuscle, Herbst
corpuscular red cell volume, mean
corrected great arteries transposition
corrected sinus node recovery time
   (CSNRT)
corrected transposition, congenital
corrected transposition of great arteries
   (CTGA)
Correra line
corridor operation in atrial fibrillation
Corrigan aortic regurgitation disease

Corrigan collapsing pulse
Corrigan disease
Corrigan pulse
Corrigan sign
Corrigan syndrome
corrugated air column
corset balloon catheter
cor sinistrum
cor taurinum
cortical intracerebral hemorrhage
cortical sign
corticale, Cryptostroma
corticobulbar disease
corticospinal disease
corticosteroid
   prenatal
   inhaled
corticosteroid-administration-related
   tuberculosis reactivation
corticosteroid in hemangioma therapy
corticosterone
cortisol production, deficient
cortisone in congenital vascular defect
   therapy
cor triatriatum
cor triatriatum dextrum
cor triloculare
cor triloculare biatriatum
cor triloculare biventriculare
corundum smelter's lung
cor venosum
cor villosum
Corvisart disease
Corvisart syndrome
Corynebacterium infection
Corynebacterium pseudotuberculosis
   infection
coryza
Cosmos pulse generator
Cosmos pulse generator pacemaker
Cosmos 283 DDD pacemaker
Cosmos II DDD pacemaker

Cossio-Berconsky syndrome
costal angle
costal cartilage
costal groove
costal interarticular cartilage
costalis, pleura
costal margin
costal margin syndrome
costal pleura
costal pleural reflection
costal pleurisy
costal retractions
costal surface of lung
costectomy
costocervical trunk of subclavian artery
costochondral joint
costochondral junction
costochondral junction syndrome
costochondritis, angina mimicked by
costoclavicular maneuver
costoclavicular test
costodiaphragmatic recess of pleura
costodiaphragmatic recesses
costolateral areas
costomediastinal recess
costophrenic angle, obliteration of
costosternal malformation
costosternal syndrome
costotome
costotransverse joint
costovertebral angle
costovertebral joint
costoxiphoid ligament
cotinine level
cottage loaf appearance (on x-ray)
cottage loaf deformity
cotton dust
cotton-mill fever syndrome
cough
   aneurysmal
   barking
   brassy

cough *(cont.)*
  bubbling
  chronic intractable
  compression
  croupy
  decubitus
  dog (compression)
  dry
  dry nonproductive
  encouraged to
  hacking
  harsh
  hollow
  loose
  mechanical
  membranous
  metallic
  Morton
  motion
  nocturnal
  nonproductive
  nonproductive dry
  productive
  rasping
  rattling
  reflex
  smoker's
  spasmodic
  Sydenham
  tea taster's
  typical regularity of
  voluntary (productive of mucus)
  wet
  whooping
  winter
  wracking
coughing
  paroxysmal
  repeated bouts of
  voluntary cough productive of
    mucus
coughing and wheezing

coughing sign
coughing up blood
cough productive of phlegm
cough productive of purulent sputum
cough productive of sputum
cough reflex
  depression of
  impaired
  inhibited
  suppressed
cough syncope
cough-thrill
Coulter counter for platelet count
coumadinization
coumarin-type anticoagulants
count
  absolute blood eosinophil
  cell
  complete blood cell (CBC)
  differential
  needle, sponge, and instrument
  platelet
  RBC (red blood cell)
  reticulocyte
  WBC (white blood cell)
counterclockwise rotation
counterclockwise superiorly oriented
  frontal QRS loop
counterimmunoelectrophoresis (CIE)
  of sputum
counter-occluder delivered into right
  atrium
counter-occluder equals buttonhole
counter-occluder threaded over loading
  wire through rubber buttonhole
counterpulsation
  balloon
  diastolic
  intra-aortic balloon (IAB)
  mechanical
  percutaneous intra-aortic balloon
    (PIBC)

countershock
  direct current electrical
  unsynchronized
coupled beats
coupled premature beats
couplet
  atrial
  ventricular
  ventricular premature contraction
coupling, excitation-contraction
coupling interval
coupling interval decrement
coup sur coup ("coo sur coo")
Cournand cardiac catheter
Cournand catheter
Cournand needle
course
  fulminant
  fulminant disease
  improving
course of the vessel
coved ST segments
covering, musculotendinous
CO_2 wave forms
Cox maze procedure
Coxiella burnetii (Rickettsia burnetii)
  infection
Coxsackie A virus
Coxsackie B virus
coxsackievirus
coxsackievirus endocarditis
coxsackievirus myocarditis
coxsackievirus pericarditis
CPAD (chronic peripheral arterial
  disease)
CPAP (continuous positive airway
  pressure)
  face mask
  nasal
CPB (cardiopulmonary bypass)
CPI (Cardiac Pacemakers, Inc.)
CPI Astra pacemaker

CPI automatic implantable defibrillator
CPI DDD pacemaker
CPI electrode lead
CPI endocardial defibrillation lead
CPI endocardial defibrillation/rate-
  sensing/pacing lead
CPI endocardial rate-sensing/pacing
  lead
CPI Endotak SQ electrode lead
CPI Endotak transvenous electrode
CPI L67 electrode
CPI external cardioverter defibrillator
  (ECD) for crinkling, patch
CPI pacemaker
CPI porous tined-tip bipolar pacing
  lead
CPI Sweet Tip lead
CPI ULTRA II pacemaker
CPI ventricular lead
CPK (creatine phosphokinase)
CPK isoenzymes (see *isoenzymes*)
C point of cardiac apex pulse
CPP (coronary artery perfusion
  pressure)
CPPV (continuous positive pressure
  ventilation)
CPR (cardiopulmonary resuscitation),
  closed chest
cps (cycles per second)
CPS (cardiopulmonary support system)
c. pulmonale (cor pulmonale)
CR Bard catheter
crackles (see also *rales*)
  auscultatory
  coarse
  diffuse
  early inspiratory
  fine
  late inspiratory
  medium
  paninspiratory
  pleural

crackling rales
Crafoord aortic clamp
Crafoord clamp
Crafoord coarctation clamp
Crafoord-Senning heart-lung machine
Crafoord thoracic scissors
cramped position
cramping, intense disabling
cramps
    calf
    muscle
Crampton test
cranial and caudal angulations
cranial angled view
cranial angulation, anteroposterior
    x-ray projection with
cranial arteritis
cranial nerve palsy
cranial vessels
cranial view
craniofacial overgrowth
cranky
crash induction of anesthesia
craterlike ulcer with jagged edges
Crawford aortic retractor
Crawford-Cooley tunneler
Crawford graft inclusion technique
Crawford suture ring
Crawford technique for thoraco-
    abdominal aneurysm
C-reactive protein
creaking friction rub
crease
    earlobe
    inframammary
creatine kinase (CK) isoenzymes
creatine phosphate
creatine phosphokinase (CPK)
creatinine concentration, 24-hour urine
creatinine estimated using modified
    Jaffé rate reaction
creatinine, urinary

creep of ventricular diastolic pressure
creeping eruption
crepitant rales
crepitation
    basal
    inspiratory
    pleural
    superficial
crepitus indux
crepitus redux
crescendo angina
crescendo-decrescendo murmur
crescendo murmur
crescendo rumble
crescendo-systolic thrill
crescendo transient ischemic attacks
crescent sign
crescentic lumen
crest
    infundibuloventricular
    supraventricular
    terminal (of right atrium)
CREST (calcinosis cutis, Raynaud's
    phenomenon, esophageal dys-
    motility, sclerodactyly, and
    telangiectasia) syndrome
CRF (chronic renal failure)
CRF (chronic reserve flow)
CRHD (chronic rheumatic heart
    disease)
cricoid cartilage
cri du chat (short arm deletion-5)
    syndrome
cricothyroid cartilage, obstetrical
    injury
cricothyroid membrane
cricothyrotomy, emergency
Crile clamp
Crile curved dissecting forceps
Crile curved forceps
Crile curved grasping forceps
Crile hemostat

Crile straight dissecting forceps
Crile straight grasping forceps
Crile-Wood needle holder
crimp
crimper
crimping
crisis (pl. crises)
  hypertensive
  hypertensive paroxysmal
  rejection
crisscross fashion
crisscross heart
crista supraventricularis
crista supraventricularis septal defect
crista terminalis atrii dextri
criteria
  Ambrose (for thrombotic lesions)
  Framingham
  Heath-Edwards
critical care unit (CCU)
critical lesion
Critikon catheter
Critikon guide wire
Croften classification for pulmonary
  eosinophilia
cromoglycate
cross- aortic
cross-clamp (noun, verb)
cross-clamp time
cross-clamping of aorta
cross-collateralization
crossed embolism
Cross-Jones disk prosthetic valve
crossover femoral-femoral bypass
crossover graft
cross-pelvic collateral vessel
cross-sectional area, luminal
cross-sectional area stenosis
cross-sectional image
cross-sectional view
crosstalk, pacemaker

croup
  catarrhal
  diphtheritic
  false
  membranous
  pseudomembranous
  spasmodic
croup syndrome
croup tent
croupous bronchitis
croupy cough
CRS (catheter-related sepsis)
CRT (cathode ray tube)
cruciate incision
Crump vessel dilator
crunch, Hamman
crura diaphragmatis
crura of the diaphragm (left and right)
cruris, angina
crus, diaphragmatic
crushing chest pain
crushing injury to chest
crushing pain
crushing substernal chest pain
Cruveilhier-Baumgarten murmur
Cruveilhier-Baumgarten syndrome
Cruveilhier nodule
Cruveilhier sign
crux (pl. cruces)
crux cordis (crux of heart)
cryoablation (see also *ablation*)
  encircling endocardial
  transmural
cryoablation catheter
cryocrit
cryolesions
cryoprecipitate
cryopreservation
cryopreserved allograft
cryopreserved homograft tissue
cryopreserved human allograft conduit

cryopreserved human aortic allograft
cryosurgery, map-guided
cryosurgical ablation
cryosurgical lesions
cryosurgical probe
cryothermia
cryptococcosis
Cryptococcus neoformans pneumonia
cryptogenic bacteremia
cryptogenic fibrosing alveolitis
cryptogenic pulmonary eosinophilia
Cryptostroma corticale
crystalloid cardioplegic solution
crystalloid fluid
crystalloid prime for heart-lung
   machine
crystals
   asthma
   Charcot-Leyden
   cholesterol
CS (coronary sinus)
CSA (cross-sectional area)
CSH (carotid sinus hypersensitivity)
C-shaped bars of cartilage
C-17 hydroxylase deficiency
CSI (coronary stenosis index)
CSICU (cardiac surgery intensive care
   unit)
CSNRT (corrected sinus node recovery
   time)
CSR (coronary sinus rhythm)
CSS (carotid sinus syndrome)
CST (contraction stress test)
C_{STAT} (static lung compliance)
CSVT (central splanchnic venous
   thrombosis)
CT (computed tomography)
CT-directed hook wire localization
CT-guided aspiration
CT-scan directed needle biopsy
CT scan, ultrafast

C3a serum level
CTGA (corrected transposition of great
   arteries)
CTR (cardiac transplant recipient)
CTR (cardiothoracic ratio)
cuboidal epithelium
cuff
   aortic
   atrial
   blood pressure
   finger
   inflow
   pneumatic
   right atrial
cuffed endotracheal tube
cuff rupture of tube
cuirasse, cor en
cuirass respirator
culprit lesion
culprit stenosis
culprit vessel
culture
   acid-fast
   sputum
culture and sensitivity, sputum
cultured for aerobes and anaerobes
cumulative effect
cuplike pockets
cupola, pleural
cup-shaped semilunar valves
Curracino-Silverman syndrome
currant jelly clot
current, alternating
current leak
current of injury
Curschmann spirals
curse, Ondine
curve
   AA
   AH
   A_1-A_2

curve *(cont.)*
  arterial dilution
  ascorbate dilution
  A2-H2
  central intra-aortic pressure
  dye
  indicator dilution
  indicator dye-dilution
  indocyanine dilution
  intracardiac dye-dilution
  left ventricular inflow velocity
  oxyhemoglobin dissociation
  Starling
  time activity (for contrast agent)
  V1-V2
  V2-A2
  venous dilution
  ventricular function
curved Cooley clamp
curved Hasson grasper
curved Kelly forceps
curved mosquito forceps
curves, catheter with preformed
curvilinear aortotomy
curvilinear defect
curvilinear lines, subpleural
Curvularia lunata
Cushing forceps
cushingoid appearance
Cushing phenomenon
Cushing, pressor response of
Cushing reflex
Cushing rongeur
Cushing syndrome
Cushing vein retractor
cushion defect
cushion, endocardial
cusp
  accessory
  anterior
  aortic
  asymmetric closure of

cusp *(cont.)*
  conjoined
  coronary
  dysplastic
  fibrocalcific
  fishmouth
  fusion of
  intact valve
  left coronary
  left pulmonary
  mitral valve
  noncoronary
  perforated aortic
  posterior
  pulmonary valve
  right coronary
  ruptured aortic
  semilunar valve
  septal
  septic perforation of
  tricuspid valve
  valve
cusp degenerator
cusp fenestration
cuspis anterior valvae atrioventricularis
  dextrae
cuspis anterior valvae atrioventricularis
  sinistrae
cuspis posterior valvae atrioventricularis dextrae
cuspis posterior valvae atrioventricularis sinistrae
cuspis septalis valvae atrioventricularis
  dextrae
cusp motion
cusp shots (films)
cut and cine film
cutaneous atrophy
cutaneous emphysema
cutaneous telangiectasia
cutaneous vascular anomaly
cutaneous vasoconstriction, peripheral

cutdown
  antecubital fossa
  brachial
  femoral
cutdown over cephalic vein
cutis laxa syndrome
cutis marmorata
cutoff
  arterial
  atherectomy
  Leather valve
  vessel (of contrast material)
  wire
Cutter aortic valve prosthesis
Cutter-Smeloff cardiac valve prosthesis
Cutter-Smeloff heart valve
cutting device
cutting mechanism was engaged
Cuvier, canal of
CV (cardioversion)
CV (closing volume)
CVA (cardiovascular accident)
CVA (cerebrovascular accident),
  posterior circulation
CVBS (congenital vascular-bone
  syndrome)
CVC (central venous catheterization)
CVIS imaging device
CVM (congenital vascular malforma-
  tion)
CvO$_2$ (mixed venous oxygen content)
CVP (central venous pressure) catheter
CVRI (coronary vascular resistance
  index)
cv wave of jugular venous pulse
cv waves, regurgitant
C wave pressure on right atrial
  catheterization
CX (circumflex)
CXR (chest x-ray), baseline
cyanide poisoning
cyanide toxicity

cyanosis
  central
  circumoral
  differential
  false
  frank
  mucous membrane
  nail bed
  perioral
  peripheral
  pulmonary
  reversed differential
  ruddy
  shunt
  slate-gray
  systemic
  tardive
  tardive pulmonary
cyanosis and clubbing
cyanosis, clubbing, or edema
  (C, C, or E)
cyanotic congenital heart disease
cyanotic heart disease
cyanotic hypoxic spells
cyanotic nail beds
Cyberlith multiprogrammable pulse
  generator
Cyberlith pacemaker
Cybertach automatic-burst atrial
  pacemaker
Cybertach 60 pacemaker
cycle
  cardiac
  length of atrial
  length of ventricular
  RR
  sinus length (SLC)
  vicious
cycle-ergometer
cycles per second (cps)
cyclical edema
cyclic idiopathic edema

cyclo-oxygenase inhibitors
cyclosporine toxicity
cyclosporin G
cylindrical bronchiectasis
cylindrical chest
cylindrical thorax
Cyriax syndrome
cyst
　alveolar
　bronchial
　bronchogenic
　bronchopulmonary
　echinococcal (of lung)
　pericardial
　Springwater
cystic emphysema

cystic fibrosis
cystic medial necrosis
cystic medionecrosis, Erdheim
cystic pulmonary emphysema
cytoimmunologic monitoring
cytology, bronchial washings
cytomegalic inclusion disease
cytomegalovirus infection
cytomegalovirus pneumonitis
cytosome

D, d

D (diaphragmatic)
D'Acosta (or Acosta) disease (acute
mountain sickness)
Da Costa syndrome (neurocirculatory
asthenia)
Dacron catheter
Dacron conduit
Dacron-covered prosthesis
Dacron graft
Dacron mesh
Dacron onlay patch-graft
Dacron outflow graft
Dacron patch graft
Dacron preclotted tightly woven graft
Dacron roof
Dacron Sauvage patch
Dacron stent
Dacron suture
Dacron tape
Dacron tube graft, albuminized woven
Dacron velour tube graft
Daig ESI-II or DSI-III screw-in lead
pacemaker
Dakin Biograft
Dale forceps
Dallas Classification System for
diagnosing myocarditis

damage
alveolar-capillary membrane
focal myocyte
myocardial wall
D'Amato sign in pleural effusion
dam, left ventricular
dampened obstructive pulse
dampened pulsatile flow
dampened wave form
damping of catheter tip pressure
Damus-Kaye-Stansel (DKS) operation
Damus-Norwood procedure
Danielson method of tricuspid valve
repair
Dardik Biograft
dark region
dark sputum
Dash rate-adaptive pacemaker
Dash single-chamber rate-adaptic
cardiac pacemaker
data acquisition
data log, ICD
Datascope DL-II percutaneous translucent balloon catheter
Datascope intra-aortic balloon pump
Datascope System 90 balloon pump
DataVue calibrated reference circle

David operation
Davidson scapular retractor
Davidson shunt
Davidson thoracic trocar
Davidson vessel clamp
Davies-Colley syndrome
Davies endomyocardial fibrosis
Davies myocardial fibrosis
Davies syndrome
Davis aneurysm clip
Davis forceps
Davis rib spreader
Davol pacemaker introducer
DBP (diastolic blood pressure)
DC (direct current)
DC cardioversion
DC defibrillator
DC electrical shock
DCA (direct current ablation)
DCA (directional coronary
    angioplasty)
DCA (directional coronary
    atherectomy)
DCM (dilated cardiomyopathy)
DCS (distal coronary sinus)
DDD mode
DDD pacemaker
DDD pacing mode
dD/dt (derived value on apex
    cardiogram)
DDM (delayed diastolic murmur)
de-airing maneuvers
de-airing of arch
de-airing of graft
de-airing procedure
de-airing site
de-airing the heart
dead space, anatomical
D-E amplitude of mitral valve
death
    aborted sudden cardiac (ASCD)
    adult sudden

death *(cont.)*
    apparent
    imminent
    infant sudden
    recurrent, not-so-sudden cardiac
    sudden
    sudden cardiac
Deaver retractor
DeBakey aortic aneurysm clamp
DeBakey arterial clamp
DeBakey arterial forceps
DeBakey Autraugrip forceps
DeBakey-Bahnson vascular clamp
DeBakey-Bainbridge clamp
DeBakey ball valve prosthesis
DeBakey-Beck clamp
DeBakey bulldog clamp
DeBakey clamps
DeBakey classification (type I, II, III)
    of aortic dissection
DeBakey coarctation clamp
DeBakey-Cooley retractor
DeBakey cross-action bulldog clamp
DeBakey curved dissecting forceps
DeBakey curved grasping forceps
DeBakey-Derra anastomosis clamp
DeBakey-Diethrich vascular forceps
DeBakey dissecting forceps
DeBakey endarterectomy scissors
DeBakey-Harken clamp
DeBakey-Howard clamp
DeBakey-Kay clamp
DeBakey patent ductus clamp
DeBakey pediatric clamp
DeBakey peripheral vascular bulldog
    clamp
DeBakey peripheral vascular clamp
DeBakey prosthetic valve
DeBakey-Reynolds anastomosis clamp
DeBakey rib spreader
DeBakey ring-handled bulldog clamp
DeBakey-Semb clamp; forceps

DeBakey straight dissecting forceps
DeBakey straight grasping forceps
DeBakey-Surgitool prosthetic valve
DeBakey tangential occlusion clamp
DeBakey technique for thoracoabdom-
    inal aneurysm
DeBakey tissue forceps
DeBakey type I aortic dissection
DeBakey valve scissors
DeBakey vascular clamp
DeBakey vascular forceps
DeBakey Vasculour prosthesis
debanding procedure
debanding, pulmonary artery
debilitation
debris
    aspiration of
    atheromatous
    atherosclerotic
    calcium
    cholesterol
    gelatinous
    grumous
    intimal
    particle
    thallium
debt
    mild oxygen
    moderate oxygen
    oxygen
    severe oxygen
debubbling procedure
debulking of aneurysm
debulking of atheroma
decannulated, decannulation
decapolar catheter
decay, free induction
deceleration-dependent heart block
deceleration, differential
deceleration time
decelerative injury
decidua

declamping
decompensated congestive heart failure
decompensation
    cardiac
    chronic respiratory
    end-stage adult cardiac
    end-stage fetal cardiac
    hemodynamic
    respiratory
    ventricular
decompress
decompression, cardiac
decompression of heart
decompression of ventricle
decompression sickness
deconditioning
decortication
    cardiac
    chemical
    heart
decortication of lung
decreased arterial hemoglobin
    saturation
decreased beta adrenergic receptor
decreased breath sounds
decreased carbon monoxide diffusion
decreased cerebral blood flow
decreased cerebral perfusion pressure
decreased closing velocity
decreased compliance
decreased diaphragmatic motion
decreased diffusing capacity
decreased dynamic compliance
decreased E-F slope
decreased exchangeable sodium
decreased exercise capacity
decreased I:E ratio
decreased inspirated oxygen tension
decreased intensity
decreased left ventricular filling on
    inspiration
decreased lung compliance

decreased P wave amplitude
decreased peripheral vascular
  resistance
decreased pulmonary vascular
  compliance
decreased stroke volume
decreased systemic resistance
decreased tidal volume
decreased venous return
decreased ventilatory capacity
decreased ventricular preload
decrease in vascular markings
decrease of blood viscosity
decrease of capillary dilatation
decremental conduction
decremental element
decremental pacing
decrescendo holosystolic murmur
decrescendo murmur
decubital ulcer
decubitus
  andral
  angina
decubitus cough
decubitus on the sound side
decubitus ulcer
deep-breathing exercises
deep calf veins
deep cardiac plexus
deep Doppler velocity interrogation
deep hypothermic circulatory arrest
deep limb lead
deep plexus
deep respirations
deep tendon reflex (DTR)
deep thrombophlebitis
deep veins
deep venous aplasia
deep venous hypoplasia
deep venous insufficiency (DVI)
deep venous thromboembolism
deep venous thrombosis (DVT)

deep visceral pain
defecation syncope
defect (see also *deformity*)
  acquired ventricular septal (AVSD)
  anastomotic
  anteroapical
  aortic septal
  aorticopulmonary
  aorticopulmonary septal
  atrial ostium primum
  atrial septal
  atrioseptal (ASD)
  atrioventricular canal
  atrioventricular septal
  AV (atrioventricular) conduction
  cardiofacial
  concomitant
  conduction
  conoventricular
  contiguous ventricular septal
  crista supraventricularis septal
  curvilinear
  cushion
  endocardial cushion
  filling (on imaging study)
  fixed
  fixed intracavitary filling
  fixed perfusion
  inferoapical
  infracristal septal
  infracristal ventricular septal
  infundibular ventricular septal
  interatrial septal (septum)
  interventricular conduction
  interventricular septal (IVSD)
  intra-atrial conduction
  intra-atrial filling
  intraluminal
  intraluminal filling
  intraventricular conduction
  junctional
  juxta-arterial ventricular septal

defect *(cont.)*
  juxtatricuspid ventricular septal
  linear
  lobulated filling
  luminal
  matched V/Q (ventilation-perfusion)
  membranous ventricular septal
  muscular ventricular septal
  nonuniform rotational (NURD)
  ostium primum
  ostium secundum
  partial AV (atrioventricular) canal
  perfusion
  peri-infarction conduction (PICD)
  perimembranous ventricular septal
  posteroapical
  postinfarction ventriculoseptal
  Rastelli type A, B, or C
    atrioventricular canal
  restrictive ventilatory
  reversible
  reversible ischemic
  reversible perfusion
  scintigraphic perfusion
  secundum and sinus venosus
  secundum atrial septal
  secundum-type atrial septal
    septal
  sinus venosus
  spontaneous closure of
  supracristal septal
  supracristal ventricular
  supracristal ventricular septal
  supracristal ventriculoseptal
  Swiss cheese ventricular septal
  transcatheter closure of atrial
    transient perfusion
  transient perfusion
  type I (supracristal) ventricular
    septal
  type II (infracristal) ventricular
    septal

defect *(cont.)*
  type III (canal type) ventricular
    septal
  type IV (muscular) ventricular
    septal
  valvular
  ventilation-perfusion
  ventricular septal or ventriculoseptal
    (VSD)
defective communication between
  cardiac chambers
defective hemoglobin synthesis
defective platelet function
defective volume regulation
defervesce, defervesced
defibrillation
  endovenous
  external
  rescue
  single pulse
  transvenous
defibrillation cathode
defibrillation coil
defibrillation electrode
defibrillation performed with lungs
  fully inflated
defibrillation shock
defibrillation threshold (DFT)
defibrillation zone
defibrillator
  AICD (automatic implantable [in-
    ternal] cardioverter-defibrillator)
  AICD-B cardioverter-
  AICD-BR cardioverter-
  AID (automatic implantable [or
    internal])
  AID-B
  automatic external (AED)
  CPI automatic implantable
  DC (direct current)
  external cardioverter
  Heart Aid 80

defibrillator *(cont.)*
  Hewlett-Packard
  implantable
  implantable cardioverter- (ICD)
  Intec implantable
  ODAM
  patient (PDF)
  transvenous lead
debrillator paddle
defibrillator pads
debrillator power source
defibrillator unit
defibrinating syndrome
defibrination
deficiency
  accessory factor
  acyl coenzyme A (acyl-CoA)
  acid lipase
  acid maltase
  $alpha_1$-antitrypsin
  alpha-galactosidase
  alpha-galactosidase A
  $alpha_1$-proteinase inhibitor (a_1PI)
  antithrombin III
  ^{11}C (C-11) hydroxylase
  ^{17}C (C-17) hydroxylase
  cardiomyopathic carnitine
  carnitine
  coagulation factor XI
  copper
  11 beta-hydroxylase
  glucocerebrosidase
  lipase acid
  lipoprotein lipase
  long chain acyl-CoA dehydrogenase
  maltase acid
  methemoglobin reductase
  multiple sulfatase
  phosphorylase kinase
  plasma coagulation factor
  plasminogen
  potassium

deficiency *(cont.)*
  protein C
  prothrombin
  17-hydroxylase
  surfactant
  systemic carnitine
  thiamine
  thyroid hormone
  vitamin B complex
  vitamin K
deficient cortisol production
deficient fibrinolysis
deficit
  base
  carbonic acid
  oxygen
  peripheral pulse
  pulse
  reversible ischemic neurologic
    (RIND)
  significant residual
  transient neurological
deflectable catheter
deflectable quadripolar catheter
deflectable-tip catheter
deflection
  delta
  His bundle
  intrinsic
  intrinsicoid
  QS
  RS
deflection of normal depolarizing wave
deflector, Cook
deflector wire
deformity (see also *defect*)
  cottage loaf
  gooseneck outflow tract
  hockey-stick tricuspid valve
  hourglass
  parachute mitral valve
  parachute-type

deformity *(cont.)*
  pulmonary valve
  rolled edge
  scimitar
  snow man
  tricuspid valve
degenerated intima, friable thickened
degeneration
  angiolithic
  atheromatous
  cardiac valve mucoid
  cardiomyopathic
  collagen
  cusp
  fatty
  fibrinoid
  glassy
  hyaline
  hydropic
  hypertensive vascular
  Mönckeberg
  mucoid medial
  mural
  myocardial
  myocardial cellular
  myocardial fibers
  myxoid
  myxomatous
  sclerotic
degeneration of mitral valve,
  myxomatous
degenerative atrioventricular node
  disease
DeGimard syndrome
deglutition syncope
degradation
  fibrinogen
  image quality
degree, noncircularity
degrees of heart block
Dehio test
dehisced

dehiscence
  perivalvular
  prosthesis
  wound
dehiscence of graft anastomosis
dehydroepiandrosterone sulfate
  (DHEA-S)
dehydrogenase, lactic
Deklene suture
Deknatel (Shur-Strip) wound closure
  tape
de la Camp sign
de Lange syndrome
delay
  atrioventricular
  conduction
  intraventricular conduction
delayed diastolic murmur (DDM)
delayed image
delayed phase of arteriogram
delayed sternal closure
delayed xenon washout
delay time, echo
Delbet sign
deleterious effect
delicate crepitation
delirium, postcardiotomy
delivered energy
Delmege sign of tuberculosis
Delrin frame of valve prosthesis,
  Dacron-covered
delta deflection
delta wave
Delta pacemaker
deltopectoral approach
deltopectoral groove
demand (standby)
demand mode of pacemaker
demand pacemaker battery
demand pulse generator unit
demarcation line
DeMartel scissors

DeMartel vascular clamp
De Martini-Balestra syndrome
dementia
  arteriosclerotic
  Binswanger
  multi-infarct
  vascular
demifacets
demise, imminent
demographic data
Demons-Meigs syndrome
Demos tibial artery clamp
de Musset sign (aortic aneurysm)
de Mussey point or sign (pleurisy)
denatured homograft
denervation, cardiac
denervation of heart
de novo angina
de novo lesion
dense adhesions
dense consolidation
dense scar
density, densities
  diffuse reticular
  discrete perihilar
  echo
  hydrogen
  increased
  mottled
  perihilar
  proton
  spin
  wedge-shaped
denudation, areas of
denude, denuding
denuded epithelium
deoxygenated blood
dep (depressed)
dependent
  pacer-
  steroid
dependent edema

dependent edema fluid, resorption of
dependent extracellular fluid accumulation
dependent rubor
dephasing, signal
depletion
  intravascular volume
  mild volume
  moderate volume
  premature battery
  profound volume
  volume
deployment
  catheter
  stent
depolarization
  atrial
  atrial premature (APD)
  cardiac
  early ventricular (preexcitation)
  His bundle–distal coronary sinus
    atrial (H-DCSA)
  His bundle–middle coronary sinus
    atrial (H-MCSA)
  premature atrial
  premature ventricular
  rapid
  ventricular
depolarization phase, diastolic
depolarization wave
deposit
  glycolipid
  hemosiderin
depressed cardiac contractility
depressed contractility
depressed diaphragm
depressed ejection fraction
depressed J point
depressed myocardial contractile
  performance
depressed right ventricular contractile
  function

depressed serum potassium
depressed T waves
depression
  cough reflex
  downhill ST segment
  hemidiaphragm
  hemodynamic
  horizontal ST segment
  marked ST segment
  myocardial
  reciprocal
  sinus node
  ST segment
depression of cough reflex
depressor anguli oris muscle
deranged left ventricular contractility
derangement
  chemical
  immunological
Dermalene suture
Dermalon suture
dermatitis, stasis
Derra commissurotomy knife
Derra valve dilator
desaturated phospholipids
desaturation, systemic arterial oxygen
descending aorta
descending aorta–pulmonary artery
  shunt
descending thoracic aorta, penetrating
  wound to
descent
  x
  X′ (X prime)
  y
Deschamps compressor
desensitizing regimen
Deseret angiocatheter
desert fever
desert rheumatism
desiccation of thrombus, laser
Desilets-Hoffman catheter introducer

desoxycorticosterone (DOC)
D'Espine sign
desquamation, epithelial
desquamative interstitial pneumonia
  (DIP)
destruction of pulmonary parenchyma
destruction of vascular bed
destructive inflammatory bronchial
  changes
detail
  exquisite
  suboptimal
detection zone
detector, cadmium iodide
detergent asthma
deterioration
  mild cardiopulmonary
  moderate cardiopulmonary
  profound cardiopulmonary
Determann syndrome
determination of all lung volumes
Detsky modified cardiac risk index
  score
De Vega prosthesis
De Vega tricuspid valve annuloplasty
development, interval (on x-ray)
deviant pathways
deviated septum
deviation
  aortic
  left axis (LAD)
  mediastinal
  right axis (RAD)
  significant axis
  tracheal
device (see also *cardiac device*)
  abdominal aortic counterpulsation
  (AACD)
  abdominal left ventricular assist
  (ALVAD)
  ablative
  Ablatr

device *(cont.)*
　biventricular assist (BVAD)
　CarboMedics valve
　Chemo-Port pervena catheter
　　system
　cutting
　CVIS imaging
　Dinamap automated blood pressure
　directional atherectomy
　Doppler
　Elecath circulatory support
　Endo Grasp
　extraction atherectomy
　HeartMate implantable ventricular
　　assist
　Herbst mandibular advancement
　Hershey left ventricular assist
　ICD-ATP (implantable cardio-
　　verter-defibrillator/atrial
　　tachycardia pacing)
　InspirEase
　intra-aortic balloon assist
　Kendall Sequential Compression
　Lebsche knife
　left ventricular assist (LVAD)
　MediPort implantable vascular
　　access
　Medtronic-Hall
　Medtronic-Hancock
　multiadjustable fitting
　Novacor left ventricular assist
　Omniscience
　PET balloon atherectomy
　Pierce-Donachy ventricular assist
　Pleur-evac
　Port-A-Cath
　pulsatile assist (PAD)
　right ventricular assist (RVAD)
　Rotablator
　rotational atherectomy
　Sarns ventricular assist
　Simpson PET balloon atherectomy

device *(cont.)*
　specimen collecting
　St. Jude
　Symbion pneumatic assist
　TEC atherectomy
　Thermocardiosystems left ventricu-
　　lar assist
　third-generation (first-, second-,
　　fourth-, etc.)
　Thoratec biventricular assist
　　(BVAD)
　Thoratec right ventricular assist
　　(RVAD)
　Thoratec ventricular assist (VAD)
　tunneling instrument
　ventricular assist (VAD)
　Wizard disposable inflation
device embolization
Devices, Ltd., pacemaker
DeVilbiss ultrasound nebulizer
devitalized tissue
devoid of circulation
DeWeese vena cava clip
dexamethasone suppression of adrenal
　tissue
Dexon suture
dextrum, cor triatriatum
Dexter-Grossman classification of
　mitral regurgitation
dextran
　high-molecular-weight
　low-molecular-weight
dextran and saline solution
dextran plasma volume extender
dextrocardia, mirror image
dextroposed aorta
dextroposition of the aorta
dextrorotatory
dextrotransposition (D-transposition)
　of great arteries
dextroversion
dextroversion of heart

DF (defibrillation)
DF lead, Telectronics endocardial
D5W, D₅W (5% dextrose in water)
DFP (diastolic filling pressure)
DFT (defibrillation threshold)
DHEA-S (dehydroepiandrosterone
    sulfate)
diabetic peripheral vascular insuffi-
    ciency
diagnosis
    clinical
    differential
    empirical
    pathologic
    postoperative
    preoperative
    presumptive
    tentative
diagnostic modality
diagnostic ST segment changes
diagnostic thoracentesis
diagonal branch of artery
diagram, Ladder
dialysis, continuous ambulatory
    peritoneal (CAPD)
diameter (or dimension)
    anteroposterior
    aortic (AD)
    aortic root
    artery
    coil-to-vessel
    increased AP (anterior-posterior)
        (of the chest)
    left anterior internal (LAID)
    left atrial
    left ventricular internal (LVID)
    luminal
    minimal luminal
    narrow anteroposterior
    right ventricular internal (RVID)
    satisfactory luminal
    skin wheal

diameter *(cont.)*
    stenosis
    transverse
    transverse cardiac
    valve
    wide luminal
diamond anastomosis principle
Diamond-Blackfan syndrome
diamond-coated burr
Diamond-Lite titanium surgical
    instrument
diamond-shaped anastomosis
diamond-shaped heart murmur
diamond-shaped sequential vein graft
diaphoresis
diaphoretic
diaphragm, diaphragms
    crura of the
    crus of the
    depressed
    elevated
    free air under the
    muscular crus of
    polyolefin rubber
diaphragmatica, pleura
diaphragm compressed downward and
    costal margin upward, exposing
    the heart
diaphragm divided at costal attachments
diaphragmatic breathing
diaphragmatic crus
diaphragmatic elevation
diaphragmatic hernia
diaphragmatic lymph nodes
diaphragmatic pacemaker
diaphragmatic pericardium
diaphragmatic pleura
diaphragmatic pleurisy
diaphragmatic surface of heart
diaphragmatic surface of lung
diaphragmatic wall myocardial
    infarction

diaphragmitis
diaphragm of stethoscope
Diasonics catheter
Diasonics transducer
diastole
  early
  late
  mid
diastolic blood pressure (DBP)
diastolic cardiac arrest
diastolic collapse of venous pulse
diastolic coronary perfusion pressure
diastolic counterpulsation
diastolic depolarization phase
diastolic diameter of left ventricle
diastolic dysfunction
diastolic filling period
diastolic gallop, prominent ventricular
diastolic gallop sound
diastolic heart failure
diastolic murmur (DM), graded from
  1 to 4
diastolic overload
diastolic perfusion pressure
diastolic perfusion time
diastolic pressure-time index (DPTI)
diastolic regurgitant velocity
diastolic reserve
diastolic rumbling murmur
diastolic thrill
diastolic velocity-time integral
DIASYS Novacor cardiac device
diathesis
  hemorrhagic
  hypertensive
diatrizoate meglumine contrast medium
diatrizoate sodium contrast medium
DIC (disseminated intravascular
  coagulation)
Dick valve dilator
dicrotic notch

dicrotic notch or wave of carotid
  arterial pulse
dicrotic pulse
diet
  AHA (American Heart Association)
  AHA low-fat
  AHA (for hypercholesterolemia)
  anticoronary
  Kempner
  Kempner rice
  low-cholesterol
  low-fat
  low in saturated fat
  low-salt
  low-sodium
  no-added-salt
  salt-restricted
  Schemm
  sodium-restricted
dietary fiber
dietary sodium restriction
dietary supplements
dietary therapy
Diethrich coronary artery instruments
diethylcarbamazine
Dietlen syndrome
difference
  aortic-left ventricular pressure
  arteriovenous oxygen (AVD O$_2$)
  AV (arteriovenous)
  discernible
  pulmonary AV
  resting AV
  systemic AV
differential cyanosis
differential deceleration
differential diagnosis
differential renal vein renin
differentiation
difficult to wean from cardiopulmonary
  bypass

difficulty in breathing
difficulty swallowing
diffuse aggressive polymorphous
  infiltrate
diffuse alveolar interstitial infiltrates
diffuse angiokeratoma disease
diffuse aortic dilatation
diffuse aortomegaly
diffuse arteriolar spasm
diffuse bilateral alveolar infiltration
diffuse cholesterol embolization
diffuse crackles
diffuse emphysema
diffuse heart block
diffuse hyperemia
diffuse hypoplasia
diffuse infiltrate
diffuse inspiratory crepitant rales
diffuse interstitial infiltrate
diffuse interstitial pulmonary fibrosis
diffuse lentiginosis
diffuse lesion
diffuse nodular densities
diffuse perivascular infiltrate
diffuse pleural thickening
diffuse pleurisy
diffuse pulmonary fibrosis
diffuse pulmonary infiltration
diffuse rales
diffuse reticular densities
diffuse reticulonodular infiltrates
diffuse ST-T depression
diffuse stenosis
diffuse subarachnoid hemorrhage
diffuse symmetric hypertrophic
  cardiomyopathy
diffuse T wave inversions
diffuse thickening of arterial intima
diffuse wheezes
diffusing capacity of alveolar capillary
  membrane

diffusing capacity of lung for CO
  (carbon monoxide) (DL_{CO})
diffusion
  decreased carbon monoxide (CO)
  impaired oxygen
dig (slang for digitalis)
dig effect
dig level
DiGeorge syndrome
digital clubbing
digitalis effect
digitalis excess
digitalis intoxication
digitalis level
digitalis toxicity
digitalization
digitalize, digitalized
digitalizing dose
digital runoff
digital storage (in cineangiography)
digital subtraction angiography (DSA)
digital subtraction pulmonary
  angiogram
digital videoangiography
digitoxicity
digoxin-specific Fab antibody
  fragments
dihydropyridine
diisocyanate asthma
Dilantin syndrome
dilatation (see also *dilation*)
  aneurysmal
  annular
  aortic root
  arterial
  balloon
  cardiac
  chamber
  diffuse aortic
  fusiform
  idiopathic pulmonary artery

dilatation *(cont.)*
  idiopathic right atrial
  intraluminal
  left ventricular
  percutaneous transluminal balloon
    (PTBD)
  poststenotic
  poststenotic aortic
  pulmonary artery
  pulmonary trunk idiopathic
  right ventricular
  sequential
  ventricular
  ventricular wall
dilatation and hypertrophy of left
  ventricle
dilatation of alveoli
dilatation of aorta
dilatation of ascending aorta
dilatation of respiratory bronchioles
dilatation of terminal bronchioles
dilatation of veins
dilated aortic root
dilated bronchi
dilated cardiomyopathy secondary to:
  chronic overload
  toxicity to doxorubicin
  toxicity to ethanol
  toxicity to uremia
dilated myocardium
dilated pulmonary artery
dilated tortuous veins
dilated vein
dilation (see also *dilatation*)
  fusiform
  multiple mural
  percutaneous balloon
  pulmonary valve stenosis
  transient left ventricular
dilation of artery by balloon catheter
dilation of bronchus
dilation of pulmonary artery

dilator
  aortic
  Brock cardiac
  Cooley valve
  Crump vessel
  Derra valve
  Dick valve
  Garrett vascular
  Gerbode valve
  Hegar
  Henley
  Hiebert vascular
  Hohn vessel
  Lucchese mitral valve
  mitral valve
  myocardial
  transventricular
  Trousseau
  Tubbs mitral valve
  UMI (not Humi)
  valve
  vein
dilator-sheath
diluent control
dilutional hematocrit
dilutional hyponatremia
dimension
  absolute artery
  aortic root
  end-systolic
  intraluminal
  intrathoracic
  left atrial
  left ventricular end-diastolic
    (LVEDD)
  left ventricular end-systolic
    (LVESD)
  left ventricular internal (LVID)
  left ventricular internal diastolic
    (LVIDD)
  left ventricular internal end-diastole
    (LVIDd)

dimension *(cont.)*
  left ventricular internal end-systole
    (LVIDs)
  left ventricular systolic (LVs)
  luminal
  right ventricular (RVD)
diminished consciousness
diminished lung volume
diminished pedal pulses
diminished systemic perfusion
diminution of pulses
diminutive vessel
dimple, blind
Dinamap automated blood pressure
  device
Dinamap blood pressure monitor and
  Oxytrak pulse oximeter
Dinamap monitor
Dinamap ultrasound blood pressure
  manometer
diode, Zener
DIP (desquamative interstitial
  pneumonia)
dip and plateau phenomenon
dip phenomenon
dip, septal
diphasic complex on EKG
diphasic postcardiotomy syndrome
diphasic P wave
diphasic T wave
diphtheritic croup
diphtheritic membrane
diphtheritic myocarditis
diplopia
Diplos M pacemaker
dipyridamole echocardiography test
dipyridamole handgrip test
dipyridamole infusion test
dipyridamole thallium imaging
dipyridamole thallium scan
dipyridamole thallium stress test

dipyridamole thallium ventriculography
dipyridamole thallium-201 scintigraphy
directable tip (of bronchoscope)
direct caval cannulation
direct current ablation (DCA)
direct current electrical countershock
direct current energy
directional atherectomy device
directional coronary angioplasty
  (DCA)
directional coronary atherectomy
  (DCA)
direct mechanical ventricular actuation
  (DMVA)
direct puncture phlebography
direct vision nasal intubation
direct vision through a mediastinoscope
Dirofilaria immitis infection
discernible difference
discernible findings
discernible venous motion
discharge, inappropriate
disc-like atelectasis
disc of endocardium
discoid shadow
discolored
discomfort
  burning
  chest
  dull substernal
  ominous chest
  precordial
  substernal burning
discordance, atrioventricular
discordant arterial connection
discordant atrioventricular connection
discordant ventriculoarterial connections
discrepancy in blood pressure in
  upper and lower extremities

discrete lesion
discrete perihilar densities
discrete pulsations
discrete sound
discrete stenosis
discrete subaortic stenosis
discriminate, discrimination
disc-type valve
disease
  acquired
  acquired heart
  acute rheumatic endocarditis
  acute rheumatic fever (ARF)
  acute rheumatic pericarditis (ARP)
  acute tuberculosis
  acyanotic congenital heart
  Adams-Stokes
  adrenal
  Albright
  alcoholic heart muscle
  allergic bronchopulmonary
    aspergillosis
  allergic bronchopulmonary fungal
  allergic myocardial granulomatous
  allergic respiratory
  allograft coronary artery
  amyloid heart
  angiokeratoma corporis diffusum
  aortic valve
  aortic valvular (AVD)
  aorto-occlusive
  aortoiliac
  aortoiliac obstructive valvular
  aortoiliac occlusive
  aortoiliac vascular
  arrhythmogenic
  arterial degenerative
  arteriosclerotic cardiovascular
    (ASCVD)
  arteriosclerotic heart (ASHD)
  arteriosclerotic peripheral vascular

disease *(cont.)*
  asbestos-related pleural
  asymptomatic left main (ALMD)
  atheromatous
  athero-occlusive
  atherosclerotic
  atherosclerotic carotid artery
    (ACAD)
  atherosclerotic pulmonary vascular
    (ASPVD)
  atypical aortic valve stenosis
  Ayerza-Arrillaga
  Bannister angioedema
  Batten
  Battey-avium complex
  Bazin
  Beau
  Becker
  Bernard-Soulier
  beryllium
  Binswanger
  bird-fancier's
  black lung
  Bornholm
  Bouillaud
  Bouveret
  branch
  bronchial type B
  budgerigar-fancier's
  Buerger
  Buerger-Gruetz
  Buerger thromboangiitis obliterans
  bullous lung
  calcified granulomatous
  California coccidioidomycosis
  carcinoid heart
  carcinoid tricuspid valve
  cardiorenal
  cardiovascular
  cardiovascular renal
  carotid occlusive

disease *(cont.)*
carotid vascular
cavitary tuberculosis
cerebellar
Chagas
cheese handler's
cheese washer's
Christmas (hemophilia B)
chronic hypertensive
chronic obstructive pulmonary
    (COPD)
chronic peripheral arterial (CPAD)
chronic rheumatic heart disease
    (CRHD)
coexisting
collagen vascular
communicative
Concato
concomitant
congenital heart (CHD)
congenital mitral valve
constrictive pericardial
contagious
COPD
cork-handler's
coronary artery (CAD)
coronary heart
Corrigan
Corrigan aortic regurgitation
corticobulbar
corticospinal
Corvisart
cyanotic congenital heart
cyanotic heart
cytomegalic inclusion
degenerative atrioventricular node
diffuse
diffuse angiokeratoma
disseminated *Mycobacterium*
    avium-intracellulare (MAI)
Döhle (Doehle)
Döhle syphilitic aortitis

disease *(cont.)*
Duroziez congenital mitral stenosis
eccentric plaque
effusive pericardial
emphysematous type A
end-stage
end-stage cardiac
end-stage cardiopulmonary
end-stage pulmonary
end-stage vascular
endocardial fibroelastosis
eosinophilic disseminated collagen
eosinophilic endomyocardial
exanthematous
extracardiac
extracranial vascular
extrapulmonary
extrapyramidal
Fabry
factor IX deficiency
Fallot
fibrocalcific rheumatic
flax-dresser's
Forbes
Friedländer (Friedlaender)
Friedländer endarteritis obliterans
functional cardiovascular
functional valve
Gairdner
gannister
Gaucher
Glanzmann
global cardiac
glycogen storage
graft occlusive
grain-handler's
great artery
Hamman
hard metal
Harley
heart
Heberden

disease *(cont.)*
Heberden angina pectoris
Heckathorn
Heller-Döhle syphilitic aortitis
hemoglobin C–thalassemia
hemoglobin E–thalassemia
hepatic veno-occlusive
Heubner
Hodgkin
Hodgson
Hodgson aortic
Horton
Huchard
hyaline membrane
hypereosinophilic heart
hyperkinetic heart
hypertensive cardiovascular
  (HCVD)
hypertensive heart (HHD)
hypertensive renal
hypertensive vascular
I-cell
idiopathic eosinophilic lung disease
idiopathic mural endomyocardial
IHD (ischemic heart disease)
iliac atherosclerotic occlusive
infectious
inflammatory aneurysmal
infrarenal aortic
inoperable
interstitial
interstitial lung disease (ILD)
intimal atherosclerotic
intrapulmonary
intrinsic
intrinsic pulmonary
iron storage
ischemic
ischemic heart (IHD)
ischemic myocardial
Kawasaki

disease *(cont.)*
Keshan
Kussmaul-Maier
kyphoscoliotic heart
latent coronary artery
latent ischemic heart
left anterior descending coronary
  artery
left main coronary artery
left main equivalent
legionnaires'
Lenegre
Letterer-Siwe
Lev
Lev acquired complete heart block
Lewis upper limb cardiovascular
Libman-Sacks
Libman-Sacks endocarditis
Löffler (Loeffler)
lower respiratory tract
Lucas-Champonnière
lunger
Lutz-Splendore-Almeida
Lyme
lymphoreticular malignant
Majocchi
maple bark stripper's
Milton
Milton angioedema
mitral valve
mitral valve stenosis (MVS)
mixed connective tissue
mixed restrictive-obstructive lung
Mönckeberg (Moenckeberg)
Mönckeberg medial sclerosis
Mondor
Mondor phlebitis
Monge
Moschcowitz
moyamoya cerebrovascular
multiple system

disease *(cont.)*
  multivalvular
  multivessel
  multivessel coronary artery
  mushroom picker's
  mushroom worker's
  necrotizing arterial
  nephrosclerosis
  nonatherosclerotic coronary artery
  nonoperable
  obstructive small airways
  occlusive
  occlusive peripheral arterial
  occult
  occupational
  one-vessel coronary artery
  Opitz
  organic heart (OHD)
  organic valve
  Osler
  Owren (Factor V deficiency)
  parenchymal
  parenchymal lung
  pericardial
  peripartal heart
  peripartum
  peripheral air-space
  peripheral arterial
  peripheral atherosclerotic
  peripheral vascular (PVD)
  Pick (of heart)
  pigeon-fancier's
  pituitary snuff-taker's
  polycystic kidney
  Pompe
  popliteal artery
  Posadas
  Posadas-Wernicke
  post-transplant coronary artery
  primary electrical
  primary myocardial

disease *(cont.)*
  pulmonary collagen vascular
    (PCVD)
  pulmonary heart
  pulmonary parenchymal
  pulmonary vascular
  pulmonary vascular obstructive
  pulmonary veno-occlusive (PVOD)
  pulseless
  Quincke angioedema
  radiation pericardial
  ragpicker's
  Raynaud
  reactive
  reactive airways (RAD)
  Reiter
  renal parenchymal
  Rendu-Osler-Weber
  renovascular
  restrictive lung
  restrictive myocardial
  rheumatic arthritis
  rheumatic chorea
  rheumatic heart (RHD)
  rheumatic mitral valve
  rheumatic valvular
  rheumatoid lung
  right coronary artery
  Roger
  Rokitansky
  Rougnon-Heberden
  San Joaquin Valley
  saphenous vein bypass graft
  Schönlein (Schoenlein)
  scleroderma heart
  silo-filler's
  single-vessel
  single-vessel heart
  sinoatrial
  sinus node
  snuff taker's pituitary

disease *(cont.)*
  Steinert
  Stokes-Adams
  Sydenham chorea
  symptomatic left main (SLMD)
  Takayasu
  thalassemia–sickle cell
  Thomsen
  three-vessel (four-, five-, etc.)
  three-vessel coronary artery
  thromboembolic
  thyrocardiac
  thyrotoxic heart
  tibial artery
  tibioperoneal occlusive
  triple coronary artery
  triple-vessel
  tsutsugamushi
  tuberculosis
  two-vessel coronary artery
  upper respiratory infection (URI)
  URI (upper respiratory infection)
  valley fever (San Joaquin Valley,
    California)
  valvular (VD)
  valvular heart
  valvulitis
  vasculo-Behçet
  veno-occlusive (VOD)
  von Willebrand (or Willebrand)
  Weil
  Wenckebach
  Werlhof
  Winiwarter-Buerger
  Wolman
  woolsorter's inhalation
disease-free vessel wall
disintegration of plaque by laser pulses
disk (see also *disc*)
  atrial
  Eigon

disk poppet
dislodgement
  complete
  lead
  partial
disobliteration, carotid
disorder
  autoimmune
  coronary vasomotion
  lysosomal storage
  nodal rhythm
  posttransplantation lympho-
    proliferative (PTLD)
  restrictive lung
disorders of conduction
disorders of impulse conduction
disorders of impulse formation
disorientation, right-left
disparate (unequal; dissimilar)
disparity
displaced apical beat
displaced to left
  apical impulse
  PMI (point of maximal impulse)
displacement
  anterior tracheal
  late systolic
  mediastinum
  ST-segment
displacement of apical beat,
  inferolateral
display
  pseudocolor B-mode
  real-time
disposable electrode
disproportion
disrupted plaque
disruption, perivalvular
dissected free
dissecting aneurysm of aorta
dissecting aortic aneurysm

dissecting aortic hematoma
dissecting sponge
dissection
  aortic (type B)
  arterial
  blunt
  carotid arterial
  cautious
  cervicocephalic arterial
  extensive
  extrapericardial
  finger
  infundibular
  intimal
  intimal-medial
  intrapericardial
  meticulous
  sharp
  spiral
  subintimal
  tedious
  thoracic aortic
  type A
  type B
  vertebral arterial
dissection flap
dissection of descending aorta
dissector
  Holinger
  Jannetta
  Lemmon intimal
  Penfield
  ring
  sponge
disseminated atheromatous
  embolization
disseminated cholesterol embolization
disseminated glial hamartoma
disseminated intravascular coagulation
  (DIC) syndrome
disseminated intravascular coagulopathy

disseminated *Mycobacterium avium-*
  intracellulare (MAI) complex
disseminated necrotizing periarteritis
disseminated tuberculosis
dissemination of organisms by bloodstream
dissociation
  atrial
  atrioventricular (AVD)
  auriculoventricular
  AV (atrioventricular)
  complete AV
  electromechanical
  Gallavardin
  incomplete atrioventricular (IAVD)
  interference
  intracavitary pressure-electrogram
  isorhythmic AV
  Mobitz-type AV
distal anastomosis, parachute technique
  for
distal aortic arch aneurysm
distal arterial bypass
distal circumflex marginal artery
distal clot
distal coronary sinus (CS)
distal graft anastomosis
distant breath sounds
distant heart tones
distended veins at 45°
distended with heparinized blood
distensibility, ventricular
distensible
distention
  atrial presystolic
  jugular vein (or venous) (JVD)
  neck vein
  passive venous
  trigeminus (of neck veins)
  venous
distention of neck veins

distichiasis-heart and vasculature
   abnormalities
distortion of ST segment
distortion, radiographic pincushion
distractibility
distress
   cardiorespiratory
   idiopathic respiratory (of newborn)
   marked respiratory
   mild respiratory
   moderate respiratory
   respiratory (of newborn)
   severe respiratory
distress at rest, respiratory
distribution
   anomalous
   binomial
   peribronchial
   perivascular
   reverse
   rimlike calcium
distributive shock
disturbance
   cardiac rhythm
   conduction
   constitutional
   electrolyte
   rhythm
   visual
disturbance of blood coagulation
disturbance of heart rhythm
diurese, diuresed
diuresis of heart failure
diuretic, diuretics
   high-ceiling
   loop
   mercurial
   osmotic
   potassium-sparing
   potassium-wasting
   thiazide

diuretic drugs
diuretic therapy
diver's syncope
divided doses
diving reflex
divisional block
dizziness, periodic
DKS (Damus-Kaye-Stansel)
DKS anastomosis
DKS procedure for congenital heart
   defects
DL_{CO} (diffusing capacity of the lung
   for carbon monoxide)
D-loop, ventricular
D-loop ventricular situs
DLP cardioplegic catheter
DLP cardioplegic needle
DM (diastolic murmur)
D-malposition of aorta
DMI (Diagnostic Medical Instruments)
   analyzer
DMI (diaphragmatic myocardial
   infarction)
DMPE (^{99m}Tc-bis-dimethylphos-
   phonoethane)
DMVA (direct mechanical ventricular
   actuation)
DNA ploidy pattern
DNAR (do not attempt resuscitation)
   orders
DNR (do not resuscitate) status
dobutamine echocardiography
dobutamine stress echocardiography
dobutamine thallium angiography
DOBV (double outlet both ventricles)
DOC (desoxycorticosterone)
DOC exchange technique
DOC guide wire extension
dock wire; docking wire
Docke diastolic murmur
Dodd perforating vein group

Dodge area-length method for
   ventricular activity
Dodge method for calculating left
   ventricular volume
Dodge method for ejection fraction
DOE (dyspnea on exertion)
Doehle (Döhle)
dog cough
Döhle (Doehle)
Döhle disease
Döhle-Heller aortitis
Döhle-Heller syndrome
Döhle syphilitic aortitis disease
dolens
   phlegmasia alba
   phlegmasia cerulea
   thrombophlebitis cerulea
DOLV (double outlet left ventricle)
dome and dart configuration on cardiac
   catheterization
dome of atrium
dome of diaphragm
dome-shaped heart
dome-shaped roof of pleural cavity
dominance
   coronary artery
   mixed
   right ventricular
   shared coronary artery
dominant, anatomically
dominant left coronary artery
dominant left coronary system
dominant right coronary artery
dominant right coronary system
doming, diastolic
doming of leaflets
doming of valve
domino procedure
Donath-Landsteiner test for
   paroxysmal cold hemoglobinuria
D1 (diagonal branch #1)

donor heart
donor heart failure
donor heart-lung block
donor organ, appropriately sized and
   matched
donor organ ischemic time
donor team
Do Not Attempt Resuscitation (DNAR)
   orders
Do Not Resuscitate (DNR) status
doom
   feeling of
   impending
Doplette
Doppler
   color flow
   continuous wave
   pulsed
   spectral
Doppler blood flow detector
Doppler blood flow monitor
Doppler blood pressure
Doppler color flow imaging,
   transesophageal
Doppler color flow mapping
Doppler color spectral analysis
Doppler coronary catheter
Doppler derived stroke distance
Doppler device
Doppler echocardiography, epicardial
Doppler fetal heart murmur
Doppler flow probe study
Doppler flow-imaging system,
   real-time, two-dimensional
Doppler flow-meter
Doppler imaging
Doppler Intra-Dop intraoperative
Doppler, intraoperative
Doppler phenomenon
Doppler pulse
Doppler shift

Doppler signal
Doppler signal enhancers
Doppler spectral analysis
Doppler study, periorbital
Doppler ultrasonic blood flow detector
Doppler ultrasonic fetal heart monitor
Doppler ultrasonic velocity detector
  segmental plethysmography
Doppler ultrasonography
Doppler velocimetry
Doppler velocity waveforms (VWFs)
Doppler venous examination
Doppler waveform analysis of blood
  vessels
Dopplette monitor
Doptone monitor of fetal heart tones
Dorendorf sign of aortic arch
  aneurysm
Dor modification
Dor reconstruction
Dor remodeling ventriculoplasty
Dorros brachial internal mammary
  guiding catheter
Dor technique
dorsal branch
dorsal pedal pulse
dorsal ramus of spinal nerve
dorsalis pedis pulse
DORV (double outlet right ventricle)
dose, doses
  digitalizing
  divided
  incremental
  loading
  maintenance
  tapering
  titrated
  tracer
dosing, titrated
Dos Santos needle for aortography
Dos Santos technique

Dotter angioplasty technique
Dotter caged balloon catheter
Dotter catheter
Dotter coaxial catheter
Dotter effect
dottering effect
Dotter Intravascular Retrieval Set
Dotter-Judkins PTA (percutaneous
  transluminal angioplasty)
Dotter method
Dotter system
Dotter technique
double-acting actuator
double aortic arch
double-barrel aorta
double-barrel lumen
double extrastimuli
double inlet left ventricle/double outlet
  both ventricles
double inlet ventricles
double-occluding clamp
double outlet both ventricles (DOBV)
double outlet left ventricle (DOLV)
double outlet left ventricle syndrome
double outlet right ventricle (DORV)
double outlet right ventricle (I–IV)
  syndrome
double pleurisy
double systolic apical impulse
double umbrella closure
double umbrella technique
double-walled fibroserous sac
double-wire atherectomy technique
doughnut configuration on thallium
  imaging
doughnut magnet
doughy mass
Douglas bag method for determining
  cardiac output
Dow method for cardiac output
Down syndrome

downhill ST segment depression
downsloping ST segment depression
downstream sampling method
downward displaced apical beat
downward displacement of apical
  impulse
downward sloping
doxorubicin cardiotoxicity
Doyen clamp grasping forceps
Doyen rib elevator
Doyen rib rasp; raspatory
dP/dt (upstroke pattern on apex
  cardiogram), peak
D point
DPTI (diastolic pressure-time index)
DPT positive skin prick test
drainage
  abscess
  anomalous pulmonary venous
  brisk
  bronchial secretions
  closed chest
  extrapleural
  pulmonary venous
  total anomalous pulmonary venous
  tube
  underwater-seal
draining vein pressure (DVP)
drain, Penrose
Drechslera hawaiiensis
drenching sweats
dressing
  Comfeel Ulcus
  Silastic tape
  stent
  Steri-Strips
  Synthaderm
  Tegaderm
  Vigilon
  Vitacuff
  wet-to-dry

Dressler fusion beat
Dressler post-myocardial infarction
  syndrome
Dressler syndrome
drifting wedge pressure
drill biopsy
drip
  I.V. (intravenous)
  postnasal
Dripps-American Surgical Association
  score to predict cardiac morbidity
drive cycle length
drive, hypoxic
Dromos pacemaker
drooping eyelid
drop attacks
drop heart
droplets, respiratory
drop test for pneumoperitoneum
drowned lung
drowsiness
drug-induced leukopenia
drug-induced orthostatic hypotension
drug-induced pericarditis
drug-induced pulmonary eosinophilia
drug-induced syncope
drug of choice
drug-refractory arrhythmia
drug-refractory tachycardia
drug-related terms (see *medication*
  entry for list of drugs)
  adrenergic blocker
  adrenergic stimulant
  adjuvant
  agonist
  alpha/beta adrenergic blocker
  aminoglycoside
  angiotensin converting enzyme
    (ACE) inhibitors
  antagonist
  anthracyclines

drug-related terms *(cont.)*
  anthraquinones
  antiadrenergic agent
  antianginal agent
  antiarrhythmic agent
  antibiotic
  anticoagulant
  antidiuretics
  antifibrinolytic
  antifilarial
  antihistamines
  antihyperlipidemic agent
  antihypertensive
  anti-infective
  anti-inflammatory
  antimicrobial
  antiparasitics
  antiplatelet
  antipruritic
  antiseptic
  antispasmodic
  antituberculosis
  antitussives
  antiviral
  bactericidal
  bacteriostatic
  beta-adrenergic receptor blocking
    agent
  beta agonist
  beta blocker
  beta blocking
  bile acid sequestrant
  bronchodilators
  calcium channel antagonist
  calcium channel blocker
  cardioselective agent
  cardioselective beta-blocker
  cardiotonic
  chronotropic agent
  corticosteroid
  cough syrup

drug-related terms *(cont.)*
  coumarin-type anticoagulant
  cyclo-oxygenase inhibitor
  decongestant
  digitalis
  diuretic
  expectorant
  ganglion blocker
  hemostatics
  histamines
  HMG-CoA reductase inhibitors
  hyperlipidemics
  hypolipidemics
  immunosuppressive
  inotropic agent
  intramuscular
  intravenous
  long-acting
  loop diuretic
  lung surfactant
  macrolide
  MAO (monoamine oxidase)
    inhibitor
  medium chain triglyceride (MCT)
  mucolytics
  neuromuscular blocking agent
  nicotinic acid
  nicotine withdrawal aid
  long-acting nitrate
  nitroglycerin
  nitrous oxide
  nonselective beta blocker
  nonsteroidal anti-inflammatory
    drugs (NSAID)
  novel plasminogen activator (NPA)
  oral
  osmotic diuretic
  phosphodiesterase inhibitor
  plasma expanders
  plasma extenders
  platelet concentrate

drug-related terms *(cont.)*
   platelet inhibitors
   potassium-sparing diuretic
   potassium-wasting diuretic
   pulmonary surfactant replacement
   quinolone antibiotic
   recombinant tissue plasminogen
      activator (rt-PA)
   respiratory stimulants
   respiratory therapy agents
   smoking deterrent
   sulfonamide
   sulfonylurea
   surfactant agents
   sympathomimetic
   sympathomimetic amine
   thiazide diuretic
   thionamides
   thrombin
   thrombolytics
   topical
   torsemide
   transdermal
   tricyclic antidepressant
   tuberculosis preparations
   vasoconstrictor
   vasoactive
   vasodilator
   vasopressor
   venous insufficiency treatment
drug-resistant tachyarrhythmia
drug therapy
drug tolerance
drumlike percussion note
Drummond marginal artery
Drummond sign of aortic aneurysm
dry air induced nasal symptoms
dry cough
dry mucous membranes
dry nonproductive cough
dry pleurisy

DSA (digital subtraction angiography)
DSAS (discrete subvalvular aortic
   stenosis)
D-shaped vessel lumen
DTAF-F (descending thoracic
   aortofemoral-femoral) bypass
D to E slope on echocardiography
DTPA, technetium bound to
DTR (deep tendon reflex)
D-transposition (dextrotransposition)
   of great arteries
dual atrioventricular node pathway
dual balloon method
dual chamber pacemaker
dual chamber pacing
dual heart rhythm
dual ventricles
Duchenne muscular dystrophy
duckbill forceps
Ducor balloon catheter
Ducor-Cordis pigtail catheter
Ducor HF (high-flow) catheter
Ducor tip
duct
   alveolar
   lymphatic
   thoracic
ductal arch
ductal constriction
ductal remnant
ductile, ductility
ductless
duct of Arantius
duct of Botallo
ductulus
ductus
   friable
   recanalized
   recurrent
   window
ductus Arantii

ductus arteriosus
  patent (PDA)
  persistent
  persistent patency of
  reversed
ductus arteriosus closure, pulmonary
  hypoperfusion unmasked by
ductus arteriosus patency
ductus bump
ductus thoracicus
ductus thoracicus dexter
ductus venosus, persistent patency of
Duffield scissors
Duffy blood antibody type
Duke bleeding time; test
dullness
  cardiac
  Gerhardt
  Grocco triangular
  left border of cardiac (LBCD)
  percussion
  shifting
  tympanitic
dullness to percussion
dull pain
dull percussion note
dull substernal discomfort
dull tympanitic resonance in pleural
  effusion
dumbbell-shaped tip
Dunlop thrombus stripper
duodenitis, hemorrhagic
duodenojejunal angle
Duostat
duplex Doppler ultrasound
duplex imaging
duplex scan (or scanning)
  color-flow
  renal
duplex ultrasound
Duran annuloplasty ring

Durapulse pacemaker
duration
  action potential (APD)
  pulse
duration of EKG wave
duration of exercise
duration of P wave
duration of QRS
Duromedics aortic valve
Duromedics prosthetic heart valve
Duroziez mitral stenosis disease
Duroziez murmur
Duroziez sign
Dusard syndrome
duskiness of skin
dusky skin color
dust
  cotton
  inhalation of environmental
dust cells
Duval-Crile lung forceps
Duval lung forceps
dV/dt (contractility)
DVI (deep venous insufficiency)
DVI pacing mode
DVI Simpson atherocath
DVP (draining vein pressure)
DVT (deep venous thrombosis)
D wave on EKG
Dyclone gargle anesthesia
dye (see also *contrast medium*)
  Cardio-Green
  Fox green
  indocyanine green
dye curve
Dynamic Air Therapy, Restcue CC
dynamic compliance
dynamic compression of airways
dynamic lung compliance (C_{dyn})
dynamic lung
dynamic pulmonary hyperinflation

dynamics, arterial wall
dysarthria
dysautonomia
dysbarism syndrome
dysbetalipoproteinemia, familial
dyscontrol, episodic
dyscrasia
   blood
   plasma cell
dysesthesia
dysfibrinogenemia
dysfunction
   autonomic
   biventricular global systolic
   cognitive
   contractile
   exercise-induced left ventricular
   focal ventricular
   global ventricular
   left ventricular (LVD)
   mitral valve (MVD)
   papillary muscle (PMD)
   regional myocardial
   sinoatrial node
   sinus node
   sleep
   ventilatory
   ventricular
dyskeratosis
dyskinesia, regional
dyskinesis
   anterior wall
   anteroapical
   left ventricular
dyskinetic cilia
dyskinetic segmental wall motion
dyslipidemia, familial genetic
dysmaturity, pulmonary
dysmodulation
dysphagia lusoria
dysphonia

dysplasia
   arrhythmogenic right ventricular
      (ARVD)
   arteriohepatic
   bronchopulmonary
   congenital polyvalvular
   endocardial
   familial arterial fibromuscular
   fibromuscular
   fibrous
   geleophysic
   perimedial
   primary chordal
   pulmonary valve (PVD)
   right ventricular
   secondary chordal
   ventricular
   ventriculo-radial
dysplastic pulmonary valve
dysplastic tricuspid valve
dyspnea
   angina-equivalent
   cardiac
   episodic
   exertional
   expiratory
   functional
   inspiratory
   mild
   nocturnal
   noncardiac
   nonexpansional
   orthostatic
   paroxysmal nocturnal (PND)
   paroxysmal wheezing
   postural
   profound
   renal
   sighing
dyspnea at rest
dyspnea on exertion (DOE)

dyspnea with cyanosis
dyspnea with tachypnea and hyper-
    ventilation
dyspneic
dysproteinemia
dysrhythmia
    cardiac
    malignant ventricular
Dysshwannian syndrome
dyssynergia
    regional
    segmental
dyssynergy

dystrophy
    asphyxiating thoracic
    Becker muscular
    Duchenne muscular
    Emery-Dreifuss muscular
    Erb limb-girdle
    infantile thoracic
    Landouzy-Dejerine
    limb-girdle
    myotonic
    progressive pulmonary
    suffocating thoracic

E, e

E (ejection sound)
EAC (expandable access catheter)
Eagle equation to predict cardiac
    morbidity
E:A ratio on echocardiogram
earlobe crease (probable risk sign for
    coronary artery disease)
early asthmatic response
early inspiratory crackles
early-onset varicose veins
early rapid repolarization
early systolic murmur
early venous filling
early ventricular depolarization
    (pre-excitation)
ear (not air) oximetry
EAS (endoscopic articulating stapler)
easily palpable carotid arterial pulse
easy fatigability
Eaton agent pneumonia
Eaton-Lambert syndrome
EBDA (effective balloon dilated area)
Eberth line
EBL (estimated blood loss)
Ebstein cardiac anomaly
Ebstein disease of tricuspid valve

Ebstein malformation
Ebstein sign
EC (ejection click)
ECA (external carotid artery)
E-CABG (endarterectomy and
    coronary artery bypass graft)
ECC (emergency cardiac care)
eccentric atherosclerotic plaque
eccentric atrial activation
eccentric coronary artery
eccentric hypertrophy
eccentric ledge
eccentric lesion
eccentric plaque disease
eccentric restenosis lesion
eccentric stenosis
eccentric tear
eccentric vessel
eccentrically placed lumen
eccentricity index
ecchymosis (pl. ecchymoses)
ECF-A (eosinophil chemotactic factor
    of anaphylaxis)
ECG or EKG (electrocardiogram)
echinococcal cysts of lung
echinococcosis

echinococcus cysts in pleura
Echinococcus granulosus infection
echo, echoes
  amphoric
  atrial
  bright, highly mobile
  dense
  homogeneous
  inhomogeneous
  linear
  metallic
  shower of
  specular
  spin
  swirling smokelike
  thick
  ventricular (on EKG)
echo (brief form for echocardiogram)
echocardiogram, -graphy
  A-mode
  akinesis on
  ambulatory Holter
  anterior left ventricular wall motion
  apical
  apical five-chamber view
  apical left ventricular wall motion
    on
  apical two-chamber view
  B bump on anterior mitral valve
    leaflet
  B-mode
  biplane transesophageal
  blood pool radionuclide
  cardiac output
  color flow imaging Doppler
  continuous loop exercise
  continuous wave Doppler
  contrast
  contrast-enhanced
  cross-sectional two-dimensional
  CW (continuous wave) Doppler
  D to E slope on

echocardiogram *(cont.)*
  dipyridamole
  dobutamine stress
  Doppler
  dyskinesis on
  E point on
  echo intensity disappearance rate on
  echo-free space on
  epicardial Doppler
  exercise
  Feigenbaum
  fetal (in utero)
  four-chamber
  hypokinesis on
  inferior left ventricular wall motion
    on
  intracardiac (ICE)
  intracoronary contrast
  intraoperative cardioplegic contrast
  late systolic posterior displacement
    on
  lateral left ventricular wall motion
    on
  left ventricular long-axis
  long-axis parasternal view
  loss of an "a" dip on
  M-mode Doppler
  myocardial contrast (MCE)
  myocardial perfusion
  parasternal long-axis view
  parasternal short-axis view
  pharmacologic stress
  postcontrast
  posterior left ventricular wall
    motion on
  postexercise
  postinjection
  postmyocardial infarction
  precontrast
  preinjection
  premyocardial infarction
  pulsed Doppler

echocardiogram *(cont.)*
  pulsed-wave (PW) Doppler
  real-time
  resting
  right ventricular short-axis
  sector scan
  septal wall motion on
    short-axis view
  signal averaged
  stress
  subcostal short-axis view
  subxiphoid view of
  three-dimensional transesophageal
  transesophageal (TEE)
  transthoracic
  2D (two-dimensional)
  two-chamber
  ventricular wall motion
echocardiogram adenosine
echocardiographic automated border
  detection
echo characteristics on ultrasound
echo contrast
echo delay time (TE)
echo density
echo-free area
echo-free space
echo-planar sequence
echogenic mass
echogenic plaque
echogenicity
echogram, mitral valve
echography, B-mode
echoicity
echolucent plaque
EchoMark angiographic catheter
echophonocardiography, combined
  M-mode
echoplanar imaging
echoreflectivity
echo reverberation

echo signature
Echovar Doppler system
ECMO (extracorporeal membrane
  oxygenation)
ECS (cardioplegic solution)
ectasia, annuloaortic
ectasia of coronary artery
ectatic emphysema
Ectocor pacemaker
ectopia cordis abdominalis
ectopia cordis, pectoral
ectopic atrial activity
ectopic atrial focus
ectopic atrial tachycardia
ectopic beat
ectopic focus (pl. foci)
ectopic impulse
ectopic lift
ectopic rest of thyroid tissue
ectopic ventricular beat
ectopic wall motion abnormality
ectopy
  asymptomatic complex (ACE)
  atrial
  bursts of ventricular
  cardiac
  frequent ventricular
  high-density ventricular
  supraventricular
  ventricular
ED (emergency department)
eddy formation
eddy sound of patent ductus arteriosus
edema
  acute pulmonary
  alveolar pulmonary
  angioneurotic
  ankle
  bland
  brawny
  bronchiolar

edema *(cont.)*
  brown
  cardiac
  cardiogenic pulmonary
  cardiopulmonary
  chemical pulmonary
  chronic
  circumscribed
  cyclic idiopathic
  cyclical
  dependent
  fingerprint
  florid
  frank pulmonary
  fulminant pulmonary
  generalized pulmonary
  giant
  gravitational
  hard
  hereditary angioneurotic (HANE)
  high-altitude pulmonary (HAPE)
  idiopathic
  intercellular
  interstitial pulmonary
  laryngeal
  leg
  localized
  lymphatic
  massive
  mild
  Milton
  mushy
  nephrotic
  neurogenic pulmonary
  noncardiac pulmonary
  noncardiogenic pulmonary
  noninflammatory
  nonpitting
  osmotic
  painless
  paroxysmal pulmonary

edema *(cont.)*
  passive
  pedal
  perihilar
  periodic
  peripheral
  perivascular
  pitting
  postoperative pulmonary
  pretibial
  pulmonary
  purulent
  Quincke
  reexpansion pulmonary
  sacral
  salt
  scalp
  solid (of lungs)
  stasis
  subglottic
  supraglottic
  terminal
  trace
  2+ pitting
  venous
  vernal (of lung)
edema fluid
edema neonatorum
edema to groins
edematous tissues
edge
  leading
  shelving
  sternal
  trailing
edge-detection angiography
Edmark mitral valve
EDRF (endothelium-relaxing factor)
EDV (end-diastolic velocity)
EDVI (end-diastolic volume index)
Edwards diagnostic catheter

Edwards-Duromedics bileaflet valve
Edwards-Kerr procedure
Edwards syndrome
Edwards woven Teflon aortic
   bifurcation graft
EF (ejection fraction)
EFE (endocardial fibroelastosis)
effect
   adverse
   Anrep
   artifact due to partial volume
   Bayliss
   Bohr
   Bowditch
   bronchodilator
   bronchomotor
   cobra head
   contractility
   copper wire
   cumulative
   deleterious
   Dotter
   dottering
   electrophysiologic
   hemodynamic
   inotropic
   jet
   osmotic
   placebo
   potassium-sparing
   proarrhythmic
   purse-stringing
   silver wire
   snowplow
   tetrodotoxin
   vasodilatory
   Venturi
effective refractory period (ERP)
efferent conduit
efficacious
efficacy of drug therapy

efficacy of treatment
efficiency, valvular
effort
   maximal inspiratory
   respiratory
   ventilatory
effort-dependent
effort syncope
effort thrombosis
effuse
effused chyle
effusion
   bloody
   cholesterol
   cholesterol pericardial
   chyliform
   eosinophilic pleural
   exudative
   hemorrhagic
   loculated
   malignant
   milky or chylous pleural
   pericardial (PE)
   pleural
   pleurisy with
   pseudochylous
   serofibrinous pericardial
   subpleural
   taut pericardial
   tiny
   turbid
effusion of blood in the pleural cavity
effusive constricting pericarditis
effusive pericardial disease
eggshell calcification
egophony at upper border of pleural
   fluid
egress of blood
Ehlers-Danlos syndrome
Eigon disk
Eikenella infection

Einthoven law for EKG
Einthoven reference lines (on EKG
  lead placement)
Einthoven triangle
Eisenmenger complex (congenital heart
  anomaly)
Eisenmenger reaction with septal
  defects
Eisenmenger syndrome
ejection, accelerated
ejection click (EC)
  palpable
  systolic
ejection fraction (EF)
  area-length method for
  basilar half
  blunted
  BSA (body surface area)
  computed
  depressed
  digital
  Dodge method for
  global
  globally depressed
  interval
  Kennedy method for calculating
  left ventricular (LVEF)
  one-third
  regional
  resting left ventricular
  right ventricular (RVEF)
  systolic
  thermodilution
  well preserved
ejection fraction acoustic quantification, left ventricular
ejectionlike systolic murmur
ejection phase indices
ejection sound (E)
  palpable aortic
  palpable pulmonic

ejection systolic murmur (ESM)
ejection time
  increased left ventricular
  prolonged
EJV (external jugular vein)
EKG or ECG (electrocardiogram)
EKG-gated multislice MRI technique
EKG-gated spin-echo MRI
EKG lead system
  Frank
  Mason-Likar
EKG rhythm strip
EKG-silent
EKG-synchronized digital subtraction
  angiography
El Gamal cardiac device
El Gamal coronary bypass catheter
Ela pacemaker
elaborate
elaboration, further
elastance
  end-systolic
  maximum ventricular (EMAX)
elastic lamina
elastic recoil
elastic recoil of artery
elastic stockings
elasticity
elasticum, pseudoxanthoma
elastomyofibrosis
Elecath circulatory support device
Elecath electrode
Elecath thermodilution catheter
elective cardiac arrest and subsequent
  reperfusion
elective replacement indicators
electrical activity, pulseless
electrical alternans
electrical axis of heart
electrical axis on EKG, J point
electrical cardioversion

electrical circulatory arrest
electrical defibrillation
electrical events of the EKG
electrical impedance
electrical inactivity
electrically conditioned and driven
    skeletal muscle
electrical potential
electrocardiogram (ECG or EKG)
    ambulatory (AECG)
    baseline
    Burdick
    computerized
    Corometrics-Aloka
    counterclockwise superiorly
        oriented frontal QRS loop
    depressed T waves on
    esophageal
    evolutionary changes on
    exercise
    fetal
    flat
    flatline
    flattened T waves on
    His bundle
    intracardiac
    intracavitary recording of
    intracoronary
    intramyocardial (during sleep)
    inverted T waves in V_3 and V_1 on
    lateral precordial leads
    Micro-Tracer portable
    normal QRS axis
    normal resting
    persistently upright T waves on
    postconversion
    pre-exercise resting supine
    precordial
    Q-S complex on
    Q waves in right precordial leads on
    resting

electrocardiogram *(cont.)*
    scalar
    serial changes in
    signal-averaged (SaECG)
    signal-averaging technique
    16-lead
    stress
    surface
    telephone transmission of
    three-channel
    three-lead
    12-lead
    upright tilt-testing
    vector
electrocardiogram leads (see *lead*)
electrocardiogram tracing
electrocardiographic gating
electrocardiographic variant
electrocardiograph machine
electrocardiography (see *electrocardio-*
    gram)
electrocardiophonogram
electrocardioscanner, Compuscan
    Hittman computerized
electrode (see also *lead*)
    "active can"
    anodal
    anterior anodal patch
    array
    Arzco TAPSUL pill
    axillary
    barbed-hook pacemaker
    Biotronik IE 65-I pacemaker
    bipolar pacemaker
    Bisping design
    bulbous-tip
    catheter
    Clark oxygen
    Cordis
    corkscrew-tip pacemaker
    CPI Endotak transvenous

electrode *(cont.)*
  CPI porous tine-tipped bipolar
    pacing
  defibrillation
  disposable
  endocardial
  endocardial pacemaker
  endocardial placement of
  Endotak
  epicardial
  epicardial pacemaker
  epicardial patch
  esophageal pill
  external adhesive patch
  flanged
  flanged Silastic tip pacemaker
  floating
  free end of
  free-floating
  hand-held
  high right atrium
  His bundle
  impedance
  J orthogonal
  J-shaped pacemaker
  Laserdish
  Medtronic bipolar
  Medtronic pacemaker
  Medtronic Transvene transvenous
  multilead
  multiple point
  myocardial
  negative pacemaker
  negative pacing
  orthogonal
  pacing
  paddle
  patch
  pectoral
  permanent pacing
  pill

electrode *(cont.)*
  platinum
  point
  porous
  porous tip
  positive pacemaker
  positive pacing
  posterior cathodal patch
  precordial surface
  quadripolar catheter
  Quinton
  recording
  ring tip
  roving hand-held bipolar
  scalp
  screw-in tip pacemaker
  sensing
  shocking
  Siemens
  Silastic
  skin
  stainless steel
  stimulating
  subcutaneous array
  subcutaneous patch
  subxiphoid
  suction-type
  sutureless myocardial
  swallowed
  target tip
  Telectronics pacemaker
  temporary pacemaker
  temporary pacing electrode
  temporary transvenous catheter
  thermistor
  thoracic
  three-turn
  tine-tipped pacemaker
  tined
  transesophageal (TEE)
  transthoracic

electrode *(cont.)*
    Transvene
    transvenous
    transvenous placement of
    tripolar transvenous screw-in
    two-turn
    unipolar coil
    unipolar pacemaker
    urethane
    Waterston pacing
    wire
electrode catheter tip
electrode gel electrode pads
electrode lead
electrode paste
electrode stimulation, transvenous
    (of atrium)
Electrodyne pacemaker
electrogram, -graphy
    coronary sinus
    CSos (coronary sinus ostium)
    esophageal
    fractionated ventricular
    His bundle (HBE)
    HRA (high right atrium)
    intra-atrial
    intracardiac
    intracavitary
    intracoronary
    right atrial
    RVA (right ventricular apical)
    sinus node
electrolyte disturbance
electrolyte imbalance
electrolytes, consisting of
    bicarbonate (bicarb; HCO_3)
    calcium (Ca)
    chloride (Cl)
    magnesium
    potassium (K)
    sodium (Na)
electromagnetic blood flow study

electromagnetic interference (EMI)
electromechanical dissociation (EMD)
    of the heart
electromechanical systole
electromechanical total artificial heart
electromechanically quiescent heart
electrophoresis
electrophysiologic effect
electrophysiologic mapping
electrophysiologic study (EPS) to
    assess ventricular arrhythmia
electrovectorcardiogram, -graphy
Elema-Schonander pacemaker
elephant on chest, feeling of
elephant trunk technique
elev (elevated)
elevated ALT (alanine aminotrans-
    ferase)
elevated AST (aspartate aminotrans-
    ferase)
elevated blood lipids
elevated diaphragms
elevated diastolic plateau
elevated gradient
elevated jugular venous pressure
elevated neck veins
elevated plasma lactate
elevated plasma renin activity,
    inappropriately
elevated pulmonary wedge pressure
elevated RT segment
elevated serum lactate level
elevated ST segment
elevated to the angle of jaw at 90°
elevated venous pressure
elevation
    central venous pressure
    diaphragmatic
    ST segment
    transient ST segment
elevation of enzymes
elevation of limb

elevation pallor of extremity
elevator
  Doyen rib
  Freer
  Matson rib
  Matson-Alexander rib
  Penfield
  rib
11-hydroxylase deficiency
elfin facies syndrome
Elgiloy frame of prosthetic valve
Elite double-loop catheter
Elite dual-chamber rate-responsive
  pacemaker
Elite guide catheter
Ellestad protocol for treadmill stress
  test
Ellestad treadmill exercise protocol
Elliotson syndrome
elliptical burr
elliptical lead
elliptical lumen
ellipticity index
Ellis-Garland line
Ellis line
Ellis sign
Ellis-van Creveld syndrome
Eloesser flap
elongated doubly pyramidal structures
elongated heart
elongation
elongation and tortuosity
elongation, aortic
elongation of globe of eye
Elsner syndrome
emaciated
EMAX (ventricular elastance,
  maximum)
embarrassment
  circulatory
  hemodynamic
  respiratory

Embden-Meyerhof-Parnas pathway
embedding of stent coils
embolectomy
  arterial
  pulmonary
  transfemoral Fogarty
emboli (pl. of *embolus*)
embolic event
embolic gangrene
embolic obstruction of pulmonary
  artery
embolic phenomenon
embolic shower
embolic stroke
embolism (also *embolus*)
  air
  amniotic fluid
  arterial
  atheromatous
  bacillary
  bland
  bone marrow
  cancer
  capillary
  cardiogenic
  catheter-induced
  cellular
  cerebral
  coronary artery
  crossed
  direct
  fat
  fibrin platelet
  foam
  gas nitrogen
  infective
  intraluminal
  massive
  miliary
  multiple
  obturating
  occluding spring

embolism *(cont.)*
  oil
  pantaloon
  paradoxical
  peripheral
  plasmodium
  polyurethane foam
  prosthetic valve
  pulmonary (PE)
  pulmonary venous-systemic air
  recurrent
  renal cholesterol
  riding
  septic
  septic pulmonary
  "shower" of
  straddling
  submassive pulmonary
  trichinous
  tumor
  venous
  visceral
embolism without infarction
embolization
  atheromatous cholesterol crystal
  balloon (therapeutic)
  balloon and coil
  cardiac tumor
  cholesterol
  chronic lung (by blood-borne eggs)
  coil (of unwanted vessel)
  coil (therapeutic)
  diffuse cholesterol
  disseminated atheromatous
  disseminated cholesterol
  massive
  septic
  Silastic bead
  stent
embolization of vascular malformation

embolization syndrome
  peripheral cholesterol
  renal cholesterol
  visceral cholesterol
  therapeutic
embolotherapy, catheter
embolus (pl. emboli) (see *embolism*)
embolus trap, Mobin-Uddin
embryonal vein
embryonic aortic arch
embryonic branchial arch
embryonic cell rests in the septum
embryonic infection
EMD (electromechanical dissociation)
  of the heart
emergency airway
emergency cardiac care (ECC)
emergency cricothyrotomy
emergent, emergently
Emerson pump
Emerson vein stripper
Emery-Dreifuss muscular dystrophy
EMF (endomyocardial fibrosis)
EMI (electromagnetic interference)
EMI-induced pacemaker failure
eminase thrombolysis
emotional angina
emphysema
  alcoholic
  alveolar
  alveolar duct
  atrophic
  bronchiolar
  bullous
  centriacinar
  centrilobular
  chronic
  chronic hypertrophic
  chronic obstructive
  compensating

emphysema *(cont.)*
  compensatory
  congenital lobar
  cutaneous
  cystic
  cystic pulmonary
  diffuse
  ectatic
  false
  focal-dust
  gangrenous
  generalized
  giant bullous
  glass blower's
  hypoplastic
  idiopathic unilobar
  infantile lobar
  interlobular
  interstitial
  intestinal
  liquefactive
  lobar
  localized obstructive
  mediastinal
  neck
  necrotizing
  neonatal cystic pulmonary
  obstructive
  oxygen-dependent
  panacinar
  panlobular
  paracicatricial
  paraseptal
  postoperative
  postsurgical
  pulmonary
  pulmonary interstitial (PIE)
  senile
  skeletal
  small-lunged
  subcutaneous

emphysema *(cont.)*
  surgical
  traumatic
  unilateral
  unilateral pulmonary
  vesicular
emphysema due to $alpha_1$-antitrypsin
  deficiency
emphysema of lungs
emphysematous bleb
emphysematous bronchitis
emphysematous bulla
emphysematous COPD (chronic
  obstructive pulmonary disease)
emphysematous expansion of left
  upper lobe
emphysematous expansion of lobe
  of lung
emphysematous lungs
emphysematous type A disease
empiric bronchodilator therapy
empiric therapy
empirical therapy
emplaced (verb)
empty beating heart
empty beating heart method
empty collapsed lung
emptying, tortuous
empyema (see also *abscess*)
  chest
  interlobar
  latent
  left-sided
  loculated
  metapneumonic
  pericardial
  pleural
  pneumococcal
  pulsating
  putrid
  right-sided

empyema *(cont.)*
  streptococcal
  synpneumonic
  thoracic
  tuberculous
empyema articuli
empyema benignum
empyema necessitatis
empyema of chest
empyema of pericardium
empyema with pachypleuritis
EMS (endoscopic multifeed stapler)
emulsified fat globules
en bloc
encapsulated bacteria
encephalopathy, hypertensive
encephalopathy, post-arrest hypoxic
encircled
encirclement
encircling endocardial cryoablation
encircling endocardial ventriculotomy
encoachment
Encor pacemaker
Encore inflation device
encroachment, luminal
en cuirasse, cor
encysted pleurisy
endarterectomized
endarterectomized segment
endarterectomy
  aortoiliac
  aortoiliofemoral
  blind
  carotid
  carotid bifurcation
  carotid eversion
  Connolly eversion
  coronary
  eversion
  extraluminal
  gas

endarterectomy *(cont.)*
  innominate
  laser
  manual core
  open
  profunda
  proximal aortic
  semiclosed
  subclavian
  transaortic
  transaortic extraction
endarterectomy and coronary artery
  bypass graft (E-CABG)
endarteritis obliterans
endartery
end diastole
end-diastolic flow
end-diastolic pressure
end-diastolic pressure-volume relation
end-diastolic velocity (EDV)
end-diastolic volume
end-expiratory lung volume (FRC)
end-expiratory pressure
end-expiratory wheezing
end-inspiratory pressure
end-inspiratory wheezes
endless loop, dual-chamber pacemaker
endoaneurysmorrhaphy
endobronchial carcinoma
endobronchial exudates
endobronchial Kaposi sarcoma
endobronchial lesion
endobronchial mucosa
endobronchial neoplasm
endobronchial obstruction
endobronchial tuberculosis
endobronchial tumor
endocardial ablation
endocardial activation mapping
endocardial catheter ablation
endocardial catheter mapping

endocardial cryoablation, encircling
endocardial cushion
endocardial cushion defect
endocardial cushion malformation
endocardial dysplasia
endocardial electrode
endocardial fibroelastosis (EFE)
endocardial fibrosis, Davies
endocardial hemorrhage, focal
endocardial lead
endocardial lesion, noninfective
endocardial mapping
endocardial pace/sense and
  defibrillation lead
endocardial plaque
endocardial pocket
endocardial resection
endocardial sclerosis
endocardial trabeculation
endocardial-to-epicardial resection
endocardiectomy
endocarditis
  atypical verrucous
  acute
  acute bacterial (ABE)
  acute infective
  acute rheumatic
  aortic valve
  atypical verrucous
  bacterial
  blastomycotic
  cachectic
  chronic
  constrictive
  coxsackievirus
  enterococcal
  fungal
  gonococcal
  histoplasmotic
  indeterminate
  infectious

endocarditis *(cont.)*
  infective
  infective aneurysmal
  Libman-Sacks
  Loeffler fibroblastic
  Loeffler parietal fibroplastic
  Löffler (Loeffler)
  malignant
  marantic
  marantic infective
  meningococcal
  monilial
  mural
  mycotic
  nonbacterial
  nonbacterial thrombotic (NBTE)
  nonbacterial verrucous
  noninfective verrucous
  nonrheumatic
  nosocomial infective
  parietal
  parietal fibroplastic
  postoperative
  prosthetic valve
  pulmonary artery catheter-
    associated
  pulmonic
  purulent
  Q fever
  rheumatic
  rickettsial
  right-side
  septic
  staphylococcal
  streptococcal
  subacute
  subacute bacterial (SBE)
  subacute infective
  syphilitic
  thrombotic
  tricuspid valve

endocarditis *(cont.)*
 tuberculous
 typhoid
 ulcerative
 valvular
 vegetative
 verrucous
 viridans
endocarditis chordalis
endocarditis infection
endocarditis lenta
endocarditis prophylaxis
endocardium
 disc of
 wafer of
endocrine neoplasia, multiple
end of atrial systole
end of systole
Endo Grasp device
endogenous hypertriglyceridemia
endogenous lipoid pneumonia
endoluminal stent
endomyocardial biopsy
endomyocardial fibrosis
 mural
 tropical
endophlebitis
end-organ
EndoSonics IVUS/balloon dilatation
 catheter
Endotak automatic internal cardioverter defibrillator (AICD)
Endotak C lead
Endotak electrode
Endotak nonthoracotomy implantable
 cardioverter-defibrillator (ICD)
Endotak SQ lead array
Endotak transvenous ICD
endothelial cells, pulmonary capillary
endothelial proliferation
endothelial surface

endothelialization of stent
endothelialization of vascular graft
endothelialized vascular grafts
endothelin-1
endothelioid cell
endothelioma
endothelium
 arterial
 pulmonary capillary
 squamous
endothelium-derived contracting factor
endothelium-derived relaxing factor
endothoracic fascia
endotoxin assay
endotoxins, gram-negative bacterial
endotracheal intubation
endotracheal tube
Endotrol tracheal tube
endovascular
endovascular infection
endovascular stented graft
endovascular ultrasonography
endovenous defibrillation
endpoint, exercise
end-pressure artifact
end-stage cardiomyopathy
end-stage cardiopulmonary disease
end-stage congestive heart failure
end-stage disease
end-stage fetal cardiac decompensation
end systole
end-systolic dimension
end-systolic elastance
end-systolic pressure-volume relation
end-systolic reversal
end-systolic volume
end-systolic volume indices
end-tidal-volume apnea
end-to-end anastomosis
end-to-side anastomosis
end-to-side portocaval anastomosis

endurance exercise
enema, Kayexalate
energy, stored
Enertrax pacemaker
engaged, cutting mechanism was
engorged collecting system
engorged tissues
engorged veins under the tongue
engorgement
    bilateral venous
    neck vessel
    pulmonary artery
    vascular
    venous
engorgement of pulmonary vessels
Engström respirator
EnGuard double-lead ICD (implantable
    cardioverter-defibrillator) system
EnGuard pacing and defibrillation
    lead system
EnGuard PFX lead electrode
enhanced
Enhanced Torque 8F guiding catheter
enhancement of Doppler flow signals
enlarged cardiac silhouette
enlarged heart
enlarged valve apparatus
enlargement (see also *hypertrophy*)
    cardiac
    chamber
    compensatory
    hilar lymph node
    mediastinal lymph node
en masse lobectomy
ensuing
enteric gram-negative bacilli
Enterobacter aerogenes bronchitis
Enterobacter agglomerans
Enterobacter cloacae
Enterobacteriaceae infection
enterococcal infection

enteropathy, protein-losing
enteroviral infection
enteroviral pericarditis
entirely chaotic pulse
entrainment
    concealed
    transient
entrance block
entrance heart block
entrapment, popliteal artery
EnTré guide wire
entry of air into pleural cavity
enucleated
enveloping fascia
environmental exposure
environmental tobacco smoking
    exposure
enzyme (see also *isoenzyme*)
    angiotensin-converting (ACE)
    cardiac
    elevated
    lysosomal
    myocardial
enzyme levels
enzyme-linked immunosorbent assay
    (ELISA)
enzyme study
EOL (end of life)
EOS (end of service)
eosinophil chemotactic factor of
    anaphylaxis (ECF-A)
eosinophil count, absolute
eosinophilia
    alveolar
    cryptogenic pulmonary
    drug-induced pulmonary
    idiopathic familial
    Löffler (Loeffler)
    profound peripheral
    prolonged pulmonary
    pulmonary

eosinophilia *(cont.)*
  pulmonary infiltration
  sputum
  tropical
eosinophilia-myalgia syndrome
eosinophilia-pulmonary tuberculosis
  syndrome
eosinophilia with asthma, pulmonary
eosinophilic asthma
eosinophilic disseminated collagen
  disease
eosinophilic endomyocardial disease
eosinophilic endomyocardial
  fibroelastosis
eosinophilic gastroenteritis, primary
eosinophilic granuloma
eosinophilic infiltrate
eosinophilic infiltration
eosinophilic leukemia
eosinophilic lung disease, idiopathic
eosinophilic pleural effusion
eosinophilic pneumonia
  acute
  chronic
  improving
  pertussoid
eosinophilic pustular folliculitis
eosinophil lung syndrome
eosinophils
EP (electrophysiology) study
eparterial bronchus
EPBF (effective pulmonary blood
  flow)
ephelides
epicanthic fold
epicardial attachment
epicardial Doppler echocardiography
epicardial Doppler flow transducer
epicardial electrode
epicardial fat, overlying
epicardial fat pad

epicardial imaging
epicardial implantation
epicardial lead
epicardial pacemaker electrode
epicardial pacemaker lead
epicardial patch cathode
epicardial reflection
epicardial space
epicardial surface
epicardial tension
epicardial vessels, vasorelaxation of
epicarditis
epicardium
epidural anesthesia
epiglottidectomy
epilepsy, laryngeal
epimyocardial rate-sensing lead
epinephrine
epipleural fibrinous exudate
episode
  anginal
  apneic
  hypercyanotic
  intermittent apneic
episode log
episode of crushing chest pain
episodic arousal
episodic bleeding
episodic dyspnea
episodic hypoxemia
epistaxis
epithelial desquamation
epithelioid cells
epithelioid hemangioendothelioma
  benign
  malignant
epithelium
  bronchiolar
  columnar
  cuboidal
  denuded

epithelium *(cont.)*
  pseudostratified columnar
  respiratory
  stratified squamous
E point of cardiac apex pulse
E point on apex cardiogram
E point on echocardiogram
E point to septal separation (EPSS)
Eppendorf catheter
EPS (electrophysiologic study) to
  assess ventricular arrhythmia
Epsilon-aminocaproic acid
EPSS (E point to septal separation)
Epstein-Barr (EB) virus infection
EPTFE (expanded polytetrafluoroethylene) vascular suture
equal in intensity
equalization of pressure
equalized diastolic pressures
equal respiratory excursions
equation
  Bernoulli
  Carter
  continuity
  Fick
  Hagenbach extension of Poiseuille
  Krovetz and Gessner
  Nernst (cardiac action potential,
    resting phase)
  Teichholz
equilibrium, acid-base
equilibrium angiocardiography,
  ambulatory
equilibrium radionuclide angiocardiography
equipment, interventional
equivalent
  angina
  metabolic
  migraine
  ventilation

equivocal exercise test
equivocal finding
equivocal results
equivocal symptoms
equivocal test
ER (emergency room)
eradication of varicose veins
Erb area
Erb limb-girdle dystrophy
Erb point (of heart)
Erdheim cystic medionecrosis
Erdheim cystic necrosis of aorta
Erdheim I syndrome
ergometer
  arm
  bicycle
  Bosch ERG 500
  Collins bicycle
  Siemens-Albis bicycle
ergometry
  arm (stress test)
  bicycle (exercise stress testing)
ergonovine infusion
ergonovine test
Ergos O_2 dual-chamber rate-responsive
  pacemaker
ERI (elective replacement indicator)
erosion
  bronchial
  graft-enteric
  plaque
erosion of bronchi by tuberculous
  lymph nodes
erosion of pulse generator pocket
ERP (effective refractory period)
  atrial
  ventricular
error, sensing
ERT (elective replacement time)
ERV (expiratory reserve volume)
erythema induratum, Bazin

erythema marginatum
erythema migrans
erythema multiforme
erythema multiforme exudativum
erythema nodosum
erythema without induration
erythematosus
    lupus
    systemic lupus (SLE)
erythroblastosis fetalis
erythrocyanosis
erythrocyte autosensitization syndrome
erythrocyte sedimentation rate (ESR)
erythrocyte sodium
erythrocytosis, stress
Erythroflex hydromer-coated central
    venous catheter
erythromelalgia
erythromycin
erythropheresis
erythropoietin
escape beat
escape interval after an Rx delivery
escape mechanism, ventricular
escape of air into lung connective
    tissue
escape pacemaker
escape rhythm
Escherichia coli (*E. coli*) pneumonia
E sign (on x-ray)
ESM (ejection systolic murmur)
Esmarch bandage
Esmarch tourniquet
esophageal adenocarcinoma
esophageal angina
esophageal atresia
esophageal balloon technique
esophageal electrocardiogram
esophageal lead
esophageal obturator airway
esophageal pain

esophageal pill electrode (disposable
    EKG lead encased in a gelatin
    capsule)
esophageal plexus
esophageal spasm mimicking angina
esophageal spasm mimicking
    myocardial infarction
esophageal temperature
esophageal varices
esophageal window
esophagitis, candidal
ESP (end-systolic pressure)
ESP/ESV ratio
ESR (erythrocyte sedimentation rate)
essential brown induration of lung
essential hypertension
essential hyponatremia
essential thrombocytosis
EST (extrastimulus testing)
Estes EKG criteria or score
estimated blood loss (EBL)
ESV (end-systolic volume)
ESVI (end-systolic volume index)
ESWI/ESVI (end-systolic wall stress
    index/end-systolic volume index)
ET (ejection time)
ethacrynic acid
ethanolaminosis
Ethibond suture
Ethicon suture
Ethiflex suture
Ethilon suture
ethmoidal sinusitis
ethmoiditis, Woakes
ethylenediaminetetraacetic acid
    disodium salt
etiology
E to A changes
E to F slope of valve
E to F slope on echocardiogram
ETT (exercise tolerance test)

eucapnic voluntary hyperventilation
eukinesis
eupnea, eupneic
euthyroid sick syndrome
euvolemic
evacuate air from the aorta
evacuated, air was
evacuation of offending pericardial
 fluid
evacuator container
evaluation of deep veins for patency
 and valvular reflux
evanescent chest pain
evanescent nature
Evans syndrome
even murmur
event
 adverse
 atrial sensed (As)
 cardinal
 embolic
 inciting
 ischemic
 morbid
 precipitating
 untoward
 ventricular sensed
event counter
event marker
eventration (peaking)
event recorder
eversion endarterectomy, Connolly
eversion technique
everting mattress sutures
everting sutures
evolution of EKG
evolutionary changes on EKG
Ewart sign
exacerbation, acute
exacerbation of chronic congestive
 heart failure

exaggerated S4
examination
 cardiac
 Doppler venous
 histologic
 lower extremity
 peripheral vascular
 physical
 pulmonary
exanthematous changes of extremities
exanthematous disease
excavatum, pectus
excellent prognosis
excess
 base
 catechol
 mineralocorticoid
 thyroid hormone
excessive bleeding
excessive salt intake
exchange
 air
 catheter
 guide wire
excimer (from "excited dimer") laser
excision(al) biopsy
excitation
 anomalous atrioventricular
 atrioventricular
 supernormal
excitation-contraction coupling
exciting factor
excrescences, Lambl
excretory intravenous pyelography
excruciating pain
excursion, excursions
 chest
 decreased valve
 equal respiratory
 full respiratory
 jugular venous

excursion *(cont.)*
  limited respiratory
  respiratory
  venous
exercise, exercises
  active
  active assisted
  active resistive
  aerobic
  breathing
  corrective
  deep-breathing
  endurance
  graduated
  injection at peak
  isometric
  isometric handgrip
  isotonic
  low-level
  peak
  relaxation
  rehabilitation
  static
  submaximal
  symptom-limited
  therapeutic
exercise capacity
  decreased
  impaired
  increased
exercise challenge
exercise duration (in minutes)
exercise echocardiography
exercise electrocardiography
exercise endpoint
exercise factor
exercise images
exercise index
exercise-induced angina pectoris
exercise-induced asthma
exercise-induced bronchoconstriction

exercise-induced left ventricular
  dysfunction
exercise-induced myocardial ischemia
exercise-inducible transient myocardial
  ischemia
exercise intolerance
exercise load (kpm/min)
exercise oximetry
exercise regimen
exercise restriction
exercise strain gauge venous
  plethysmography
exercise stress test, positive
exercise stress testing protocol (see
  protocol)
exercise stress-redistribution
  scintigraphy
exercise testing protocol (see *protocol*)
exercise thallium-201 stress test
exercise thallium-201 tomography
exercise therapy
exercise tolerance
  decreased
  increased
  improving
exercise tolerance test (ETT), graded
exertional angina
exertional capacity
exertional chest pain
exertional dyspnea
exertional pain
exertional syncope
exertion, pain precipitated by
exhalation, forced
exhaling into the atmosphere
exit heart block, sinoatrial
exogenous glucocorticoid
exogenous invasion
exogenous mineralocorticoid
exogenous pneumonia
Exosurf

expandable access catheter (EAC)
expanded polytetrafluoroethylene
(ePTFE) vascular graft
expanded reinforced polytetrafluoroethylene (ER-PTFE) vascular graft
expanders, plasma
expanding valvotome
expansile aortic segment
expansion
complete stent
emphysematous
lung
rapid fluid
stent
expansion of upper lobe, emphysematous
expectorant drugs
expectorate (verb)
expectoration of blood
expectoration of bloody sputum
expeditious
expiration
forced
grunting
prolonged
sighing
tidal
whining
expiratory attenuation
expiratory dyspnea
expiratory flow limitation
expiratory grunting
expiratory phase
expiratory rales
expiratory reserve volume (ERV)
expiratory resistance
expiratory rhonchi, coarse sibilant
expiratory slowing
expiratory wheezes
expiratory whining
expired gas

explanted
exponential simultaneous waveforms,
truncated
exposure
ambient ozone
asbestos
environmental
environmental tobacco
smoking
extraperitoneal
extrathoracic
in utero
intraperitoneal
passive smoking
second-hand smoke
exposure to cold, pain precipitated by
exposure to irritants
exposure to isocyanate
Express over-the-wire balloon catheter
Express PTCA catheter
exquisite detail
exquisite pain
exsanguinate, exsanguinated
exsanguinating hemorrhage into
pleural space
exsanguination
fatal
massive
partial
extended collection device
extension
basal
intracavitary (of tumor)
hilar
medial
parenchymal
parietal
extension tubing
extensive dissection
external adhesive patch electrode
external cardiac cooling

external cardiac massage
external carotid artery
external carotid steal syndrome
external defibrillation
external iliac stenosis
external jugular veins
external jugular venous cannula
external penetrating wound of lung
extirpation of saphenous vein
extirpation of valve
extra-adrenal pheochromocytoma
extracardiac anomalies
extracardiac collateral circulation
extracardiac conduit
extracardiac disease
extracardiac right-to-left shunt
extracardiac systolic arterial murmur
extracavitary-infected graft
extracavitary prosthetic arterial graft
extracellular fluid
extracellular fluid volume
extracorporeal carbon dioxide (CO_2)
    removal technique
extracorporeal circulation
extracorporeal circulation using heart-
    lung machine
extracorporeal circulatory support
extracorporeal hepatic assistance
extracorporeal membrane oxygenation
    (ECMO)
extracorporeal ultrafiltration
extracranial carotid artery athero-
    sclerosis
extracranial carotid system
extracranial cerebral circulation
extracranial cerebral system
extracranial-intracranial bypass
extract, lyophilized allergen
extraction atherectomy device
extraction catheter atherectomy,
    transcutaneous

extraction catheter, transluminal
extraction endarterectomy, transaortic
Extractor three-lumen retrieval balloon
extradural vertebral plexus of veins
extraluminal endarterectomy
extrapericardial dissection
extrapericardial patch placement
extraperitoneal exposure
extrapleural drainage
extrapleural hemorrhage
extrapolate
extrapolation
extrapulmonary disease
extrapulmonary tuberculosis
extrapyramidal disease
extraskeletal osteosarcoma of the heart
extrastimulation
extrastimulus (pl. extrastimuli)
    critically timed
    double
    multiple
    paired
    premature
    single
    triple
extrastimulus pacing
extrastimulus technique
extrastimulus testing (EST)
extrasystole
    atrial
    atrioventricular (AV)
    infranodal
    interpolated
    junctional
    nodal
    nonpropagated junctional
    premature ventricular
    retrograde
    ventricular
extrasystolic arrhythmia
extrathoracic exposure

extrathoracic obstruction
extravasated blood
extravasated red blood cells
extravasation of blood
extravasation of erythrocytes into
   alveoli
extravasation of fluid in alveoli
extravasation of intravascular contents,
   secondary
extravascular granulomas
extravascular mass
extravascular pressure
extremities
   blue
   cold
   cyanotic
   mottled
   numb
   tingling
extrinsic allergic alveolitis
extrinsic asthma
extrinsic compression
extrinsic compression of trachea

extrinsic lesion
extrinsic sick sinus syndrome
extubate, extubated
extubation
exuberant atheroma formation
exudate
   bloody
   endobronchial
   epipleural fibrinous
   fibrinous
   mucopurulent
   retinal
   sanguineous
   serous
   sticky
   tenacious bronchial
exudation of fibrin-rich fluid
exudative consolidation
exudative effusion
exudative pericardial fluid
exudative pleurisy
exudative tuberculosis
exude

F, f

Fab fragment, antimyosin
Fabry disease
face, hypercalcemic
face mask CPAP (continuous positive
  airway pressure)
facial freckling, myxoma syndrome
  with
facies
  asymmetric crying
  elfin
  mitral
  mitrotricuspid
  moon
facies anterior cordis
facies costalis pulmonis
facies diaphragmatica cordis
facies diaphragmatica pulmonis
facies dolorosa
facies inferior cordis
facies interlobares pulmonis
facies mediastinalis pulmonis
facies sternocostalis cordis
facilitate
faciobrachial symptoms
factitial
factitious symptoms

factor, factors (see also *coagulation
  factors of blood*)
antihemophilic blood coagulation
atrial natriuretic (ANF)
blood coagulation
cardiac risk (see *cardiac risk*)
Christmas blood coagulation
circular shape
coagulation
cobra venom (for myocardial
  ischemia)
endothelium-derived contracting
endothelium-derived relaxing
  (EDRF)
endothelium-relaxing
exciting
exercise
Hageman
histamine-releasing
inciting
myocardial depressant
platelet activating
platelet-derived growth
precipitating
predisposing
rheumatoid arthritis

factor *(cont.)*
  risk
    tumor necrosis, alpha (TNFa)
    von Willebrand (also Willebrand)
    von Willebrand blood coagulation
  factor IV platelet
  factor IX deficiency
  factor III platelet deficiency syndrome
Fahr-Volhard syndrome
FAI (functional aerobic impairment)
failure
  acute congestive
  acute heart
  acute renal
  acute ventilatory
  backward heart
  battery
  biventricular heart
  cardiac
  chronic renal
  chronic respiratory
  circulatory
  compensated congestive heart
  congestive heart (CHF)
  decompensated congestive heart
  diastolic heart
  donor heart
  end-stage congestive heart
  end-stage liver
  fetal heart
  forward heart
  heart
  heart forward
  heart power
  high-output cardiac
  high-output circulatory
  high-output heart
  hypoxemic respiratory
  intrauterine cardiac
  intrauterine heart
  left heart

failure *(cont.)*
  left ventricular
  left-sided congestive heart
  low-output heart
  pacemaker battery
  peripheral circulatory
  postoperative renal
  primary bioprosthetic valve
  pulmonary
  pump
  refractory congestive heart
  refractory heart
  respiratory
  right heart
  right-sided congestive heart
  right ventricular
  systolic heart
  ventilatory
failure of match test at 3 inches
failure to capture
failure to sense
faint breath sounds
faint, common
faint friction rub
fainting spell
Fallot disease
Fallot pentalogy (tetralogy of Fallot
  plus atrial septal defect)
Fallot syndrome
Fallot tetralogy
Fallot trilogy in congenital cyanotic
  heart disease
false A_2
false aneurysm, late
false bruit
false bundle-branch block
false channel
false croup
false cyanosis
false emphysema
false lumen

false-positive test result
false sac
familial amyloidosis
familial annuloaortic ectasia
familial aortic dissection
familial arterial fibromuscular
   dysplasia
familial arteriopathy
familial atresia
familial cardiomegaly
familial cardiomyopathy
familial chylomicronemia
familial dysautonomia
familial dysbetalipoproteinemia
familial elevated triglycerides
familial endocardial fibroelastosis
familial fibromuscular dysplasia of
   arteries
familial genetic dyslipidemia
familial hyperbetalipoproteinemia
familial hypercholesterolemia
familial hyperchylomicronemia
familial hyperlipidemia
familial intracranial hemangioma
familial intracranial hemorrhage
familial myxoma of the heart
familial pulmonary hypertension
familial varicose veins
family history of heart disease
family history of hypertension
family history of myocardial infarction
Family Index of Life Events (FILE)
fan-shaped view
Fanconi-Hegglin syndrome
FAP (femoral artery pressure)
far field
farmer's lung
fascia (pl. fasciae)
   anterior
   enveloping
   extrapleural

fascia (cont.)
   Gerota
   obturator
   pectoralis
   posterior
   prepectoral
   superficial
   thoracic
fascicles
fascicular bundles
fascicular heart block
fascicular heartbeat
fasciculations
fasciculoventricular bypass fiber
fasciculoventricular bypass tracts
fasciotomy, anterior compartment
fashion
   antegrade
   retrograde
FAST (flow-assisted, short-term)
FAST balloon catheter
fast-flow lesions
fast-flow malformation
fast-flow vascular anomaly
Fast-Pass lead pacemaker
fast-pathway conduction
fat
   animal (in diet)
   epicardial
   mediastinal
   monounsaturated
   overlying epicardial
   polyunsaturated
   preperitoneal
   properitoneal
   saturated
   unsaturated
fatal exsanguination
fat embolism syndrome (FES)
fatigability, easy
fatigue, progressively severe

fat removed from anterior surface of
   pericardium
fat-suppressed breathhold technique
fatty acids
fatty bone marrow
fatty degeneration
fatty streak atherosclerosis
Favaloro-Morse rib spreader
Favaloro sternal retractor
favorable prognosis
FBN1 gene
FBN2 gene
FDG (fluorodeoxyglucose)
FDP (fibrin degradation products)
fear of impending death (or doom)
   from angina
feasible alternatives
feature, conspicuous
febrile agglutinins
$FeCO_2$ (fraction of expired CO_2)
Federici sign
feeders
feeder veins
feeding mean arterial pressure
   (FMAP)
feeling of impending doom prior to
   myocardial infarction
feet, cold
$FEF_{25-75\%}$ (forced midexpiratory flow)
Feigenbaum echocardiogram
F-18 2-deoxyglucose uptake on PET
   scan
Feldaker syndrome
felt bolster, Teflon
felt strip
feminine aorta, small
femoral above-knee popliteal bypass
femoral approach for cardiac catheterization
femoral artery cutdown
femoral artery pressure

femoral artery, superficial
femoral-femoral bypass graft
femoral-femoral crossover
femoral-peroneal in situ vein bypass
   graft
femoral-popliteal bypass surgery
femoral-popliteal Gore-Tex graft
femoral pulse
femoral thrombophlebitis
femoral vein percutaneous insertion
femoral vein, superficial
femoral venoarterial bypass
femoral venous approach
femoris, profunda
femoroaxillary bypass
femorodistal bypass
femorodistal popliteal bypass graft
femorofemoral approach
femorofemoral bypass
femorofemoral subcutaneous suprapubic graft
femorofemoropopliteal
femoroperoneal bypass graft
femoropopliteal atheromatous stenosis
femoropopliteal bypass surgery
femoropopliteal thrombosis
femoropopliteal vein graft
femorotibial bypass graft
fem-pop (slang for femoral-popliteal)
   bypass
fenestra (pl. fenestrae)
fenestrated Fontan procedure
fenestration
   aortopulmonary
   apical
   cusp
   interchordal space
fenestration of dissecting aneurysm
Ferguson forceps
ferruginous bodies
ferrule (on pacemaker wires)

FES (fat embolism syndrome)
fetal bradycardia
fetal cardiac anomalies
fetal cardiac arrhythmia
fetal echocardiography in utero
fetal heart failure
fetal hydrops (hydrops fetalis)
  nonimmune
  nonimmunological
fetal ultrasonography
fetal umbilical vein injection under
  sonographic guidance
fetalis, hydrops
fetid bronchitis
FEV (forced expiratory volume)
FEV_1 (forced expiratory volume in
  1 second)
FEV_1/FVC (forced vital capacity)
  ratio
FEV_3 (forced expiratory volume in
  3 seconds)
FEV_t (forced expiratory volume,
  timed)
fever
  acute rheumatic (ARF)
  Animal House (organic dust
    syndrome)
  atropine
  brassfounder's
  cotton-mill
  desert
  drug
  foundryman's
  hay
  hectic
  histamine
  low-grade
  mahogany
  metal fume
  Monday
  parrot

fever (cont.)
  perennial
  pneumonic lung
  polymer fume
  Pontiac
  Q
  rheumatic
  Rocky Mountain spotted
  rose
  San Joaquin Valley
  spiking
  threshing
  valley
fever and chills
fevers, chills, and sweats
FFA (free fatty acid) scintigraphy,
  labeled
FFP (fresh frozen plasma)
FHC (familial hypertrophic cardiomyopathy)
fiber, fibers
  accelerating
  atrio-Hisian; atriohisian
  Brechenmacher
  bulbospiral
  bystander
  cardiac accelerator
  cardiac depressor
  cardiac muscle
  cardiac pressor
  collagenous
  depressor
  dietary
  fasciculoventricular bypass
  fasciculoventricular Mahaim
  impulse conducting
  intercostal bundle
  James
  Kent
  Mahaim
  Mahaim and James

fiber *(cont.)*
  muscle
  nodoventricular bypass
  Purkinje
fiberbronchoscope, -scopy
fiberoptic angioscopy
fiberoptic bronchoplasty
fiberoptic bronchoscope, -scopy
fiber-shortening velocity (VCF)
fibrillate
fibrillating heart, hypothermic
fibrillation
  atrial (AF)
  auricular
  idiopathic ventricular
  reversible ventricular
  ventricular (VF)
fibrillation-flutter
fibrillation rhythm
fibrillator, electric
fibrillator source
fibrillatory impulse
fibrillin gene mutation
fibrin bodies of pleura
fibrin clot
fibrin degradation products (FDP)
fibrin glue, autologous
fibrin glue sealant
fibrinogen
  radiolabeled
  technetium 99m-labeled
fibrinogen degradation
fibrinogen-fibrin conversion syndrome
fibrinoid degeneration
fibrinoid necrosis
fibrinolysis
  deficient
  physiologic
fibrinolysis of thrombi
fibrinolytic system
fibrinolytic therapy

fibrinopeptide A
fibrinopurulent pleurisy
fibrinous pleurisy
fibrinous bronchitis
fibrinous chorditis
fibrinous exudate
fibrinous pericarditis
fibrinous pleurisy
fibrinous pleuritis
fibrinous split products
fibrin platelet emboli
fibrin products
fibrin-rich exudate
fibrin-rich thrombus
fibrin split products
fibrin-stabilizing blood coagulation
  factor
fibrocalcific cusps
fibroelastoma of heart valve
fibroelastoma, papillary
fibroelastosis
  adult
  endocardial
  familial endocardial
  primary endocardial
  secondary endocardial
  subendocardial
fibrofatty yellow plaque
fibrogenic dust disease
fibroid lung
fibroid myocarditis
fibroma of heart
fibromuscular dysplasia, familial
  arterial
fibromuscular ridge
fibronectin concentration
fibroplasia
  intimal
  medial
fibrosa, intervalvular
fibrosarcoma of heart

fibrosclerotic
fibroserous pericardial sac
fibrosi cordis, annuli
fibrosiderosis
fibrosing alveolitis associated with
    systemic sclerosis
fibrosing lung diseases
fibrosis
    African endomyocardial
    asbestos-induced pleural
    bauxite (of lung)
    bundle branch
    confluent
    cystic
    Davies endocardial
    Davies endomyocardial
    diatomite
    diffuse interstitial pulmonary
        (DIPF)
    diffuse pulmonary
    endocardial
    endomyocardial (EMF)
    graphite
    His-Purkinje system
    idiopathic pulmonary (IPF)
    interstitial
    interstitial diffuse pulmonary
    interstitial prematurity
    interstitial pulmonary
    intra-alveolar
    mediastinal idiopathic
    myocardial
    nodal
    nonnodular
    perialveolar
    perianeurysmal retroperitoneal
    periaortic
    peribronchial
    perielectrode
    perivascular
    plexiform

fibrosis *(cont.)*
    postinflammatory pulmonary
    postradiation
    progressive interstitial pulmonary
    pulmonary interstitial idiopathic
    pulmonary vein
    radiation
    retroperitoneal
    rheumatic
    tropical endomyocardial
fibrosis and inflammation, periaortic
fibrosis of pericardium
fibrosum, pericardium
fibrotic distortion of valve
fibrotic honeycombing
fibrotic mitral valve
fibrotic nodules
fibrotic plaques
fibrotic scarred media
fibrous cord
fibrous dysplasia
fibrous hyperplasia
fibrous mediastinitis
fibrous pericarditis
fibrous pericardium
fibrous plaque atherosclerosis
fibrous pleural adhesions
fibrous ring
fibrous skeleton of heart
fibrous tab
fibrous trigone, left
Fick cardiac output index
Fick cardiac output method
    assumed
    direct
Fick equation or formula
Fick method for calculating cardiac
    output
Fick oxygen method of cardiac output
Fick principle of cardiac output
Fiedler myocarditis

Fiedler syndrome
field
    bloodless
    collapsed lung
    far
    high-power
    low-power
    lung
    near
    rf (radio frequency)
    surgical
field-dependent
fifth intercostal space
fifth left interspace
fifth rib
figure-3 sign
figure-of-8 suture
filiform pulse
filipuncture
fillet the wound tract open
filling
    augmented
    capillary
    decreased left ventricular
    left atrial
    left ventricular
    passive
    period of rapid ventricular
    period of reduced ventricular
    period of ventricular
    rapid (RF)
    retrograde
    right atrial
    right ventricular
    ventricular
filling defect (on x-ray)
filling of right ventricle, augmented
filling phase, rapid
filling pressure
filling rate, peak
films, manual subtraction

filter
    bird's nest percutaneous IVC
    bird's nest vena caval
    caval
    Gianturco-Roehm bird's nest vena
      caval
    Greenfield vena caval
    Kimray-Greenfield caval
    Mobin-Uddin umbrella
    Mobin-Uddin vena caval
    percutaneous inferior vena cava
      (IVC)
    prophylactic IVC
    Simon nitinol percutaneous IVC
    umbrella
    Venatech percutaneous IVC
filtration rate, reduced glomerular
final rapid repolarization
Finapres blood pressure monitor
finding, findings
    auscultatory
    cardinal
    characteristic
    concomitant
    equivocal
    no discernible
    ominous
    pathognomonic
    salient physical
    scanty
    spurious
fine crackles
fine crepitant rales
fine needle biopsy
fine rales
fine-speckled appearance
fine wheezes
Finesse cardiac device
Finesse large-lumen guiding catheter
finger clubbing
finger cuff

finger dissection divides costal
   attachments of diaphragm
finger fracture dissection
fingertip sign
fingerlike projection
finned pacemaker lead
Finochietto forceps
Finochietto retractor
Finochietto rib spreader
Finochietto thoracic scissors
FiO$_2$ (forced inspiratory oxygen)
firing of ectopic atrial focus
firm mass
first branch of artery
first component
first-degree atrioventricular (AV)
   heart block
first diagonal branch
first intercostal space
first obtuse marginal artery
first order chordae
first-pass imaging
first-pass radionuclide exercise angiocardiography
first-pass study
first septal perforator
first-stage Norwood operation
Fischer sign
Fisher exact test
fish-flesh appearance
fishhook lead
fishmeal worker's lung
fishmouth configuration of mitral
   valve
fishmouth stenosis
Fisoneb nebulizer
Fissinger-Rendu syndrome
fissure
   horizontal
   lung
   oblique

fist palpation
fistula
   aortic sinus
   aortic sinus to right ventricle
   aortocaval
   aortoenteric
   aorta-left ventricular
   aortopulmonary
   aorta-right ventricular
   arteriovenous (AVF)
   AV (arteriovenous)
   Brescio-Cimino AV
   bronchocutaneous
   bronchopleural
   cameral
   carotid artery-cavernous sinus
   carotid cavernous
   cerebral arteriovenous
   chylous
   coil closure of coronary artery
   congenital pulmonary
   coronary
   coronary arteriosystemic
   coronary arteriovenous
   coronary artery cameral
   coronary artery to right ventricular
   coronary artery-pulmonary artery
   coronary-cameral
   coronary-pulmonary
   graft-enteric
   hepatic arteriovenous
   hepatopleural
   intrapulmonary arteriovenous
   mediastinal
   microvenoarteriolar
   paraprosthetic-enteric
   persistent bronchopleural
   pleural
   pulmonary arteriovenous
   radial artery to cephalic vein
   thoracic

fistula *(cont.)*
 tracheobronchial
 tracheoesophageal
fistulectomy
 bronchocutaneous
 bronchopleuromediastinal
 bronchovisceral
 laryngeal
 laryngotracheal
 thoracicoabdominal
 thoracicogastric
 thoracicointestinal
 tracheoesophageal
Fitzgerald aortic aneurysm forceps
FIVC (forced inspiratory vital
 capacity)
five-second breathhold
fixed airway obstruction
fixed aortic ejection click
fixed area of narrowing in large airway
fixed defect
fixed intracavitary filling defect
fixed mass
fixed pulmonary valvular resistance
fixed-rate pacing
fixed rate permanent pacemaker
fixed splitting of heart sound
FL4 guide
flabby heart
Flack node
Flack sinoatrial node
flail chest
flail mitral leaflet
flail mitral valve
flank incision
flap
 dissection
 Eloesser
 intimal
 muscle
 necrotic

flap *(cont.)*
 pedicle
 pericardial
 pleural
 scimitar-shaped
 Waldenhausen subclavian
flaplike valves
flap valve ventricular septal defect
flaring of the alae nasi
FLASH (fast low-angle shot) cardiac
 MRI study
flashlamp-pulsed dye laser
flat chest
flat-hand test
flat lined (verb)
flat neck veins
flat P wave
flat percussion note
flat ST segment depression
flattened T waves
flattening of chest wall
flattening of ST segment
flax-dresser's disease
Fleischner sign
Fletcher coagulation factor
Flexguard tip catheter
Flexguide intubation guide
Flex guide wire
flexibility
flexible angioscope
flexible cardiac valve
flexible fiberoptic bronchoscopy
flexible J guide wire
flexible steerable guide wire
flexible suction cannula
Flexon steel suture
FL4 guide
flip-flop of heart
flip-flop sensation in chest
flip, LDH_1
flipped LDH

flipped LD_1/LD_2 ratio
flipped T wave
floating leaflets
flopping in chest
floppy aortic valve
floppy mitral valve syndrome
floppy tongue
floppy valves
floppy valve syndrome
flora
   multiple unidentified respiratory
     (MURF)
   normal
Florence flask appearance
Flo-Rester vessel occluder
florid cardiac tamponade
florid edema
florid Hantavirus pulmonary syndrome
florid Marfan syndrome
flotation catheter
flow
   antegrade
   antegrade blood
   antegrade diastolic
   aortic (AF)
   backward
   blood
   cerebral blood (CBF)
   chronic reserve
   collateral
   collateral blood
   compromised
   coronary blood
   coronary reserve (CRF)
   dampened pulsatile
   decreased cerebral blood
   effective pulmonary blood (EPBF)
   effective pulmonic
   forward
   Ganz method for coronary sinus
   great cardiac vein (GCVF)

flow *(cont.)*
   high velocity
   intercoronary collateral
   laminar
   left-to-right
   maximum midexpiratory
   midexpiratory tidal
   mitral valve
   myocardial blood (MBF)
   peak
   peak expiratory (PEF)
   peak tidal expiratory flow
   pulmonary blood (PBF)
   pulmonic output
   pulmonic versus systemic
   redistribution of pulmonary
     vascular
   regional myocardial blood
   regurgitant
   regurgitant systolic
   restoration of
   retrograde
   retrograde systolic
   reversed vertebral blood (RVBF)
   sluggish
   systemic blood (SBF)
   systemic output
   tissue
   total cerebral blood (TCBF)
   transmitral
   tricuspid valve
   turbulent blood
   turbulent intraluminal
flow-compromising lesion
flow-directed catheter
flow-guided Inoue balloon
flow-limited expiration
flow mapping technique
flowmeter
   blood
   Doppler

flowmeter *(cont.)*
  Narcomatic
  Parks 800 bidirectional Doppler
  pulsed Doppler
  Statham electromagnetic
flow rates, rapid inspiratory
flow redistribution
Flowtron DVT (deep venous
  thrombosis) pump system
Flowtron intermittent compression
  garment
flow velocity profile
flow velocity signals
flow void
flow-volume curve
flow-volume loop (in spirometry
  reports)
flow-volume, tidal inspiratory
flu exposure
Fluckiger syndrome
fluctuant
fluffy infiltrate
fluid
  crystalloid
  dependent edema
  evacuation of offending pericardial
  extracellular
  exudative pericardial
  Fluosol-DA 20% oxygen-transport
  hemorrhagic
  increased interstitial
  interstitial
  parenteral
  pericardial
  pleural
  serosanguineous
  straw-colored
  subpulmonic
  tissue
  transudative pericardial
  turbid

fluid accumulation, dependent extracellular
fluid accumulation in tissues
fluid balance
fluid challenge
fluid collection, loculated
fluid expansion, rapid
fluid extravasation
fluid-filled mass
fluid flow between capillaries and
  interstitial tissue
fluidification
fluid intake, restricted
fluid level
fluid overload
fluid resorption
fluid restriction
fluid resuscitation
fluid retention
fluid volume, extracellular
fluid volume, increased extracellular
flu-like illness
flu-like symptoms
fluorescein angiography
fluorescence spectroscopy
fluorodeoxyglucose (FDG) radioactive
  tracer
fluorography, spot-film
fluoroscope, fluoroscopy
  biplane
  C-arm digital
  chest
fluoroscopic control, advanced under
fluoroscopic guidance
fluoroscopic road-mapping technique
  in angioplastic vascular procedures
Fluosol (artificial blood)
Fluosol oxygen transport medium and
  plasma expander
Fluosol-DA 20% oxygen-transport
  fluid

flush
    bright red
    circumoral
    heparinized saline
    malar
flush aortogram
flushed
flush method of taking blood pressure
    in infants
flushing of catheter
flutter
    atrial (AFl)
    auricular
    coarse atrial
    impure
    mediastinal
    pure
    ventricular
flutter-fibrillation
fluttering of valvular leaflet
fluttering sensation
flu vaccine
fluximetry
fluxionary hyperemia
FMAP (feeding mean arterial
    pressure)
foam embolus
foamy appearance of exudate
foamy exudate in the air spaces
foamy lipoid material
focal changes
focal dilatations of air spaces
focal-dust emphysema
focal eccentric stenosis
focal endocardial hemorrhage
focal interstitial infiltrate
focal intimal thickening
focal moderate rejection
focal myocyte damage
focal neurologic signs
focal perivascular infiltrate

focal stenosis
focal wall motion abnormality
focus, foci
    Assmann
    atrial
    ectopic
    junctional
    radiolucent
    Simon
Foerster forceps
Fogarty adherent clot catheter
Fogarty arterial embolectomy catheter
Fogarty balloon catheter
Fogarty balloon catheterization
Fogarty-Chin clamp
Fogarty-Chin extrusion balloon
    catheter
Fogarty embolectomy, transfemoral
Fogarty forceps
Fogarty HydroGrip clamp
Fogarty occlusion catheter
Fogarty venous thrombectomy
    catheter
Foix-Alajouanine syndrome
fold
    epicanthic
    pericardial
    Rindfleisch
    ventriculoinfundibular
folic acid deficiency anemia
fomites
Fontan anastomosis of atrial
    appendage to pulmonary artery
Fontan-Kreutzer repair, modified
Fontan modification of Norwood
    procedure for hypoplastic left-sided
    heart syndrome
Fontan operation for tricuspid atresia
    and pulmonary stenosis
Fontan operation, takedown of
Fontan repair

foot cradle
foramen of Morgagni
foramen ovale
foramen ovale, patent
foramen secundum
Forbes disease
force
   contractile
   lateral anterior
   reciprocal
   reserve
   rest
   stroke
Force balloon dilatation catheter
forced exhalation
forced expiratory volume (FEV)
forced expiratory volume in 1 second
   (FEV$_1$)
forced expiratory volume in 3 seconds
   (FEV$_3$)
forced inspiratory oxygen (FiO$_2$)
forced midexpiratory flow
   (FEF$_{25-75\%}$)
forced vital capacity (FVC)
force-frequency relation
forceful heartbeat
forcefully wedged
forceful parasternal motion
force-length relation
force of contraction
forceps
   Adson
   alligator
   Allis
   artery
   Babcock
   Bailey aortic valve cutting
   Bengolea artery
   biopsy
   biopsy cup
   Bloodwell

forceps *(cont.)*
   blunt
   Boettcher artery
   bottle nose
   bronchus
   Brown Adson
   Brunschwig artery
   bulldog
   Carmalt artery
   cone nose
   Cooley-Baumgarten aortic
   Cooley vascular
   Crile
   curved Kelly
   curved mosquito
   Cushing
   Dale
   Davis
   Debakey
   DeBakey arterial
   DeBakey Autraugrip
   DeBakey-Diethrich vascular
   DeBakey dissecting
   DeBakey-Semb
   DeBakey tissue
   DeBakey vascular
   Doyen
   duckbill
   Duval-Crile lung
   Duval lung
   Effler-Groves
   Ferguson
   Finochietto
   Fitzgerald aortic aneurysm
   Foerster
   Fogarty
   Foss
   Gemini thoracic
   Gerald
   Gerbode
   grasping

forceps *(cont.)*
   Halsted
   Harrington-Mixter thoracic
   Harrington thoracic
   Hayes Martin
   Heiss artery
   hemoclip-applying
   hemostatic
   Hendrin
   Hopkins aortic
   jeweler's
   Johns Hopkins
   Johnson thoracic
   Jones IMA
   Julian thoracic
   Karp aortic punch
   Kocher
   Koeberlé
   Lahey thoracic
   Lees artery
   Lejeune thoracic
   Lillehei valve
   Mayo Péan
   Meeker
   micro
   Mixter
   mosquito
   NIH mitral valve
   Ochsner
   O'Shaughnessy artery
   Overholt thoracic
   Péan
   Pennington
   Phaneuf artery
   Potts bronchus
   Potts bulldog
   Potts-Smith tissue
   Potts thumb
   Potts vascular
   Price-Thomas bronchial
   Randall stone

forceps *(cont.)*
   Rochester-Mixter artery
   Ruel
   Rumel thoracic
   Russian tissue
   Samuels
   Sarot artery
   Selman vessel
   Semb
   Singley
   Snowden-Pencer
   sponge
   spoon
   straight biopsy cup
   straight-end cup
   Thomas Allis
   thumb
   tissue
   tonsillar
   toothed Adson tissue
   torsion
   Tuttle thoracic
   up-biting biopsy cup
   up-biting cup
   Westphal
   Yasargil artery
force-velocity relation
forcipressure
foreign-body aspiration
foreign body in respiratory
   passages
foreign body reaction
foreign body upper airway obstruction
foreshortening, annular
forestall
form, wave
format
   hemodynamic
   slice
   three-dimensional
   two-dimensional

formation
   eddy
   exuberant atheroma
   honeycomb
   thrombus
formation of blood clots within leg
   veins
forme fruste (pl. formes frustes)
forme tardive
formidable risk
formula (see also *equation*, *method*)
   Bazett
   Boyd
   Cannon
   Fick
   Ganz coronary sinus flow
   Gorlin
   Gorlin valve area
   Hakki
   Hamilton-Stewart
   Yeager
Forney syndrome
Forrester syndrome
Forrester Therapeutic Class
40 joule rescue shock
45° position
forward failure
forward flow
forward flow of velocity
forward heart failure
forward triangle method
forward velocity (on Doppler)
fossa
   antecubital
   cardiac
   oval (of heart)
   popliteal
fossa ovalis
fossa ovalis cordis
fossae ovalis, limbus
Foss forceps

foul-tasting sputum
four-chamber apical view
four-chamber plane on echocardiography
Four Corners virus
Fourier analysis of electrocardiogram
Fourier transform
fourth intercostal space
fourth left interspace
foveated chest
Fowler position
Fox green dye
F point of cardiac apex pulse
fraction (see also *ejection fraction*)
   beta lipoprotein
   blood plasma
   depressed ejection
   ejection
   MB
   plasma
   regurgitant
fractional area
fractional inspired oxygen concentration)
fractional myocardial shortening
fractional shortening (of left ventricle)
fraction of expired carbon dioxide
   ($FeCO_2$)
fracture
   annular
   laryngeal
   lead
   pacing lead
   plaque
fractured ribs
fracturing, plaque
fragility, capillary hereditary
fragmentation
fragments, Fab
Framingham criteria for heart failure
Framingham data

frank blood
Frank capillary toxicosis
frank cyanosis from hypoxemia
frank edema
Frank EKG lead system placement
frank hemorrhage
Frank lead
frank pulmonary edema
frank rigors
Frank sign
Frank-Starling law of the heart
Frank-Starling mechanism or principle
Frank-Starling relationship
Frank vectorcardiogram (VCG)
Frank XYZ orthogonal lead system
Fräntzel murmur (Fraentzel)
frappage
Frater stitch or suture
fraught with error
fraying of the edges
Frazier suction tip or tube
FRC (functional residual capacity)
freckling, myxoma syndrome with
    facial
Fredrickson and Lees classification of
    hyperlipoproteinemia (type I-V)
free air passage
free air under the diaphragm
free end of electrode
free-floating electrode
freehand aortic valve homograft
free induction decay
freeing up of adhesions
freely movable mass
free pericardial space
Freer elevator
free tie
free wall
    posterior
    ventricular
free wall tract

fremitus
    bronchial
    friction
    pectoral
    pericardial
    pleural
    rhonchal
    tactile
    tussive
    vocal (VF)
French 5 angiographic catheter
French MBIH catheter
French scale for caliber of catheter
frequency
    angina with recent increase in
    resonant
    respiratory
frequency analysis of Doppler signal
frequent sneezing
frequent ventricular ectopy
fresh frozen plasma (FFP)
fresh frozen plasma infusion
Freund anomaly
FR4 guiding catheter
friability
friable ductus
friable lesion
friable mass
friable mucosa
friable thickened degenerated intima
friable tumor
friable vegetations
friable wall
friction between pleural and
    pericardial surfaces
friction fremitus
friction rub
    coarse
    creaking
    faint
    grating

friction rub*(cont.)*
  harsh
  loud
  pericardial
  pleural
  scratchy
  shuffling
  soft
Friedel Pick syndrome
Friedländer (Friedlaender)
Friedländer bacillus
Friedländer disease
Friedländer pneumonia
Friedländer endarteritis obliterans
  disease
Friedreich ataxia
Friedreich ataxic cardiomyopathy
Friedreich phenomenon
Friedreich sign
Frimodt-Moller syndrome
frog breathing
frond-like appearance
frontal plane loop
frontal plane on EKG
frontotemporal muscle
frothy fluid
frothy mixture
frothy sputum
Frouin, quadrangulation of
Frouin technique
FRP (functional refractory period)
  atrial
  ventricular
FSV (forward stroke volume)
fucosidosis
fugax, amaurosis
fulcrum, left ventricular
fulguration during electrophysiologic
  study
fulguration, endocavitary
full-blown cardiac tamponade

fullness, periorbital
full pause
full respiratory excursions
full-thickness button of aortic wall
full-thickness Carrel button
full-thickness infarction of ventricular
  septum
full-volume loop spirometry
fully implanted ventricular assist device
fulminant, acute eosinophilic
  (pneumonia-like syndrome)
fulminant course of disease
fulminant pulmonary edema
fulminant tuberculosis
fumes
  metal
  polytetrafluoroethylene
  Teflon-fluon
  toxic
function
  compromised ventricular
  depressed right ventricular
    contractile
  exercise LV
  global left ventricular
  global systolic left ventricular
  global ventricular
  left atrial (LA)
  left ventricular (LV)
  left ventricular systolic/diastolic
  left ventricular systolic pump
  myocardial contractile
  regional left ventricular
  regional ventricular
  reserve cardiac
  rest LV (left ventricular)
  rest RV (right ventricular)
  right atrial (RA)
  right ventricular (RV)
  right ventricular systolic/diastolic
  ventricular contractility (VCF)

functional aerobic impairment (FAI)
functional classification of congestive
   heart failure
functional dyspnea
functional heart murmur
functional impairment
functional reentry
functional refractory period (FRP)
functional residual capacity (FRC)
funduscopic
funduscopy
fungal endocarditis
fungal hyphae and spores
fungal infections of the lungs
fungal myocarditis
fungal pericarditis
fungal pneumonia
fungal smear
fungus-laden straw
funic souffle
funicular souffle

funnel chest
funnel chest syndrome
Fürbringer sign (Fuerbringer)
furosemide inhalation
furrier's lung
fused commissures
fused papillary muscle
fusiform aneurysm
fusiform bronchiectasis
fusiform dilatation or dilation
fusiform narrowing of arteries
fusiform shadow
fusion
   commissural
   leaflet
fusion beat
fusion QRS complex
fuzzy echo
FVC (forced vital capacity)
f wave of jugular venous pulse

G, g

Gairdner disease
Gaisböck syndrome (Gaisboeck)
galactosidase deficiency, alpha-
Galaxy pacemaker
Gallavardin dissociation
Gallavardin murmur
Gallavardin phenomenon
Gallavardin syndrome
gallop
  atrial
  diastolic
  early diastolic
  late diastolic
  low-frequency
  mid diastolic
  murmur, or rub (GMR)
  presystolic
  presystolic atrial
  prominent ventricular diastolic
  protodiastolic
  S_3 (third heart sound)
  S_4 (fourth heart sound)
  summation (S_3 and S_4)
  systolic
  ventricular
  ventricular diastolic
gallop rhythm

gallop sound
gamma camera
ganglion, ganglia
ganglion blocker
ganglionectomy, left stellate
gangrene
  atherosclerotic
  embolic
  lung
  presenile
  pulmonary
  Raynaud
  static
  thrombotic
  venous
gangrenous emphysema
gangrenous lung tissue
gannister disease
Ganz-Edwards coronary infusion
  catheter
Ganz formula for coronary sinus flow
gap, auscultatory
Garcia aorta clamp
Gardner-Diamond syndrome
gargle, Dyclone
gargoylism
Garland triangle

garment
Flowtron intermittent compression
Jobst
pneumatic antishock (PASG)
pneumatic foot compression
Garrett dilator
Garrett retractor
Garrett vascular dilator
Gärtner (Gaertner) phenomenon
gas, gases
alveolar
arterial blood (ABG)
expired
hypoxic-hypercapnic
inspired
gas accumulation under serous tunic
of intestine
gas chromatography
gas endarterectomy
gas exchange, pulmonary
gas nitrogen embolism
gasping for breath
gasping respirations
gastric contents, pulmonary aspiration
of
gastric window
gastritis, hemorrhagic
gastrocardiac syndrome
gastrocnemius muscle
gastroenteritis, primary eosinophilic
gastroepiploic artery
gastroepiploic artery graft
gastrohepatic omentum
gas volumes, thoracic
gated blood (pool) cardiac wall
motion study
gated blood pool ventriculogram
gated cardiac blood pool imaging
gated equilibrium blood pool scanning
gated inflow technique
gated magnetic resonance imaging

gated radionuclide ventriculography
gated view (in MUGA, multiple gated
acquisition scan)
GateWay Y-adapter rotating hemostatic valve
gating, echocardiographic
gating of heartbeats
Gaucher disease
gauge, strain
gauze, Surgicel
GCVF (great cardiac vein flow)
GEA (gastroepiploic artery) graft
gel
EKG
electrode
Lectron II electrode
gelatin compression boot
gelatinous debris
gelatinous mottled sputum
Gelatin Resorcine Formal biological
glue injection
Gelfilm
Gelfoam
Gelfoam soaked in thrombin
Gelpi retractor
Gemini DDD pacemaker
Gemini thoracic forceps
gene
FBN1 (implicated in Marfan
syndrome)
fibrillin
microfibrillar protein fibrillin
gene mutation, fibrillin
General Electric pacemaker
General Electric Pass-C echocardiograph machine
generalized alveolitis
generalized arteriosclerosis
generalized capillary leak
generalized emphysema
generalized pulmonary edema

generator (see also *pacemaker*)
asynchronous
Aurora pulse
bipolar
Chardack-Greatbatch implantable
    cardiac pulse
Cosmos pulse
Cyberlith multi-programmable
    pulse
fixed rate
implantable pulse
intrapleural pulse
Jewel pulse
lithium-powered pulse
Medtronic demand pulse
multiprogrammable pulse
PCD pulse
physiologic
Programalith III pulse
pulse
Spectrax SXT pulse
subpectoral pulse
Telectronics PASAR antitachy-
    cardia pulse
unipolar programmable rate-
    responsive
Ventak PRX pulse
Ventak P2 pulse
Ventak pulse
ventricular demand
ventricular inhibited pulse
Ventritex Cadence
Versatrax pulse
GenESA pharmacological stress test
genetic dyslipidemia, familial
Genisis pacemaker
Gensini catheter
Gensini scoring of coronary artery
    disease
Gentle-Flo suction catheter
Gerald forceps

Gerbode dilator
Gerbode forceps
Gerbode mitral valvulotome
Gerbode patent ductus clamp
Gerbode valve dilator
Gerhardt sign
Gerhardt triangle
German measles
Gerota fascia
GE single-photon emission computer-
    ized tomography
GE Starcam single-crystal tomograph-
    ic scintillation camera
Gey solution
Ghajar guide for intraventricular
    catheter placement
Ghon complex
Ghon lesion
Ghon tubercle
ghosts, alveolar cell
giant A waves
giant bullous emphysema
giant capillary hemangioma with
    thrombocytopenia and purpura
giant cavernous hemangioma
giant cell aortitis
giant cell arteritis
giant cell carcinoma
giant cell interstitial pneumonia (GIP)
giant cell myocarditis
giant cells
    Langhans
    multinucleate
giant edema
giant left atrium
giant platelets
Gianturco embolization coils
Gianturco occlusion coils
Gianturco-Roehm bird's nest vena
    caval filter
Gianturco-Roubin flexible coil stent

Gianturco wool-tufted wire coil stent
Gibbon and Landis test for peripheral
  circulation
Gibson murmur
Giertz rongeur
gigantism of pulmonary acini
Gigli saw
Gill-Jonas modification of Norwood
  procedure
GIP (giant cell interstitial pneumonia)
giving up/given up syndrome
gland
  alveolar
  paramediastinal
  thymus
Glanzmann disease
Glasgow sign
glass blower's emphysema
Glenn anastomosis
Glenn operation for congenital
  cyanotic heart disease
Glenn procedure
Glenn shunt
GLH (Green Lane Hospital)
GLH insertion method
GLH syndrome
Glidewire guide wire
gliding and rotatory movements
global cardiac disease
global cerebral hypoperfusion
global ejection fraction
global hypokinesis
global left ventricular dysfunction
globally depressed ejection fraction
global myocardial ischemia
global systolic left ventricular dysfunction
global ventricular dysfunction
global ventricular function
global wall motion abnormality
globoid heart

globular chest
globular sputum
globulin
  antihemophilic (AHG)
  antithymocyte
  rabbit antithymocyte (RATG)
globus hystericus
globus sensation
glomectomy, carotid
glomeriform arteriovenous anastomosis
glomeriform arteriovenular anastomosis
glomus jugulare
glossopharyngeal breathing
glossopharyngeal neuralgia
glossopharyngeal syncope
gloved finger signs
Glover coarctation clamp
Glover patent ductus clamp
Glover vascular clamp
Gluck rib shears
glucocerebrosidase deficiency
glucocorticoid, exogenous
glucocorticoid-remediable hyperaldosteronism
glue
  adjunctive biological
  autologous fibrin
  fibrin
glutamic oxaloacetic transaminase
  (GOT)
glutaraldehyde-stabilized human
  umbilical cord vein graft
glutaraldehyde-tanned bovine collagen
  tubes for grafts
glutaraldehyde-tanned bovine valve
  prosthesis
glutaraldehyde-tanned porcine heart
  valve
glycogen storage disease
glycogenosis, cardiac
glycolipid deposit

glycolysis
glycoproteinosis
glycosides, cardiac
glycosphingolipid metabolism
glycyrrhetinic acid
GMR (gallop, murmur, or rub)
goblet cells
Goethlin test
Goetz cardiac device
Golaski knitted Dacron graft
gold-195m radionuclide
Goldblatt clamp to produce hypertension experimentally
Goldblatt hypertension
Goldblatt phenomenon
Goldenhar syndrome
Goldman cardiac risk index score
Goldman class or score
gonococcal endocarditis
gonococcal pericarditis
Gonzales blood group
good caliber
good cholesterol
Goodale-Lubin cardiac catheter
Goodpasture syndrome
goose flesh
Goosen aortotome
Goosen vascular punch
gooseneck deformity of outflow tract (on x-ray)
Gore-Tex bifurcated vascular graft
Gore-Tex cardiovascular patch
Gore-Tex catheter
Gore-Tex limb
Gore-Tex shunt
Gore-Tex soft tissue patch
Gore-Tex surgical membrane
Gore-Tex vascular graft
Gorlin catheter
Gorlin formula for aortic valve area
Gorlin hydraulic formula for mitral valve area

Gorlin method for cardiac output
Gorlin pacing catheter
Gorlin syndrome
Gosling pulsatility index
Gott shunt
Gott shunt/butterfly heart valve
Gould PentaCath 5-lumen thermodilution catheter
Gould Statham pressure transducer
Gouley syndrome
Gowers syndrome
gracile habitus
gracilis, habitus
grade 2/6 systolic ejection murmur
grade 2-3/6 ("grade two to three over six") (or II-III/VI) murmur
gradient
    alveolar-arterial oxygen tension
    aortic outflow
    aortic valve (AVG)
    aortic valve peak instantaneous
    arteriovenous pressure
    brain-core
    coronary perfusion
    diastolic
    elevated
    end-diastolic aortic–left ventricular pressure
    holosystolic
    instantaneous
    left ventricular outflow pressure
    maximal estimated
    mean mitral valve
    mean systolic
    mitral valve
    negligible pressure
    outflow tract
    peak diastolic
    peak instantaneous
    peak pressure
    peak right ventricular–right atrial systolic

gradient *(cont.)*
  peak systolic (PSG)
  peak-to-peak pressure
  pressure-flow
  pulmonary artery diastolic and
    wedge pressure (PADP-PAWP)
  pulmonary artery to right ventricle
    diastolic
  pulmonary outflow
  pulmonic valve
  residual
  right ventricular to main pulmonary
    artery pressure
  stenotic
  subvalvular
  systolic
  transaortic systolic
  translesional
  transmitral
  transmitral diastolic
  transpulmonic
  transstenotic pressure
  transtricuspid valve diastolic
  transvalvar
  transvalvular
  transvalvular pressure
  tricuspid valve
  ventricular
gradient across valve
gradient-echo imaging sequence
gradient-echo pulse sequence
gradient-echo sequence imaging
graduated exercises
graft
  albumin-coated vascular
  albuminized woven Dacron tube
  allograft
  aorta to left anterior descending
    saphenous vein bypass
  aortic allograft
  aortic homograft
  aortic tube

graft *(cont.)*
  aortobifemoral bypass
  aortobiprofunda bypass
  aortocoronary bypass
  aortocoronary saphenous vein
    bypass
  aortocoronary snake
  aortofemoral
  aortofemoral bypass (AFBG)
  ascending aorta–abdominal aorta
    bypass
  autogenous
  autogenous saphenous vein
  autologous
  autologous patch
  autologous reversed vein
  axillary-axillary bypass
  axillary-femorofemoral bypass
  axillobifemoral bypass
  axillofemoral bypass
  below-knee popliteal to distal
    peroneal reversed vein
  bifurcated
  bifurcated vascular
  bifurcation
  Biograft
  BioPolyMeric
  Björk-Shiley
  bovine allograft
  bovine heterograft
  brachioaxillary interposition
    bypass
  Cabrol I tube
  Cabrol-II interposition coronary
    prosthetic
  cardiac allograft
  carotid-carotid venous bypass
  collagen-impregnated knitted
    Dacron velour
  composite
  composite valve
  composite vein

graft *(cont.)*
 compressed Ivalon patch
 conduit
 Cooley woven Dacron
 coronary artery bypass (CABG)
 crossover
 cryopreserved human aortic
  allograft
 Dacron knitted
 Dacron onlay patch
 Dacron outflow
 Dacron patch
 Dacron preclotted
 Dacron tightly woven
 Dacron tube (or tubular)
 Dacron velour
 Dacron velour tube
 de-aired
 diamond-shaped sequential vein
 double velour knitted
 Edwards woven Teflon aortic
  bifurcation
 endothelialization of vascular
 endothelialized vascular
 endovascular stented
 expanded polytetrafluoroethylene
  (ePTFE) vascular
 expanded reinforced polytetrafluoroethylene (ER-PTFE)
  vascular
 extracardiac
 extracavitary prosthetic arterial
 extracavitary-infected
 extrathoracic carotid subclavian
  bypass
 femoral-distal popliteal bypass
 femoral-distal vein
 femoral-femoral bypass
 femoral-peroneal in situ vein
  bypass
 femorofemoral subcutaneous
  suprapubic

graft *(cont.)*
 femoroperoneal bypass
 femorotibial bypass
 gastroepiploic artery
 GEA (gastroepiploic artery)
 glutaraldehyde-stabilized human
  umbilical cord vein
 glutaraldehyde-tanned bovine
  carotid artery
 glutaraldehyde-tanned bovine
  collagen tubes for vascular
 glutaraldehyde-tanned porcine
  heart valve
 Gore-Tex
 Gore-Tex bifurcated vascular
 Gore-Tex jump
 Hancock pericardial valve
 Hancock vascular
 Hemashield
 hepatorenal bypass
 hepatorenal saphenous vein bypass
 heterograft
 heterologous
 homograft
 horseshoe tubular
 HUV (human umbilical vein)
  bypass
 IEA (inferior epigastric artery)
 iliac-renal bypass
 ilioprofunda bypass
 IMA (internal mammary artery)
 infected
 infrainguinal vein bypass
 in situ
 in situ vein
 internal saphenous vein
 internal mammary artery (IMA)
 internal saphenous vein
 internal thoracic artery (ITA)
 interposition
 Ionescu-Shiley pericardial valve
 Ionescu-Shiley vascular

graft *(cont.)*
  ITA (internal thoracic artery)
  jump
  kinking of
  knitted
  knitted Dacron
  knitted Dacron arterial
  knitted double velour Dacron patch
  LIMA (left internal mammary artery)
  Meadox Microvel
  Microvel double velour
  modified human umbilical vein (HUV)
  noncavitary prosthetic
  nonreversed saphenous vein
  nonvalved
  Ochsner
  occluded
  onlay
  outflow
  patch
  patent
  Plasma TFE vascular
  popliteal-blind peroneal
  popliteal-distal bypass
  porcine xenograft
  preclotted
  preclotted patch
  prosthetic patch
  PTFE (polytetrafluoroethylene)
  pulmonary autograft
  radial artery
  saphenous vein (SVG) bypass
  Sauvage
  sequential
  sequential bypass
  snake
  splenorenal arterial bypass
  St. Jude composite valve
  stabilized human umbilical vein
  straight

graft *(cont.)*
  straight tubular
  supraceliac aorta-femoral artery bypass
  supraceliac aorta-visceral artery bypass
  supraceliac aortic bypass
  supraceliac aortofemoral bypass
  synthetic
  Teflon
  thoracic aorta-femoral artery bypass
  thrombosed
  transluminally placed stented tube
  tubular
  umbilical vein
  unilateral aortofemoral
  valved
  vascular
  vein patch
  ventriculoarterial
  woven Dacron
  woven Dacron tube
  wraparound
  Y
  Y-shaped
graftable
graft ACE fixed-wire balloon catheter
GraftAssist vein and graft holder
graft dependent
graft endocarditis
graft-enteric erosion
graft-enteric fistula
graft entrapment
graft erosion into bowel lumen
graft excision
grafting (see *graft*)
graft insertion site
graft material, synthetic (see *prosthesis*)
graft occlusion

graft occlusive disease
graft-patch
graft patency
graft preservation
  complete
  partial
graft replacement of descending aorta
graft-seeking catheter
graft shrinkage
graft stenosis
graft trimmed on the bias
Graham-Burford-Mayer syndrome
Graham Steell heart murmur
grain-handler's disease
grain-handler's lung
gram-negative bacterial endotoxins
gram-negative cocci
gram-negative sepsis
gram-positive cocci
Gram stain
Grancher sign
Grancher triad
Grant aneurysm clamp
granular cell tumor of the heart
granular pharyngitis
granulated
granulation stenosis
granulation tissue
granules, aggregated eosinophil
granulocytic leukemia
granuloma
  coccidioidal
  eosinophilic
  extravascular
  lethal midline
  noncaseating
  tuberculous
granulomatosis
  allergic
  allergic angiitis and
  bronchocentric
  Langerhans cell

granulomatosis *(cont.)*
  necrotizing respiratory
  organic
  Wegener
granulomatous and necrotizing replacement of bronchial epithelium
granulomatous disease, allergic
  myocardial
granulomatous inflammation of
  bronchi
granulomatous myocarditis
granulomatous pneumonitis
granulomatous reaction
granulomatous rhinitis
graphite fibrosis of lung
grasping forceps
grass
  June
  Timothy
GRASS (gradient recalled acquisition
  in steady state)
grating bruit
grating friction rub
Graupner method
grave prognosis
gravido-puerperal cardiomyopathy
gravitational edema
gray hepatization of lung
grayish sputum
great arteries, complete transposition
  of the
great artery disease
great artery, overriding
great cardiac vein
great cardiac vein flow
great coronary vein
great saphenous vein
great vessel, orientation of
great vessels transposition
greater cardiac vein
greater saphenous system
greater saphenous vein

Green retractor
green sputum
Greene sign
Greenfield filter
Greenfield IVC (inferior vena cava)
    filter
Greenfield vena caval filter
Gregg-type cannula
Gregoire blue syndrome
Gregory baby profunda clamp
Gregory carotid bulldog clamp
Gregory external clamp
Gregory forceps
Gregory stay suture
grim prognosis
GRIP torque device
grippe
grippy feeling
Grocco sign of pleural effusion
Grocco triangular dullness
groin area
Grollman catheter
Grollman pigtail catheter
groove
    anterior interventricular
    atrioventricular (AV)
    deltopectoral
    interatrial
    interventricular
    posterior interventricular
    Waterston
Groshong double-lumen catheter
Gross coarctation occlusion clamp
grossly audible wheezing
Grossman scale for regurgitation
Grossman sign
ground glass appearance of lungs
ground glass infiltrates in lungs
ground plate
grounding lead
Grover clamp

growth factor, platelet-derived
growth retardation
Gruentzig (Grüntzig)
grumose (or grumous) material
grumous debris
grunting
    expiratory
    minimal expiratory
    respiratory distress with
grunting expiration
grunting murmur
grunting respirations
Grüntzig (Gruentzig)
Grüntzig angioplasty technique
Grüntzig balloon catheter angioplasty
Grüntzig Dilaca catheter
Grüntzig technique for PTCA
Gsell-Erdheim syndrome
G suit (for syncope)
Guangzhou GD-1 prosthetic valve
guanine nucleotide binding protein
guanine nucleotide regulatory proteins
guarded prognosis
Guardian AICD (automatic implant-
    able cardioverter-defibrillator)
Guardian ICD (implantable cardio-
    verter-defibrillator)
Guardian pacemaker
guarding
guidance
    fluoroscopic
    under fluoroscopic
guide
    ACS LIMA
    Amplatz tube
    Arani
    FL4
    Flexguide intubation
    Muller catheter
    Pilotip catheter
    steerable wire

guide wire
  ACS (Advanced Catheter Systems)
  Amplatz Super Stiff
  angiographic
  atherolytic
  atherolytic reperfusion
  Bentson floppy-tip
  Critikon
  Flex
  flexible
  flexible J
  floppy
  floppy-tipped
  Hi-Per Flex
  Hi-Torque Flex-T
  Hi-Torque Floppy (HTF)
  Hi-Torque Intermediate
  Hi-Torque Standard
  high torque
  high-torque floppy
  hydrophilic
  Hyperflex
  J
  J tip
  J-tipped exchange
  J-tipped spring
  Linx exchange
  Magnum
  Medrad
  PDT

guide wire *(cont.)*
  preformed
  Redifocus
  Rosen
  Schwarten LP
  shapeable
  Sof-T
  soft-tipped
  Sones
  SOS
  steerable
  straight
  TAD
  Teflon-coated
  transluminal angioplasty
  USCI
  VeriFlex
  Wholey Hi-Torque Floppy
  Wholey Hi-Torque Modified J
  Wholey Hi-Torque Standard
guide wire exchanged
guiding catheter
guiding shots
guillotine, rib
Gunn crossing sign
gusset, woven Dacron
Gutgeman clamp
guy suture
guy-wire support for mitral valve
  leaflet

H, h

habitus
   asthenic
   body
   gracile
   large
habitus gracilis
hacking cough
haematobium, Schistosoma
Haemonetics Cell-Saver System
Haemophilus infection
Haemophilus influenzae (*H. influenzae*)
Haemophilus influenzae bronchitis
Haemophilus influenzae laryngitis
Haemophilus influenzae pneumonia
Hagar probe
Hageman blood coagulation factor
Hageman factor
Hageman factor activation
Haight-Finochietto rib retractor
Haight rasp
Haight rib spreader
Haimovici arteriotomy scissors
hair growth
   decreased lower leg
   distribution of
hair loss
Hakki formula

Haldane-Priestley tube
Hale syndrome
half-hitch knots
Hall cutter
Hall-effect position sensor
Hall-Kaster mitral valve prosthesis
Hall-Kaster tilting-disk valve
   prosthesis
Hall prosthetic heart valve
Hall sign
Hall sternal saw
Hall valve disruption
Halo catheter
halothane
Halsted forceps
hamartoma
   cardiac
   chondromatous
Hamburg classification of congenital
   vascular defect
Hamilton-Stewart formula for
   measuring cardiac output
Hamman crunch
Hamman disease
Hamman murmur
Hamman pneumopericardium sign
Hamman-Rich syndrome

hammocking of leaflet
hammocking of mitral valve
hammock mitral valve
hammock valve
Hampton hump
Hanafee catheter
Hancock aortic bioprosthesis
Hancock aortic punch
Hancock bioprosthesis
Hancock bioprosthetic valve
Hancock conduit
Hancock mitral valve prosthesis
Hancock M.O. II porcine bioprosthesis
Hancock pericardial prosthetic valve
Hancock porcine heterograft valve
Hancock porcine prosthetic heart
  valve
Hancock valved conduit
Hancock valve prosthesis
Hancock vascular graft
hand-agitated contrast medium
hand-agitated solution with microbubbles
hand-bagging of oxygen
handgrip exercise test
H&H (hemoglobin and hematocrit)
hand-heart syndrome
hand-held mapping probe
hand-held nebulizer
hand-held retractor
hand injection
hand-made injection
hand-shaped bend
hand turgor
HANE (hereditary angioneurotic
  edema)
hanging drop test for pneumoperitoneum
hangout interval
hangout of dicrotic notch in
  pulmonary arterial pressure
Hank balanced salt solution

Hantavirus pulmonary syndrome
HAPE (high-altitude pulmonary
  edema)
Harbitz-Mueller syndrome
hard metal disease
hard, pitting edema
hardening of arteries
Harkavy syndrome
Harken auricle clamp
Harken prosthetic valve
Harken rib spreader
Harley paroxysmal hemoglobinuria
harmonious aortic root
Harrington-Mayo thoracic scissors
Harrington-Mixter thoracic forceps
Harrington retractor
Harrington thoracic forceps
Harrison groove
harsh cough
harsh friction rub
harsh murmur
Hartzler ACX-II or RX-014 balloon
  catheter
Hartzler angioplasty balloon
Hartzler LPS dilatation catheter
Hartzler Micro II balloon
Hartzler Micro XT dilatation catheter
Hartzler rib retractor
Harvard ventilator
harvest of donor organs for
  transplantation
harvested vein
harvester lung
harvesting, vein
harvesting vein, tissue, or organ from
  donor for transplantation
Hatle method to calculate mitral valve
  area
Hayem-Widal acquired hemolytic
  anemia
Hayem-Widal syndrome
Hayes Martin forceps

hay fever
Haynes 25 material for prosthetic
  valve construction
HBE (His bundle electrogram)
HBO (hyperbaric oxygen)
HBP (high blood pressure)
HC or HCM (hypertrophic cardio–
  myopathy)
HCT or Hct (hematocrit)
HCVD (hypertensive cardiovascular
  disease)
H-DCSA (His bundle-distal coronary
  sinus atrial) depolarization
HDL (high-density lipoproteins)
HDM (house dust mites)
HDM bronchial provocation test
HDM challenge
headache after cocaine use
head-down tilt test
headhunter catheter
head-up tilt test
healing infarct
heart
  abdominal
  air-driven artificial
  Akutsu total artificial
  alcoholic
  ALVAD (intra-abdominal left
    ventricular assist device)
  artificial
  angiosarcoma of
  armored
  artificial
  athlete's
  athletic
  axis of
  balloon-shaped
  Baylor total artificial
  beer
  beriberi
  boat-shaped
  bony

heart *(cont.)*
  booster
  boot-shaped (on x-ray)
  bovine
  bread-and-butter
  bulb of
  cardiogenic shock
  cervical
  chaotic
  conical
  crisscross
  dome-shaped
  donor
  drop
  dynamite
  electrical axis of
  electromechanical artificial
  electromechanically quiescent
  elongated
  empty
  encased
  enlarged
  extracorporeal
  extracorporeal artificial
  failing
  fat
  fatty
  fibroid
  fibroma of
  flabby
  flask-shaped
  frosted (frosting; icing)
  globoid
  hairy
  hanging (suspended)
  holiday
  Holmes
  horizontal
  hyperdynamic
  hyperkinetic
  hyperthyroid
  hypertrophied

heart *(cont.)*
  hypoplastic
  hypoplastic left
  hypothermic
  icing (frosting)
  intermediate
  intracorporeal artificial
  irritable
  ischemic
  Jarvik 7 or 8 artificial
  Jarvik 7-70 artificial
  left (atrium and ventricle)
  Liotta total artificial (TAH)
  luxus
  lymphosarcoma of
  malposition of the
  massively enlarged
  mean electrical axis of
  mechanical
  mildly enlarged
  movable
  myxedema
  myxoma of
  nervous
  nonshocked
  normothermic fibrillating
  nutrition
  one-ventricle
  orthotopic biventricular artificial
  orthotopic univentricular artificial
  ovoid
  ox
  paracorporeal
  parchment
  pear-shaped
  pectoral
  pendulous
  Penn State total artificial
  permanent artificial
  Phoenix total artificial
  pulmonary
  Quain fatty

heart *(cont.)*
  recipient
  resting
  rhabdomyoma of
  right (atrium and ventricle)
  round
  sabot
  semihorizontal
  semivertical
  single-outlet
  skin (peripheral blood vessels)
  snowman (on x-ray)
  soft
  soldier's
  spastic
  stiff
  stone
  superoinferior
  suspended
  Symbion J-7 70 mL total artificial
  Symbion Jarvik-7 artificial
  systemic
  tabby cat
  teardrop
  temporary artificial
  three-chambered
  thrush breast
  tiger
  tiger lily
  tobacco
  total artificial (TAH)
  transplanted
  transverse
  Traube
  triatrial
  trilocular
  univentricular
  University of Akron artificial
  upstairs-downstairs
  Utah artificial
  Utah TAH (total artificial heart)
  venous

heart *(cont.)*
  venting of
  vertical
  wandering
  water-bottle
  wooden shoe
Heart Aid 80 defibrillator
heart and great vessels
heart and hand syndrome
heart and lung transplantation
heart apex
heart assist system
heart attack (myocardial infarction)
heartbeat (see also *beat*)
  coupling
  dropped
  fascicular
  fluttering
  forceful
  irregular
  irregularly irregular
  pounding
  racing
  rapid
  regular
  regularly irregular
  skipping
heart block (see *block*)
  atrioventricular
  bifascicular
  bundle branch
  complete
  complete atrioventricular
  complete congenital
  congenital
  deceleration-dependent
  diffuse
  entrance
  exit
  first-degree atrioventricular (AV)
  incomplete atrioventricular (AV)
  intraventricular

heart block *(cont.)*
  Mobitz type I
  Mobitz type II
  myofibrillar intraventricular
  peri-infarction
  secondary atrioventricular
  sinoatrial
  sinoauricular
  surgically induced complete
  trifascicular
  2:1 atrioventricular
  Wenckebach's incomplete
    atrioventricular (AV)
heartburn (pyrosis; water brash)
heartburn type of pain
heart catheterization
  femoral
  transseptal
  transvenous
heart contraction
  isometric
  isotonic
heart decortication
heart disease
  amyloid
  atherosclerotic
  cyanotic congenital
  neonatal
  nutritional
heart failure
  acute
  backward
  chronic
  compensated congestive
  congestive
  decompensated congestive
  diastolic
  donor
  fetal
  forward
  Framingham criteria for
  high-output

heart failure *(cont.)*
  intrauterine
  left-sided
  low-output
  refractory
  right-sided
  systolic
heart failure cells
heart failure from thiamine deficiency
heart forward failure
heart-hand II syndrome
heart in sinus rhythm
heart-lung bloc
heart-lung machine
  Crafoord-Senning
  Mayo-Gibbon
heart-lung transplant (transplantation)
heart massage
HeartMate battery-operated portable
  system
HeartMate implantable left ventricular
  assist device (LVAD)
HeartMate implantable ventricular
  assist device
heart murmur (see *murmur*)
heart overload
heart power failure
heart prosthesis
heart pump, BVS (biventricular support) system
heart rate (see also *rate*)
  intrinsic
  resting
  target
heart rate reserve mechanism
heart rate response
heart rhythm, dual
heart remnant
heart sac
heart sound (see *sound*)
heart tamponade
heart tones (sounds)

heart transplant or transplantation
  heterotopic
  orthotopic
heart transplant rejection
heart valve (see *valve*; *prosthesis*)
heart wall at risk for injury from
  infarction
heartwire, bipolar temporary
heat-expandable stent
heated humidified oxygen
Heath-Edwards classification of
  pulmonary vascular disease
Heath-Edwards criteria
heating, nonablative
heat intolerance
heave
  left lower parasternal
  parasternal
  substernal
  sustained left ventricular
heave and lift
heaviness, chest
heaving of chest wall
heaving precordial motion
heavy chain, myosin
Heberden angina pectoris disease
Heberden sign
Heberden syndrome
Heckathorn disease
Heckathorn factor VIII deficiency
hectic flush
heelstick hematocrit in neonates
Hegar dilator
Hegglin syndrome
Heifitz clip
Heim-Kreysig sign
Heineke-Mikulicz maneuver
Heineke-Mikulicz procedure
Heinz body
Heiss artery forceps
helical coil stent
helical-tip Halo catheter

helium-filled balloon catheter
Helistat absorbable collagen hemostatic sponge
Helitene absorbable collagen hemostatic agent
Heller-Döhle (Doehle)
Heller-Döhle syphilitic aortitis disease
Heller esophagocardiomyotomy
Helminthosporium
helplessness
Hemaflex PTCA sheath with obturator
hemangioendothelioma, malignant
hemangiolymphangioma
hemangioma
  bulky
  cardiac
  cavernous
  deep
  extremity
  familial intracranial
  fibrofatty
  giant cavernous
  intramuscular
  lung
  problematic
  proliferative
  proliferative phase
  subcutaneous
  verrucous
hemangioma-thrombocytopenia syndrome
hemangiomatosis, pulmonary capillary
hemangioma with platelet trapping
hemangiopericytoma
Hemaquet catheter introducer
Hemaquet PTCA sheath with obturator
Hemaquet sheath
Hemaquet sheath introducer
Hemashield graft
Hemashield woven vascular graft

hematemesis
hematest positive, trace
hematocrit (HCT)
  dilutional
  heelstick
  Wintrobe
hematogenous dissemination from lungs
hematogenous metastasis
hematogenous pulmonary involvement
hematoma
  acute intramural
  aneurysmal
  dissecting aortic
  intramural
  intrarenal
  mural
  pericardial
  perirenal
  retroperitoneal
  subcapsular
hematoma cap
  azygos
  left pleural apical
hematopoiesis
hematopoietic cells
hematoporphyrin derivative (HPD)
Hemex prosthetic valve
hemianesthesia
hemiarch
hemiaxial view (x-ray)
hemiazygos vein
hemiblock (left or right)
  anterior
  anterior-posterior
  bundle branch
  left anterior-superior (LASH)
  left posterior (LPH)
hemicardium
hemic calculus
hemicranial pain

hemidiaphragm, attenuation by
hemidiaphragm depression
hemi-Fontan operation
hemihypertrophy
hemilaryngectomy
hemi-Mustard pericardial baffle
hemiparesis
  contralateral
  ipsilateral
hemithorax (pl. hemithoraces)
hemithymectomy
hemitruncus
hemitruncus repair
hemochromatosis, idiopathic
hemoclip, Samuels
hemoconcentration
HemoCue photometer for hemoglobin
  determination
hemodilution, intentional transoperative
hemodynamic assessment
hemodynamic changes
hemodynamic data
hemodynamic depression
hemodynamic effect
hemodynamic embarrassment
hemodynamic factors
hemodynamic findings
hemodynamic format
hemodynamic impairment
hemodynamic instability
hemodynamic monitoring, continuous
hemodynamic overload
  acute
  chronic
hemodynamic pathogenesis of
  vascular-bone syndromes
hemodynamic pattern
hemodynamic picture
hemodynamic profile
hemodynamic results
hemodynamic significance

hemodynamic support
hemodynamically significant findings
hemodynamically significant lesion
hemodynamically stable
hemodynamics, cardiovascular
hemofiltration
hemoglobin (Hb, Hgb)
  abnormal
  glycosylated
  low
  normal
  pyridoxilated stroma-free (SFHb)
  recombinant (rHb1.1)
  stroma free (SFHb)
hemoglobin A
hemoglobin and hematocrit (H&H)
hemoglobin C
hemoglobin C–thalassemia disease
hemoglobin electrophoresis
hemoglobin E–thalassemia disease
hemoglobin S (sickle hemoglobin)
hemoglobinopathies
hemolysis
hemolytic anemia
Hemopad absorbable collagen
  hemostat
hemoperfusion
hemopericardium
hemophilia
  classical
  vascular
hemophilia A (factor VIII deficiency)
hemophilia B (factor IX deficiency)
Hemophilus (see *Haemophilus*)
hemopleuropneumonia syndrome
hemopneumothorax
hemoptysis
Hemopump, Nimbus
hemorrhage
  anastomotic
  arterial
  capillary

hemorrhage *(cont.)*
  chronic parenchymal
  diffuse subarachnoid
  Duret
  exsanguinating (into pleural space)
  external
  extrapleural
  familial intracranial
  focal endocardial
  frank
  internal
  intracranial
  intramural arterial
  intraplaque (IPH)
  intrapleural
  intrapulmonary
  intraventricular (IVH)
  life-threatening
  massive exsanguinating
  meningeal
  nontraumatic epidural
  parenchymal
  peribronchiolar
  postoperative mediastinal
  pulmonary
  salmon-patch
  splinter
  subarachnoid (SAH)
  venous
hemorrhage in plaque
hemorrhage into atheromatous plaque
hemorrhage per rhexin
hemorrhagic bronchitis
hemorrhagic bronchopneumonia
hemorrhagic consolidation
hemorrhagic diathesis
hemorrhagic disorder
hemorrhagic duodenitis
hemorrhagic fluid
hemorrhagic gastritis
hemorrhagic pericarditis
hemorrhagic pleurisy

hemorrhagic shock
hemorrhagic telangiectasia, hereditary
hemorrhagic zone, pyramidal
hemosiderin deposit
hemosiderin, phagocytized
hemosiderosis
  idiopathic pulmonary
  pulmonary idiopathic
  transfusional
hemostasis was achieved
hemostat (see also *forceps*)
  collagen
  Crile
  Hemotene absorbable collagen
  Kelly
  Kocher
  Mayo
  microfibrillar
  mosquito
  Woodward
hemostatic agent
  Helitene absorbable
  Instat collagen absorbable
hemostatic material, Tissucol fibrin-
  collagen
hemostatic sponge
  Collastat
  Helistat absorbable collagen
  Hemotene absorbable collagen
hemothorax
Hendrin ductus clamp; forceps
Henle-Coenen test
Henle elastic membrane
Henle fenestrated membrane
Henle loop
Henle membrane
Henley dilator
Henley vascular clamp
Henoch-Schönlein purpura
heparin
  low-dose
  neutralize the effects of

heparin admininstration
heparin anticoagulation, systemic
heparinization
  adequate
  post-PTCA
  systemic
  total body
heparinized blood
heparinized saline flush
heparinized saline solution
heparin lock for administering
  medication
heparin lock introducer
heparin neutralized with protamine
  sulfate
heparinoid compound
heparin rebound
heparin not reversed
heparin reversed with protamine
hepatic arteriovenous fistula
hepatic congestion
hepatic necrosis
hepatic vein pulsation
hepatic vein thrombosis
hepatic veno-occlusive disease
hepatization
  gray
  red
hepatoclavicular view
hepatojugular reflux
hepatomegaly, pulsating
hepatopleural fistula
hepatorenal bypass graft
hepatorenal saphenous vein bypass
  graft
Herbst appliance, removable
Herbst corpuscles
Hercules power injector
hereditary angioedema
hereditary angioneurotic edema
  (HANE)
hereditary capillary fragility

hereditary hemolytic anemia
hereditary hemorrhagic diathesis
hereditary hemorrhagic telangiectasia
hereditary lymphedema
hereditary ovalocytosis
hereditary pseudohemophilia
hereditary sideroblastic anemia
hereditary spherocytosis
Hering-Breuer inverted oculocardiac
  reflex
Hering, nerve of
Hering phenomenon
hermetically sealed standby pacemaker
hernia
  diaphragmatic
  inguinal
  intrapericardial diaphragmatic
  mediastinal
  umbilical
Hershey left ventricular assist device
Hespan (hetastarch) plasma volume
  expander
Hess capillary test
hetastarch (Hespan)
heterogeneity, temporal
heterogeneous appearance
heterograft (see also *graft*)
  bovine
  porcine
  xenograft
heterologous graft
heterologous surfactant
heterophile antibodies
heterotaxy
  abdominal
  visceral
heterotaxy syndrome
heterotopic heart transplantation
Hetzel forward triangle method for
  cardiac output
Heubner disease
Hewlett-Packard color flow imager

Hewlett-Packard defibrillator
Hewlett-Packard transducer
Hewlett-Packard ultrasound unit
HFD40 (duration of terminal QRS
    high frequency signal)
HFJV (high-frequency jet ventilation)
HFLA duration
HFQRSD (duration of high frequency
    QRS)
HFRMS (voltage of terminal QRS
    high frequency signal)
Hgb (hemoglobin)
HHD (hypertensive heart disease)
HH' interval
hiatus, tendinous
hibernation, myocardial
Hickman indwelling right atrial
    catheter
Hidalgo catheter
Hiebert vascular dilator
high-altitude pulmonary edema
    (HAPE)
high-amplitude impulse
high arched palate
high blood pressure (HBP)
high defect in atrial septum
high-density lipoprotein (HDL)
high filling pressure
high-flow, low-resistance pattern
high-frequency nebulizer
high-frequency jet ventilation (HFJV)
high-grade lesion
high-grade obstructive lesion
high-grade stenosis
high interstitial pressure
high lateral wall myocardial infarction
high left main diagonal artery
high-low (see *Hi-Lo*)
high minute ventilation
high-output circulatory failure
high-output heart failure
high pacing thresholds

high-pitched ejection murmur
high-pitched opening snap
high-pitched rhonchi
high-pitched signal
high-power field
high-rate detect interval
high-rate pacing
high-rate ventricular response, atrial
    fibrillation with
high reflectivity
high-resolution computed tomography
    scan
high-resolution magnification
high right atrium
high right atrium electrode
high-speed burr
high-speed rotation dynamic
    angioplasty catheter
high take-off of left coronary artery
high torque (see *Hi-Torque*)
high-velocity jet
hilar adenopathy
hilar area
hilar artery
hilar haze
hilar lymphadenopathy
hilar lymph node enlargement
hilar mass
hilar prominence
hilar shadows (on x-ray)
Hill sign
Hi-Lo Jet tracheal tube
hilum of lung
hilus (hilum)
hilus tuberculosis
Himmelstein sternal retractor
Himmelstein valvulotome
Hines and Brown test
H. influenzae organism
hinge, annulocuspid
hip claudication
Hi-Per cardiac device

Hi-Per Flex guide wire
Hippel-Lindau syndrome
hippocratic sound
His bundle ablation
His bundle deflection
His bundle electrogram, -graphy
    (HBE)
His, bundle of
Hislop-Reid syndrome
His-Purkinje conducting system
His-Purkinje system (HPS)
His-Purkinje system fibrosis
histamine acid phosphatase
histamine challenge
histamine concentration
histamine control
histamine flush
histamine receptors
His-Tawara atrioventricular bundle
His-Tawara atrioventricular node
histiocytoid cardiomyopathy
histiocytosis X
histocompatibility antigen
histogram, plasma
histologic examination
histomorphometric analysis of biopsy
    specimen
Histoplasma myocarditis
histoplasmosis
histoplasmotic endocarditis
history
    antecedent
    family
    pack-a-day smoking
    pack-year smoking
    remote
    salient
Hi-Torque Flex-T guide wire
Hi-Torque Floppy (HTF) guide wire
Hi-Torque Intermediate guide wire
Hi-Torque Standard guide wire
HIV (human immunodeficiency virus)

HIV infection
HLA-B27 antigen
HLA typing
HLHS (hypoplastic left heart syn-
    drome)
HLP (hyperlipoproteinemia)
H-MCSA (His bundle-middle coro-
    nary sinus atrial) depolarization
HMG CoA reductase inhibitor
H-mode echocardiography
HOC or HOCM (hypertrophic
    obstructive cardiomyopathy)
hockey-stick appearance of catheter tip
hockey-stick deformity of cusp (on
    echocardiogram)
hockey-stick deformity of tricuspid
    valve
hockey-stick incision, midline
Hodgkin disease
Hodgkin-Key murmur
Hodgson aneurysmal dilatation of the
    aorta
Hodgson aortic disease
Hodgson disease
Hoen nerve hook
Hohn vessel dilator
holder
    needle
    prosthetic valve
    valve
    wire needle
Holger-Nielsen artificial respirations
holiday heart syndrome
Holinger dissector
hollow chest syndrome
hollow cough
hollow tunneler
Holmes heart
Holmes syndrome
holmium laser
holmium yttrium aluminum garnet
    (Ho:YAG) laser

holmium:YAG laser for angioplasty
holosystolic mitral valve prolapse
holosystolic murmur
Holter monitor
Holter monitoring, continuous
Holter shunt
Holter tubing
Holter valve
Holt-Oram atriodigital dysplasia
Holt-Oram syndrome
Holzknecht space
Homans sign
Hombach lead placement system
homoartery
homocystinuria, congenital
homocystinuria syndrome
homogeneity
homogeneous appearance
homogeneous echo
homogeneous material
homogeneous perfusion
homogeneous thallium distribution
homograft
   cryopreserved
   denatured
   freehand aortic valve
homograft conduit
homograft reaction
homograft root replacement
homologous blood transfusion
homonymous hemianopia
homotransplantation
honeycomb formation
honeycomb lung
honeycombing (cysts)
honeycombing, fibrotic
honk
   late systolic
   precordial
honking murmur
hood forceps
hooding, interchordal

hood of graft
hood punch
hook
   Adson
   fishhook
   Hoen nerve
   Krayenbuehl vessel
   nerve
   Selverstone cardiotomy
   tracheal
   valve
hook scissors
hook wire localization, CT-directed
Hoover sign
hopelessness
Hope murmur
Hope sign
Hopkins aortic clamp
Hopkins forceps
horizontal chin cleft
horizontal fissure of lung
horizontal long-axis slice
horizontal mattress suture
horizontal plane loop
horizontal ST segment depression
hormone
   adrenocorticotropic
   antidiuretic
   somatotropin-releasing
Horner syndrome
horseshoe configuration on thallium
   imaging
horseshoe-shaped syncytium
horseshoe tubular graft
Horton disease
Horton giant cell arteritis
host, nonimmunocompromised
hostile
hot spots (on technetium pyrophosphate scan)
hourglass deformity
hourglass-shaped lesion

house dust mite
housing and pusher plate
Howell coronary scissors
Howell-Jolly body
Howell test for hemoglobin
Ho:YAG (holmium yttrium aluminum
garnet) laser
HPD (hematoporphyrin derivative)
H-PCSA (His bundle-proximal coro-
nary sinus atrial depolarization)
h peak of jugular venous pulse
H'P interval
h plateau of jugular venous pulse
HPS (His-Purkinje system)
H-Q interval
H-QRS interval
HR (heart rate) (beats/min)
HRA (high right atrium)
H spike and H' spike
HTN or Htn (hypertension)
hub of balloon lumen
hub of needle
Huchard continued arterial
hypertension
Huchard disease
Huchard essential hypertension
Huchard sign
hue, violaceous
Hufnagel aortic clamp
Hufnagel prosthetic valve
Hughes-Stovin syndrome
hum
buzzing venous
cervical venous
venous
human immunodeficiency virus (HIV)
human leukocyte antigen B27
human parvovirus (HPV)
Human Surf
humidifier lung
humming rhonchi
humoral response

hump, Hampton
Humphries aortic clamp
hunger, air
Hunter canal
Hunter operation for correction of
aneurysm
Hunter-Sessions balloon
Hunter-Sessions inferior vena cava
balloon occluder
Hunter syndrome
Hunter tendon rod insertion for deep
venous insufficiency (DVI)
Hurler syndrome
Hurwitz thoracic trocar
Hutchinson-Gilford progeria syndrome
Hutinel-Pick syndrome
HUV (human umbilical vein) bypass
graft
H-V (His-ventricular) interval
HV-1 patch lead
h wave of jugular venous pulse
H waves
Hx (history)
hyalin nodules
hyaline cartilage
hyaline change
hyaline degeneration
hyaline membrane disease
hyaline necrosis
hyaline thrombi
hyalinization
arteriolar
subendothelial
hyaluronidase
HydraCross TLC PTCA catheter
hydrate, hydrated
hydration
hydrocyanic acid release
hydrogen density
hydropericardium
hydrophilic guide wire
hydropic degeneration

hydropneumothorax
hydrops
  nonimmune fetal
  nonimmunological fetal
hydrops fetalis (fetal hydrops)
hydrostatic pressure of the blood
hydrothorax
hydroxyl radical
hydroxylase deficiency
hydroxyurea
hyparterial bronchi
hyperabduction maneuver
hyperactive carotid sinus reflex
hyperacute rejection
hyperadrenergic orthostatic
  hypotension
hyperaeration
hyperaldosteronism
  glucocorticoid-remediable
  idiopathic
  indeterminate
hyperalphalipoproteinemia
hyperamylasemia
hyperbaric chamber
hyperbaric oxygen
hyperbasemia
hyperbetalipoproteinemia, familial
hyperbilirubinemia
hypercalcemia-supravalvular aortic
  stenosis
hypercalcemic face
hypercapnia
  progressive
  well-compensated
hypercapnic acute asthma
hypercarbia (hypercapnia)
hypercholesterolemia
  familial
  polygenic
hyperchylomicronemia, familial
hypercoagulability

hypercoagulable state
hypercyanotic angina
hypercyanotic episode
hypercyanotic spell
hyperdynamic apical impulse
hyperdynamic AV fistulae
hyperdynamic heart syndrome
hyperdynamic impulse
hyperdynamic PMI
hyperdynamic right ventricular
  impulse
hyperdynamic state
hyperechoicity
hyperemia
  active
  arterial
  collateral
  diffuse
  fluxionary
  passive
  reactive
  venous
hyperemia of mucous membranes
hypereosinophilic syndrome, idiopathic
hyperestrogenemia
hyperextension of neck
Hyperflex guide wire
Hyperflex steerable wire
hyperfunction, adrenal gland
hypergammaglobulinemia
hyperhidrosis
hyperinflation, dynamic pulmonary
hyperinsulinemia
hyperintense
hyperkalemia
hyperkalemic crystalloid cardioplegic
  solution for heart-lung machine
hyperkinesia, compensatory
hyperkinetic circulation
hyperkinetic heart disease
hyperkinetic heart syndrome

hyperkinetic hypertension
hyperkinetic PMI (point of maximal
   impulse)
hyperkinetic segmental wall motion
hyperlipidemia
   carbohydrate-inducible
   combined
   familial
   familial combined
   mixed
   multiple lipoprotein-type
   remnant
hyperlipoproteinemia (HLP), Fredrickson and Lees classification of
   (type I-V)
hyperlucency
hyperlucent lung
hypermagnesemia
hypernephroma, metastatic to heart
hyperosmotic solution
hyperostosis associated with venous
   malformation
hyperoxaluria
hyperoxia
hyperparathyroidism, primary
hyperpermeability, capillary
hyperpiesia
hyperpiesis
   adrenocortical
   arterial fibromuscular
   congenital adrenal
   congenital segmental renal
   fibrous
   intimal
   medial
   neointimal
hyperplastic lesion
hyperpnea
   paroxysmal
   unloaded
hyperreactivity to isocyanate vapor

hyperreninemia
hyperresonance
hyperresonant percussion note
hyperresponsiveness
   airway
   allergen-induced bronchial
   persistent bronchial
hypersecretion
   ACTH
   mucus
hypersensitive carotid sinus syndrome
hypersensitive xiphoid syndrome
hypersensitivity angiitis
hypersensitivity
   carotid sinus (CSH)
   paraaminosalicylic acid
hypersensitivity pneumonia
hypersensitivity pneumonitis
hypersensitivity reaction
hypersensitivity vasculitis
hypertension (HTN, Htn)
   accelerated
   acquired
   adrenal
   aortic coarctation-related
   arterial (AHT)
   Baumgarten portal
   benign
   borderline
   complicated
   continued arterial
   disproportionate femoral systolic
   essential
   familial pulmonary
   glucocorticoid-induced
   Goldblatt
   Huchard essential
   hyperkinetic
   hypoxic pulmonary
   idiopathic
   intermittent

hypertension *(cont.)*
  intracranial
  labile
  long-standing
  low-renin
  low-renin essential
  malignant
  mineralocorticoid-induced
  obesity-related
  occult
  oral contraceptive-induced
  pale
  paroxysmal
  poorly controlled
  portal
  posterior fossa
  precapillary pulmonary
  pregnancy-induced
  pregnancy-related
  primary
  primary pulmonary (PPH)
  profound
  proximal
  pulmonary (PHTN)
  pulmonary arterial
  pulmonary thromboembolic
  pulmonary venous
  red
  refractory
  renal
  renin-dependent
  renovascular
  secondary
  surgically curable
  sustained
  symptomatic
  systemic
  systemic venous
  systolic
  thromboembolic pulmonary
  untreated
  vascular

hypertension *(cont.)*
  venous
  volume-dependent
  white-coat (fear of doctors)
hypertension exacerbated by dialysis
hypertension secondary to excessive
  licorice ingestion
hypertension variant, Baumgarten
  portal
hypertensive cardiomegaly
hypertensive cardiopathy
hypertensive cardiovascular disease
hypertensive crisis
hypertensive diathesis
hypertensive emergency
hypertensive encephalopathy
hypertensive heart disease
hypertensive ischemic ulcer
hypertensive left ventricular
  hypertrophy
hypertensive paroxysmal crisis
hypertensive renal disease
hypertensive retinopathy
hypertensive vascular degeneration
hypertensive vascular disease
hyperthyroidism
hyperthyroidism-induced atrial
  fibrillation
hypertonic airways
hypertonic saline challenge
hypertonicity
hypertrichosis of skin
hypertriglyceridemia
  carbohydrate-induced
  endogenous
  familial
  sporadic
hypertrophic cardiomyopathy (HC)
hypertrophic obstructive cardiomyopathy (HOC or HOCM)
hypertrophic pulmonary osteoarthropathy

hypertrophic rhinitis
hypertrophic subaortic stenosis
hypertrophied arterioles
hypertrophied heart
hypertrophied intima
hypertrophied myocardium
hypertrophy
  adaptive
  asymmetric septal (ASH)
  biatrial
  biventricular
  cardiac
  concentric left ventricular
  eccentric
  eccentric left ventricular
  four-chamber
  hypertrophic
  left atrial
  left ventricular (LVH)
  lipomatous (of the interatrial
    septum)
  myocardial cellular
  panchamber
  right atrial
  right ventricular (RVH)
  scalenus anticus muscle
  type A (B or C) right ventricular
  unilateral
  ventricular
  Wigle scale for ventricular
hypertrophy of bone
hypertrophy of cardiac muscle fibers
hypertrophy of muscle
hypertrophy of myocardium
hyperuricemia
hypervagotonia
hypervascular arterialization
hyperventilation
  coughing
  eucapnic voluntary
  psychophysiologic
hypervolemia

hyphae
hypoadrenergic orthostatic hypotension
hypoaeration
hypoalbuminemia
hypoaldosteronism, hyporeninemic
hypobarism-acute mountain sickness
hypobasemia
hypocalcemia
hypocapnia
hypocapnic
hypocarbia (hyocapnia)
  alveolar
  arterial
hypochromic anemia
hypochromic microcytic anemia
hypocontractility
hypoechogenic
hypoechoic layer
hypoechoic mantle
hypofunction, adrenal gland
hypogastric artery
hypogastric system
hypogenetic lung syndrome
hypoglossus
hypoglycemia
hypointense
hypokalemia, iatrogenic
hypokalemia-induced arrhythmia
hypokinesia, hypokinesis
  apical
  cardiac
  diffuse
  diffuse ventricular
  global
  hypokinetic
  inferior wall
  regional
  septal
hypokinetic left ventricle
hypokinetic segmental wall motion
hypolucency of lung
hypomagnesemia

hyponatremia
  dilutional
  essential
hypo-osmolality, cellular
hypoparathyroidism
hypoperfusion
  acute alveolar
  apical
  global cerebral
  peripheral
  pulmonary
  resting regional myocardial
  septal
  systemic
hypopharynx
hypophosphatemia
hypoplasia
  alveolar
  annular
  aortic arch
  aortic tract complex
  arterial
  ascending aorta
  congenital isolated
  deep venous
  diffuse
  left ventricle
  left ventricular
  pulmonary artery
  right ventricular
  transverse aortic arch
  ventricular
hypoplasia of aortic annulus
hypoplasia of aortic isthmus
hypoplasia of artery
hypoplasia of vein
hypoplastic aorta syndrome
hypoplastic aortic arch
hypoplastic emphysema
hypoplastic heart
hypoplastic heart ventricle
hypoplastic horizontal ribs

hypoplastic left (or left-sided) heart
  syndrome (HLHS)
hypoplastic left ventricle syndrome
hypoplastic right heart
hypoplastic subpulmonic outflow
hypoplastic tricuspid orifice
hypopnea, obstructive
hypopotassemia
hypoproteinemia
hypoprothrombinemia
hyporeninemic hypoaldosteronism
hyporeninism
hyposensitive carotid sinus syndrome
hyposensitization
hypostatic bronchopneumonia
hypostatic congestion
hypostatic pneumonia
hypostatic pulmonary insufficiency
hypotension
  chronic orthostatic
  drug-induced orthostatic
  exercise-induced
  exertional
  hyperadrenergic orthostatic
  hypoadrenergic orthostatic
  idiopathic orthostatic
  orthostatic
  orthostatic primary
  permanent idiopathic
  postural
  stress-induced
  sympathicotonic orthostatic
  vascular
hypotension unresponsive to volume
  administration
hypotensive response to saralasin
hypothermia
  deep
  endogenous
  local
  mild whole body
  moderate whole body

hypothermia *(cont.)*
  myocardial
  profound
  surface-induced deep
  systemic and topical
  topical
  total body
hypothermia blanket
hypothermic arrest
hypothermic cardioplegic arrest
hypothermic cardiopulmonary bypass
hypothermic circulatory arrest,
  profound (PHCA)
hypothermic fibrillating heart
hypothermic perfusion
hypothermic, profoundly
hypothyroidism
hypotonicity
hypoventilation
  alveolar
  central
  congenital central
  idiopathic
  primary alveolar
hypovolemia, hypovolemic
hypovolemic shock

hypoxanthine
hypoxemia
  arterial
  episodic
  refractory
hypoxemia at rest
hypoxemic respiratory failure
hypoxemic spell
hypoxia
  arterial
  cerebral
  chronic
  myocardial
  relative
hypoxia-ischemia
hypoxic drive
hypoxic-hypercapnic gas
hypoxic pulmonary hypertension
hypoxic pulmonary vasoconstriction
hypoxic spell
hysteresis
  AV (atrioventricular) delay
    (AVDH)
  rate
hysterical syncope
hystericus, globus

I, i

IAB (intra-aortic balloon) catheter
IABP (intra-aortic balloon pump)
IAS (interatrial septum)
iatrogenic avulsion
iatrogenic hypokalemia
iatrogenic puncture
IAVB (incomplete atrioventricular block)
IAVD (incomplete atrioventricular dissociation)
ICA (internal carotid artery)
ICD (internal cardioverter-defibrillator) inappropriate activation of tiered-therapy
ICD-ATP (implantable cardioverter-defibrillator/atrial tachycardia pacing) device
ICD data log
ICD interrogation, transtelephonic
ICE (intracardiac echocardiography)
I-cell disease
ice-pick view on M-mode echocardiogram
ice, topical
ICEG or ICEGM (intracardiac electrogram)

ICHD pacemaker code
ichorous pleurisy
ICS (intracellular-like, calcium-bearing crystalloid solution)
icteric sputum
ICU (intensive care unit)
ICUS (intracoronary ultrasound)
IDC (idiopathic dilated cardiomyopathy)
Ideal cardiac device
idiopathic benign pericarditis
idiopathic bradycardia
idiopathic cardiomegaly
idiopathic cardiomyopathy
idiopathic dilated cardiomyopathy
idiopathic eosinophilic lung disease
idiopathic familial eosinophilia
idiopathic fibrosing alveolitis
idiopathic fibrosis, pulmonary interstitial
idiopathic hemochromatosis
idiopathic hyperaldosteronism (IHA)
idiopathic hypereosinophilic syndrome
idiopathic hypertrophic cardiomyopathy
idiopathic hypertrophic subaortic stenosis (IHSS)

idiopathic hypoventilation
idiopathic mural endomyocardial
    disease
idiopathic obstructive sleep apnea
idiopathic orthostatic hypotension
idiopathic pleural calcification
idiopathic pulmonary arteriosclerosis
    (IPA)
idiopathic pulmonary fibrosis
idiopathic pulmonary hemosiderosis
    (IPH)
idiopathic regressing arteriopathy
idiopathic restrictive cardiomyopathy
idiopathic thrombocytopenic purpura
idiopathic unilobar emphysema
idiopathic ventricular fibrillation
idiopathic ventricular tachycardia
idioventricular rhythm (IVR),
    accelerated
IDL (intermediate density lipoprotein)
IDM (immediate diastolic murmur)
IDSA (intraoperative digital subtrac-
    tion angiography)
IEA (inferior epigastric artery) graft
I:E ("I to E") (inspiratory–expiratory)
    ratio
^{125}I (I 125) fibrinogen scan
IgE level
IHA (idiopathic hyperaldosteronism)
IHSS (idiopathic hypertrophic
    subaortic stenosis)
intra-atrial conduction delay
IJV (internal jugular vein)
ILBBB (incomplete left bundle branch
    block)
iliac artery angioplasty
iliac artery system
iliac atherosclerotic occlusive disease
iliac fossa
iliac-renal bypass graft
iliac stenosis, external
iliac vessel

iliocaval compression syndrome
iliocaval junction
iliocaval tree
iliofemoral bypass
iliofemoral thrombophlebitis
iliofemoral vein thrombosis
iliopopliteal bypass
ilioprofunda bypass graft
ill-defined chest pain
ill-defined mass
illness, flu-like
Illumen-8 guiding catheter
IMA (inferior mesenteric artery)
IMA (internal mammary artery)
IMA graft
IMA pedicle
IMA retractor
image, images (see also *imaging*)
    artifact
    attenuated
    bull's eye
    coronal
    cross-sectional
    delayed
    initial
    intermediate
    sagittal
    silhouette
    tomographic
    T1-weighted
    T2-weighted
    ultrasonic tomographic
image quality degradation
imaging (see also *scan*)
    antifibrin antibody
    cardiac blood pool
    color flow
    C-11 (^{11}C) acetate
    dipyridamole thallium
    Doppler color flow
    duplex
    echoplanar

imaging *(cont.)*
    ED (end-diastolic)
    exercise
    four-hour delayed thallium
    gated cardiac blood pool
    gradient-echo sequence
    indium-111 (^{111}In) antimyosin
    infarct avid
    magnetic resonance (MRI)
    multiple gated equilibrium cardiac
        blood pool
    myocardial perfusion
    postexercise
    radioisotope
    real-time
    redistribution myocardial
    redistribution thallium-201
    regional ejection fraction (REFI)
    rest
    rest myocardial perfusion
    rest thallium-201 myocardial
    rubidium-82
    resting
    stress
    stress thallium-201 myocardial
    technetium (Tc 99m) myocardial
    technetium (Tc 99m) pyrophos-
        phate myocardial
    thallium myocardial perfusion
    thallium-201 myocardial
    timed
    transesophageal Doppler color flow
    ultrafast
imaging agent (see *contrast medium*)
imbalance
    acid-base
    electrolyte
    ventilation-perfusion (V/Q)
    ventilatory capacity-demand
IMI (inferior myocardial infarction)
immediate diastolic murmur (IDM)
immediate intervention

imminent death
imminent demise
immobilization
immobilized
immotile cilia syndrome
immunoassay, reverse
immunoblastoid lymphocytes
immunoblot assay, three-antigen
    recombinant
immunodeficiency with thrombo-
    cytopenia and eczema
immunohemolytic anemia
immunologic deficiencies
immunologic injury
immunologic markers
immunological derangement
immunomodulate
immunoscintigraphy
immunosuppress
immunosuppressive agent
immunosuppressive drug
immunosuppressive induction
immunosuppressive therapy
immunotherapy
impaction, mucoid (in bronchi)
impaired consciousness
impaired exercise capacity
impaired filling pressures
impaired oxygen diffusion
impaired venous return
impaired ventilation-perfusion
impairment
    circulatory
    functional
    inspiratory muscle function
    motor
    renal function
    sensory
impairment of contractility
impedance
    acoustic
    aortic

impedance *(cont.)*
  electrical
  lead
  pacemaker lead
  pulmonary arterial input
  pulmonary vascular bed
  vascular
impedance electrodes
impedance phlebography
impedance plethysmography (IPG)
impede filling
impediment
impending closure
impending doom, feeling of
impending infarction
impending myocardial infarction
imperfecta, osteogenesis
imperforate aneurysm
impinges
impinging
implant threshold
implantable automatic atrial cardioverter-defibrillator
implantable cardioverter-defibrillator
  (ICD)
  Cadence
  Cadence biphasic
  PCD
implantable circulatory support device
implantable system
implantation
  cardioverter/defibrillator
  epicardial
  intrapleural pulse generator
  pacemaker
  permanent pacemaker
  subxiphoid
  subpectoral pulse generator
  transvenous
implantation response
implanted pacemaker

impotence
Impragraft
impulse
  absent apical
  apical
  atrial filling
  bifid precordial
  cardiac
  cardiac apex
  double systolic apical
  downward displacement of apical
  ectopic
  episternal
  fibrillatory
  high-amplitude
  hyperdynamic
  hyperdynamic apical
  hyperdynamic right ventricular
  jugular venous
  juxta-apical
  late systolic
  left parasternal
  left ventricular
  mild systolic
  palpable apical
  paradoxic apical
  point of maximal (PMI)
  precordial
  prolonged left ventricular
  prominent systolic venous
  right parasternal
  sustained apical
  systolic
  undulant
impulse-conducting system of heart
IMV (intermittent mandatory
  ventilation)
inactive mode
inactivity, electrical
inadequate cardiac output
inadequate numbers of platelets

inadequate oxygenation of blood
inadequate runoff
inadequate visualization
inappropriate activation of ICD
inappropriate discharges
inappropriately elevated plasma renin
   activity
inaudible
incentive spirometer, -metry
incessant tachycardia
incision
   anterolateral
   arteriosubmammary
   cervical extension
   collar
   commissural
   cruciate
   Denis Browne abdominal
   flank
   inguinal crease
   intercostal
   left paramedian
   longitudinal
   median sternotomy
   midline hockey-stick
   midline sternotomy
   oblique abdominal
   oblique subcostal
   parasternal
   periosteal
   pleuropericardial
   posterior parietal peritoneal
   posterolateral
   posterolateral thoracotomy
   pterional
   quasitransmural endocardial
   rib-resecting
   stab wound
   stepladder
   sternotomy
   submammary

incision *(cont.)*
   subxiphoid
   suprasternal notch
   thoracicoabdominal
   thoracoabdominal
   thoracotomy
   transverse
   transverse submammary
   trap-door
   visceral rotation
   xiphoid to os pubis
   xiphopubic midline
incision of aorta
incisura
   aortic
   pulmonary artery
incisura apicis cordis
incisura of carotid arterial pulse
inciting event
inciting factors
inclination of the treadmill
inclusion technique of aortic grafting
inclusion technique of Bentall
incoherence, magnetic resonance spin
incompetence
   aortic
   aortic valve
   chronotropic
   communicating vein
   mitral valve
   postphlebitic
   pulmonary
   traumatic tricuspid
   tricuspid valve
   valve
   valvular
incompetence of communicating vein
incompetent valve
incomplete atrioventricular block
   (IAVB)
incomplete Kartagener syndrome

index *(cont.)*
  mean ankle-brachial systolic
    pressure
  mean wall motion score
  mitral flow velocity
  myocardial infarction recovery
    (MIRI)
  myocardial jeopardy
  myocardial O_2 demand
  Nakata
  O_2 consumption
  penile brachial pressure (PBPI)
  postexercise (PEI)
  predicted cardiac
  profundal popliteal collateral
  pulmonary arterial resistance
  pulmonary blood volume (PBVI)
  pulmonic output
  pulsatility
  QOL (quality of life)
  regurgitant
  resting ankle-arm pressure (RAAPI)
  right and left ankle
  stroke (SI)
  stroke volume (SVI)
  stroke work (SWI)
  systemic arteriolar resistance
  systemic output
  systolic pressure-time
  tension-time (TTI)
  thoracic
  venous distensibility (VDI)
  wall motion score
  Wood units
index of runoff resistance
indicator dilution curve
indicator-dilution method for cardiac
  output measurement
indicator fractionation principle
indices (see *index*)
indirect blood supply
indium-labeled antimyosin antibodies

indium 111 (^{111}In)
indium 111 antimyosin antibody
indium 111 radioisotope
indium 111 scintigraphy
indium 111 labeled antimyosin antibody MRI
indocyanine dilution curve
indocyanine green dye for detection of
  intracardial shunt
indocyanine green dye method for
  cardiac output measurement
indolent bacterial infection, chronic
indolent infection in pleural space
indolent ulcer
indomethacin
induced thrombosis of aortic
  aneurysm
inducibility basal state
inducibility, VT (ventricular tachycardia)
inducible
induction
  immunosuppressive
  sputum
induction anesthesia
indurated mass
indurated tissue
induration
  brawny
  brown pulmonary
  erythema without
indurative mediastinitis
indurative pleurisy
induratum, Bazin erythema
inefficiency, ventilatory
inelastic pericardium
inequality, ventilation-perfusion
inexorable progression
in extremis
Inf (infarction)
infant, profoundly obtunded
infantile histiocytoid cardiomyopathy

infantile lobar emphysema
infantile pneumonia
infantile syndrome
infantile thoracic dystrophy
infarct (see also *infarction*)
  anemic
  bland
  embolic
  focal skin
  healing
  hemorrhagic
  livedo reticularis-digital
  red
  thrombotic
  transmural
  transmural myocardial
  uninfected
infarct avid imaging (hot spot scan,
  technetium pyrophosphate scan)
infarct expansion
infarctectomy
infarcted heart muscle
infarcted lung segment
infarcted segment of lung
infarction (see also *infarct*)
  acute myocardial (AMI)
  age indeterminate
  anterior myocardial (AMI)
  anterior-wall myocardial
  anteroinferior myocardial
  anterolateral myocardial
  anteroseptal myocardial
  apical myocardial
  arrhythmic myocardial
  atherothrombotic
  atherothrombotic brain
  atrial
  Battey-avium complex
  cardiac
  cerebral
  concomitant

infarction *(cont.)*
  diaphragmatic myocardial (DMI)
  evolving myocardial
  extensive anterior myocardial
  full-thickness
  high lateral myocardial
  hyperacute myocardial
  impending
  impending myocardial
  inferior myocardial (IMI)
  inferolateral myocardial
  inferoposterolateral myocardial
  intestinal
  intraoperative myocardial
  lacunar
  lateral myocardial
  mesenteric
  myocardial (MI)
  myocardial (see *myocardial infarction*)
  non-Q wave myocardial
  nonarrhythmic myocardial
  nonfatal myocardial
  nontransmural myocardial
  old myocardial
  papillary muscle
  posterior myocardial
  posteroinferior myocardial
  postmyocardial
  postmyocardiotomy
  pulmonary
  Q wave myocardial
  recent myocardial
  right ventricular
  segmental bowel
  septal myocardial
  septic pulmonary
  severe
  silent myocardial
  sinoatrial node
  subacute myocardial

infarction *(cont.)*
  subendocardial (SEI)
  subendocardial myocardial
  transmural myocardial
infarctionlike
infarction of the lung
infarctoid cardiopathy
infarct size limitation
Infasurf
Infatabs
infected lead
infected thrombosed graft
infection
  anaerobic lung
  Ancylostoma braziliense
  Ancylostoma duodenale
  Ascaris lumbricoides
  Ascaris suum
  aspergillosis
  atypical tuberculosis
  bacterial
  Brugia malayi
  chronic indolent bacterial
  Clonorchis sinensis
  clostridial
  complicating
  concurrent
  *Corynebacterium pseudo-
    tuberculosis*
  cytomegalovirus
  Dirofilaria immitis
  Echinococcus granulosus
  endovascular
  Enterobacteriaceae
  enterococcal
  enteroviral
  Epstein-Barr virus
  Haemophilus
  HIV
  intestinal parasitic
  Kingella
  Legionella pneumophila

infection *(cont.)*
  mediastinal
  meningococcal
  Mycobacterium avium-intracellulare
    (MAI)
  Mycobacterium avium complex
    (MAC)
  Mycobacterium simiae
  mycobacterial
  Mycoplasma pneumoniae
  Necator americanus
  Neisseria
  nocardiosis
  nosocomial lung
  nosocomial opportunistic
  opisthorchiasis
  opportunistic
  Paragonimus westermani
  parasitic
  polymicrobial
  primary prosthetic graft
  Pseudomonas aeruginosa
  Rickettsia burnetii
  Schistosoma
  secondary bacterial
  self-limited (limiting) respiratory
  spirochetal
  Staphylococcus aureus
  Strongyloides stercoralis
  superimposed bronchial
  suppurative pulmonary
  Toxocara
  Treponema pallidum
  Trichinella spiralis
  tubercular
  tuberculosis
  viral
  viridans streptococcal
  Wuchereria bancrofti
  Yersinia
infectious disease
infectious insult

infective aneurysmal endocarditis
infective embolism
infective endocarditis, marantic
infective myocarditis
infective pericarditis
infective rhinitis
infective silicosis
infective thrombosis or thrombus
inferior basal segment
inferior border of heart
inferior border of lung
inferior border of rib
inferior bronchi
inferior ligaments
inferior lobe of lung
inferior margin of superior rib
inferior mediastinum
inferior mesenteric artery
inferior pulmonary ligament
inferior pulmonary vein
inferior thyroid vein
inferior tip of the scapula
inferior vena cava (IVC)
inferior vena cava orifice
inferior vena cava syndrome
inferior wall akinesis
inferior wall hypokinesis
inferior wall MI (myocardial
  infarction)
inferobasal
inferolateral displacement of apical
  beat
inferolaterally
inferolateral wall myocardial infarction
inferomedially
inferoposterior wall myocardial
  infarction
inferoposterolateral
infestation
  metazoal
  parasitic
  Plasmodium falciparum

infestation *(cont.)*
  protozoal
  roundworm
  Toxocara canis
infiltrate, infiltration
  aggressive interstitial
  aggressive perivascular
  apical
  basilar
  basilar zone
  bilateral interstitial pulmonary
  bilateral upper lobe cavitary
  bronchocentric inflammatory
  butterfly pattern of
  cavitary
  consolidated
  diffuse
  diffuse aggressive polymorphous
  diffuse alveolar interstitial
  diffuse bilateral alveolar
  diffuse interstitial
  diffuse perivascular
  diffuse reticulonodular
  eosinophilic
  fluffy
  focal interstitial
  focal perivascular
  ground glass
  interstitial
  interstitial nonlobar
  invasive angiomatous interstitial
  lung
  lymphocytic
  massive
  micronodular
  migratory
  mononuclear
  multifocal aggressive
  mural
  patchy, migratory
  peripheral
  pulmonary

infiltrate *(cont.)*
  pulmonary eosinophilic
  pulmonary parenchymal
  reticulonodular
  retrocardiac
  strandy
  sulfasalazine-induced pulmonary
  transient
infiltration of pulmonary parenchyma
infiltrative cardiomyopathy
Infiniti catheter from Cordis
inflamed edematous medium-sized
  bronchi
inflamed pleura
inflamed throat
inflammation
  alveolar septal
  fibrinous
  granulomatous (of bronchi)
  mucosal
inflammation and fibrosis, periaortic
inflammation of a vein
inflammation of cardiac muscle
inflammation of heart muscle
inflammatory adhesions
inflammatory aortoarteritis,
  nonspecific
inflammatory exudate
inflammatory granulomatous reaction
inflammatory myocarditis
inflammatory polypoid mass
inflammatory reaction
inflammatory response syndrome,
  systemic
inflammatory response, whole body
inflated to 300 mm Hg, tourniquet
inflation
  sequential balloon
  simultaneous balloon
inflow cuff
inflow disease progression

inflow tract of left ventricle
influenza
influenzal myocarditis
infra-apical
infra-auricular
infracardiac type total anomalous
  venous return
infraclavicular
infraclavicular pocket
infracolic midline
infracristal ventricular defect
infracristal ventricular septal defect
infradiaphragmatic vein
infragenicular popliteal artery
infragenicular position
infrageniculate artery
infrainguinal bypass stenosis
infrainguinal revascularization
infrainguinal vein bypass graft
infrainguinal vein graft
inframammary crease
inframammary syndrome
inframyocardial
infrapopliteal vessel
infrapulmonary position
infrarenal abdominal aorta
infrarenal aortic disease
infrarenal aortic repair
infrarenal stenosis
infrasternal angle
infundibular atresia
infundibular chamber
infundibular dissection
infundibular pulmonary stenosis
infundibular resection
infundibular septum, parietal extension
  of
infundibular stenosis, subpulmonic
infundibular subpulmonic stenosis
infundibulectomy, right ventricular
infundibuloventricular crest

infundibulum
  os
  right ventricular
infusion
  fresh frozen plasma
  isoproterenol
  packed red blood cells
  prostaglandin
  retrograde coronary sinus
  saralasin
  volume
  whole blood
infusion line, peripheral intravenous
ingestion
  chronic excessive licorice
  chronic salicylate
  salicylate
inguinal crease incision
inguinal region
inhalation
  furosemide
  methacholine chloride
  smoke
  toxic gas
  toxic vapor
inhalation aerosol, pirbuterol acetate
inhalation aspirin challenge
inhalation bronchial challenge testing
inhalation by slow inspiration
inhalation challenge, methacholine
inhalation of beryllium dust
inhalation of dust particles
inhalation of environmental dusts
inhalation of radioactive xenon gas
inhalation pneumonia
inhalation tuberculosis
inhaled bronchodilator
inhaled corticosteroids
inhaler, metered-dose
inherently unstable condition
inhibited respiration

inhibition
  lipoprotein plasminogen
  myopotential
  prostaglandin synthesis
inhibitor
  HMG-CoA reductase
  monoamine oxidase (MAO)
  phosphodiesterase
  thrombus
inhibitor of platelet aggregation
initial shock
injection
  bolus
  double
  hand
  intra-amniotic
  intra-arterial
  intramuscular (I.M.)
  intramuscular fetal
  intraperitoneal fetal
  intravascular
  intravenous (I.V.)
  intravenous bolus
  intravenous fetal
  manual
  opacifying
  power
  sclerosing
  selective
  serial
  straight AP pelvic
injection at peak exercise
injection port
injection test for pneumoperitoneum
injector
  Hercules power
  Medrad power angiographic
  pressure
injury
  blunt
  brachial plexus

injury *(cont.)*
  concomitant tracheal
  crushing
  decelerative
  immunologic
  intercostal nerve
  obstetrical
  penetrating lung
  pulmonary parenchymal
  radial vascular thermal
  rapid deceleration
  subendocardial
  through-and-through
Injury Scale, Abbreviated
Injury Severity Score (ISS)
inner bright layer
innermost intercostal muscles
innocent heart murmur
innocuous
innominate (*not* innominant)
innominate artery arteritis
innominate artery buckling
innominate artery kinking
innominate artery, penetrating injury to
innominate artery stenosis
innominate (brachiocephalic) veins
Innovator Holter system
inoperable disease
inotropes
inotropic activity of drug
inotropic activity of the heart,
  increased
inotropic agent
inotropic effect
inotropic state
inotropic stimulation
inotropic support
inotropic therapy
Inoue balloon catheter
insertion
  chordal
  percutaneous (via femoral vein)

insidious onset
insidious progression
in situ bypass
in situ graft
in situ grafting
in situ vein graft
inspiration, inhalation by slow
inspiration phase
inspiratory augmentation of A_2-P_2
  interval (heart sounds)
inspiratory crepitation
inspiratory dyspnea
inspiratory-expiratory breath sounds
inspiratory-expiratory (I:E) ratio
inspiratory flow rates, rapid
inspiratory flow-volume, tidal
inspiratory increase in venous pressure
inspiratory maneuvers, repetitive
  maximal (against closed shutter)
inspiratory muscle function impairment
inspiratory phase
inspiratory prolongation of interval
inspiratory rales
inspiratory reserve volume (IRV)
inspiratory retraction
inspiratory rhonchi, post-tussive
inspiratory spasm
inspiratory wheeze
InspirEase device
inspired air
inspissated mucus
instability
  hemodynamic
  ischemic
  ventricular electrical
instantaneous gradient
Instat collagen absorbable hemostatic
  agent
INSTAT MCH (microfibrillar
  hemostat)
in-stent balloon redilation
instrument, tunneling

instrumentation
insufficiency
  acute cerebrovascular
  acute coronary
  aortic (AI)
  aortic valve
  arterial
  autonomic
  basilar artery
  brachial-basilar
  cardiac
  cardiopulmonary
  chronic venous
  congenital pulmonary valve
  coronary
  hypostatic pulmonary
  mitral (MI)
  myocardial (MI)
  nonocclusive mesenteric arterial
  nonrheumatic aortic
  postirradiation vascular
  post-traumatic pulmonary
  pulmonary (PI)
  pulmonary valve
  renal
  respiratory
  Sternberg myocardial
  transient ischemic carotid
  tricuspid (TI)
  valvular
  valvular aortic
  venous
  vertebrobasilar arterial
insufficiency of aortic valve
insufficient pulmonary arterial flow
insulating pad to retard premature
  rewarming
insult
  aortic
  infectious
  toxic
intact Medtronic xenograft valve

intact valve cusp
intact ventricular septum
Intact xenograft prosthetic valve
intake, restricted fluid
Intec implantable defibrillator
integral
  aortic flow velocity
  pulmonary flow velocity
integrated bipolar sensing
integrity of the suture line violated
intense disabling cramping
intensity
  angina with recent increase in
  decreased
  equal in
  maximal
  signal
  variable
intensity of heart sounds
intensive care unit (ICU)
intentional transoperative hemodilution
interatrial baffle
interatrial baffle leak
interatrial communication
interatrial groove
interatrial septal defect
interatrial septum, lipomatous hypertrophy of the
interatrial transposition of venous
  return
interbronchial mass
intercaval band
intercellular edema
intercellular space
interchondral joint
interchordal hooding
interchordal space fenestration
intercommunicating channels
intercoronary anastomosis
intercoronary collateral flow
intercoronary steal syndrome
intercostal artery

intercostal bundle fibers
intercostal incision
intercostal lymph nodes
intercostal muscle
intercostal nerve injury
intercostal neuromuscular bundle
intercostal retraction on inspiration
intercostal space
　　left fifth
　　ninth
　　right first
　　right second
intercostal vein
intercostal vessels
interdiction
interdigitating coil stent
interface
　　air (on x-ray)
　　catheter-skin
　　media-adventitia
interference dissociation
interferon level
interfibrosis
interlobar empyema
interlobar fissure
interlobar pleurisy
interlobar septa
interlobular emphysema
interlobular pleurisy
interlobular septa
interlobular vessels
intermedia, angina
intermediate artery
intermediate coronary syndrome
intermediate-density lipoprotein
intermediate heart
intermediate images
intermediate tuberculin test
Intermedics epicardial pacing lead
Intermedics patch leads
Intermedics Quantum pacemaker
intermedius, bronchus

intermittent apneic episodes
intermittent cannon a waves on jugular
　　venous pulse tracing
intermittent claudication
intermittent junctional bradycardia
intermittent mandatory ventilation
　　(IMV)
intermittent occlusion
intermittent positive pressure breathing
　　(IPPB)
intermittent venous claudication
internal caliber
internal capsule intracerebral hemor-
　　rhage
internal carotid artery
internal clot
internal elastic lamina
internal intercostal membrane
internal intercostal muscles
internal jugular approach for cardiac
　　catheterization
internal jugular bulb
internal jugular triangle
internal jugular vein
internal jugular venous cannula
internal mammary artery (IMA)
internal pacemaker
internal saphenous vein grafting
internal thoracic artery
internal thoracic vein
internodal pathway
internodal tract
interpleural analgesia
interpleural space
interpolated ventricular premature
　　complex
interposition graft
interrenal stenosis
interrogation
　　color-duplex
　　pulse Doppler
　　transtelephonic ICD

interrupted aortic arch
interrupted pledgeted sutures
interruption, aortic arch
interscapulovertebral arterial bruit
interspace
 fifth left
 fourth left
 second left
 third left
interstitial arteriosclerotic nephritis
interstitial diffuse pulmonary fibrosis
interstitial edema
interstitial emphysema
interstitial fibrosis
interstitial fluid
interstitial infiltrate
 diffuse alveolar
 invasive angiomatous
interstitial lung disease (ILD),
 rheumatoid-arthritis-associated
interstitial markings, increased
interstitial nonlobar infiltrates
interstitial plasma cell pneumonia
interstitial pneumonia air leak
interstitial pneumonia, lymphoid
interstitial prematurity fibrosis
interstitial pulmonary edema
interstitial pulmonary fibrosis
interstitial scarring
interstitial space
interstitial tissues
interstitium
Intertach pacemaker
interval
 A-A
 A_1-A_2
 abbreviated
 A-C
 acquired prolonged Q-T
 Ae-H
 A-H
 A_2 incisural

interval *(cont.)*
 A_2/MVO (aortic valve closure to
 mitral valve opening)
 A_2 to opening snap
 atrial escape (AEI)
 atrioventricular
 AV (atrioventricular)
 AV delay (AVDI)
 cardioarterial
 confidence
 coupling
 escape
 fixed coupling
 flutter R
 H-Ae
 hangout
 H-H'
 H1-H2
 H'P
 H-Q
 H-QRS
 H-V
 inspiratory prolongation
 interectopic
 isoelectric
 long Q-T
 lower rate
 P-A
 pacemaker escape
 P-H
 P-P
 P-R
 preejection
 prolongation of QRS
 prolonged
 prolonged P-R
 prolonged Q-T
 Q to first sound
 Q-T
 Q-H
 QRS
 QRST

interval *(cont.)*
  Q-S$_1$
  Q-S$_2$
  Q-T
  Q-Tc
  Q-U
  right ventricular systolic time
    (RVSTI)
  R-P
  R-R
  S-QRS
  S$_1$-S$_2$
  S$_1$-S$_3$
  S$_2$OS (second sound to opening
    snap)
  short P-Q
  short P-R
  spike-Q
  ST
  systolic time (STI)
  upper rate
  V-A
  varying P-R
  V-H
interval development (on x-ray)
interval intra-atrial conduction
intervention
  immediate
  surgical
  therapeutic
interventional EP (electrophysiology)
interventional equipment
interventional procedure
interventricular (IV)
interventricular conduction delay
interventricular groove
  anterior
  posterior
interventricular septal defect
interventricular septum
interventricular sulcus, posterior
interventricular vein, posterior

intestinal emphysema
intestinal parasitic infection
intima
  diffuse thickening of arterial
  friable thickened degenerated
  hypertrophied
  tunica
intimal atherosclerotic disease
intimal debris
intimal dissection
intimal fibroplasia
intimal flap
intimal hyperplasia
intimal irregularity
intimal-medial dissection
intimal proliferation
intimal tear
intimal thickening
intimate attachment of diseased vessel
intimomedial thickness
intolerance
  exercise
  heat
in toto
intoxication, potassium
intra-abdominal arterial bypass graft
intra-acinar pulmonary arteries
intra-adrenal pheochromocytoma
intra-alveolar fibrosis
intra-amniotic injection
intra-aortic balloon assist
intra-aortic balloon counterpulsation
intra-aortic balloon double-lumen
  catheter
intra-aortic balloon pump (IABP)
intra-arterial filling defects
intra-arterially
intra-arterial thrombus
intra-articular ligament
intra-atrial baffle
intra-atrial baffle operation
intra-atrial conduction defect

intra-atrial conduction interval
intra-atrial electrogram
intra-atrial filling defect
intra-atrial reentrant tachycardia
intra-atrial reentry
intra-atrial thrombi
intracardiac baffle
intracardiac calcium
intracardiac echocardiography (ICE)
intracardiac electrogram
intracardiac mass
intracardiac pressure in Doppler
echocardiogram
intracardiac repair
intracardiac right-to-left shunt
intracardiac shunt
intracardiac shunting
intracardiac thrombus
Intracath catheter
intracavitary clot formation
intracavitary electrogram
intracavitary extension of tumor
intracavitary filling defect
intracavitary pressure-electrogram
dissociation
intracerebral hemorrhage
basilar
bulbar
cerebellar
cerebral
cerebromeningeal
cortical
internal capsule
intrapontine
pontine
subcortical
ventricular
intracoronary ethanol ablation
intracoronary stent placement
intracoronary stenting
intracoronary thrombolytic therapy
intracoronary ultrasound (ICUS)

intracranial berry aneurysm
intracranial hemorrhage
intracranial hypertension
intracranial pressure, increased
intracranial tuberculoma
intractable heart failure
intractable bleeding disorder
intradiaphragmatic aortic segment
intraerythrocytic *Babesia*
intra-Hisian (or intrahisian) AV block
intra-Hisian (or intrahisian) delay
intraluminal defect
intraluminal dimension
intraluminal filling defect
intraluminal flow, turbulent
intraluminal sutureless prosthesis
intraluminal thrombus, laminated
intramural arterial hemorrhage
intramural coronary artery aneurysm
intramural hematoma, acute
intramuscular aortic segment
intramuscular fetal injection
intramuscular hemangioma
intramuscular ketamine
intramyocardial electrocardiography
during sleep
intramyocardially
intranodal block
Intra-Op autotransfusion
intraoperative arteriography
intraoperative autologous transfusion
(IOAT)
intraoperative digital subtraction
angiography (IDSA)
intraoperative hypotension
intraoperative laser ablation
intraoperative laser photocoagulation
of ventricular tachycardia
intraoperative myocardial infarction
intraoperative testing
intraosseous vascular malformations
intrapericardial bleeding

intrapericardial dissection
intrapericardial ligation
intrapericardial patch lead placement
intrapericardial poudrage
intrapericardial pressure
intraperitoneal exposure
intraperitoneal fetal injection
intraperitoneal migration of pacemaker
intrapleural hemorrhage
intrapleural implantation of pulse
    generator
intrapleurally
intrapleural pressure
intrapontine intracerebral hemorrhage
intrapulmonary disease
intrapulmonary hemorrhage
intrapulmonary pressure
intrapulmonary shunt (or shunting)
intrarenal hematoma
intraretinal microangiopathy (IRMA)
intrathoracic airways obstruction
intrathoracic dimension
intrathoracic Kaposi sarcoma
intrathoracic pressure
intrathoracic upper airway obstruction
intrauterine cardiac failure
intrauterine growth retardation
    (IUGR)
intrauterine heart failure
intravascular clotting process
intravascular coagulation, disseminated
intravascular coagulation of blood
intravascular contents, secondary
    extravasation of
intravascular filling defect
intravascular fragmentation of red
    blood cells
intravascular mass
intravascular oxygenator (IVOX)
    artificial lung
intravascular polymorphonuclear
    leukocytosis

intravascular pressure
intravascular prosthesis
intravascular sickling, lung
intravascular space
intravascular stenting
intravascular thrombosis
intravascular ultrasound (IVUS)
intravascular volume depletion
intravascular volume status
intravascularly volume depleted
intravenous (I.V. or IV)
intravenous bolus
intravenous bolus injection
intravenous coronary thrombolysis
intravenous fetal injection
intravenous fluorescein angiography
    (IVFA)
intravenous infusion line, peripheral
intravenous line
intravenous pyelogram, -graphy (IVP)
    excretory
    rapid-sequence
intravenous TKO (to keep open [the
    vein, needle, or catheter])
intraventricular aberration
intraventricular block, conduction
    delay
intraventricular conduction abnormality
intraventricular conduction defect
intraventricular conduction delay
intraventricular hemorrhage (IVH)
intraventricular right ventricular
    obstruction
intraventricular systolic tension
intraventricular tunnel repair
Intrepid PTCA catheter
intrinsic asthma
intrinsic deflection
intrinsic disease
intrinsic heart rate
intrinsic positive end-expiratory
    pressure

intrinsic pulmonary disease
intrinsic sensing
intrinsic sick sinus syndrome
intrinsic stenotic lesions
intrinsic vein graft lesion
intrinsic vein graft stenosis
intrinsicoid deflection
introduced, catheter
introducer
    Becton-Dickinson
    Check-Flo
    Cook
    Desilets-Hoffman catheter
    electrode
    Hemaquet catheter
    Hemaquet sheath
    heparin lock
    Littleford-Spector
    LPS Peel-Away
    Mullins catheter
    Pacesetter
    peel-away
    percutaneous lead
    permanent lead
    Tuohy-Borst
introducer sheath
intubate
intubated
intubation
    blind nasal
    direct vision nasal
    direct vision orotracheal
    endotracheal
    orotracheal
intussusception of vein
in utero exposure
invaginate
invagination
invariability of cardiac dullness during
    phases of respiration
invariable

invasion
    exogenous
    mediastinal
invasive angiomatous interstitial
    infiltration
invasive cardiology
inverse inspiratory/expiratory time
    ratio
inversion
    diffuse T wave
    isolated ventricular
    T wave
inversus
    situs
    situs viscerum
inversus totalis, situs
inverted P wave
inverted T waves in V_1 and V_3
inverted terminal T wave
inverted U wave
inverted Y configuration
in vivo balloon pressure
involvement of lingula
IOAT (intraoperative autologous
    transfusion)
Ioban prep
iodine (see *contrast medium*)
Ionescu-Shiley bioprosthetic valve
Ionescu-Shiley bovine pericardial
    valve
Ionescu-Shiley heart valve
Ionescu-Shiley low-profile prosthetic
    valve
Ionescu-Shiley pericardial xenograft
    valve
Ionescu-Shiley standard pericardial
    prosthetic valve
Ionescu-Shiley valve prosthesis
Ionescu-Shiley vascular graft
Ionescu tri-leaflet valve
ionic potassium

IPA (idiopathic pulmonary arteriosclerosis)
IPG (impedance plethysmography)
IPH (idiopathic pulmonary hemosiderosis)
IPH (intraplaque hemorrhage)
IPPA (iodine-123 phenylpentadecanoic
  acid)
IPPB (intermittent positive pressure
  breathing)
ipsilateral hemispheric carotid TIA
  (transient ischemic attack)
ipsilateral nonreversed greater
  saphenous vein bypass
IRBBB (incomplete right bundle
  branch block)
Irex Exemplar ultrasound
IRMA (intraretinal microangiopathy)
iron-deficiency anemia
iron overloading
iron storage disease
irradiation pneumonia
irregular hazy luminal contour
irregular heartbeat
irregular mass, polypoid calcified
irregular rhythm, sinusoidal
irregularity
  diffuse
  intimal
  luminal
  pulse
irregularly irregular cardiac rhythm
irreversible airways obstruction
irreversible ischemia
irreversible narrowing of the
  bronchioles
irreversible organ failure
irrigation, saline
irritability
  atrial
  myocardial
  ventricular

irritable heart
irritant-induced asthma
irritants
  exposure to
  nonspsecific
  respiratory
irritation, bronchial
IRV (inspiratory reserve volume)
Isch (ischemia)
ischemia
  brachiocephalic
  cardiac
  carotid artery
  cerebral
  coronary
  exercise-induced
  exercise-induced myocardial
  exercise-induced transient
    myocardial
  global myocardial
  hypoxia-
  irreversible
  limb-threatening
  myocardial
  nonlocalized
  peri-infarction
  provocable
  regional myocardial
  regional transmural
  remote
  reversible
  segmental
  silent
  silent myocardial
  subendocardial
  transient cerebral
  transient myocardial
  vertebral-basilar
  vertebrobasilar
  zone of
ischemic cardiomyopathy
ischemic changes, persistence of

ischemic congestive cardiomyopathy
ischemic contracture
ischemic decompensation
ischemic disease
ischemic episode
ischemic event
ischemic heart disease (IHD)
ischemic heart disease syndrome
ischemic instability
ischemic necrosis
ischemic-reperfusion injury
ischemic rest pain
ischemic segment (on echocardiogram)
ischemic ST segment changes
ischemic time
ischemic ulcer, hypertensive
ischemic viable myocardium
ischemic zone
ischemically mediated mitral
   regurgitation
isocapnic hyperventilation-induced
   bronchoconstriction
isoelectric at J point
isoelectric line
isoelectric period
isoelectric ST segment
isoenzyme
  cardiac
  CK
  CK-BB (CK$_1$)
  CK-MB
  CK-MM (CK$_3$)
  CPK
  CPK-MB (CK$_2$)
  LDH$_1$ (LDH1)
  LDH$_2$ (LDH2)
  Regan
  serial cardiac
isolated diffuse myocarditis
isolated heat perfusion of an extremity
isolated ventricular inversion

isolation, respiratory
isomerism, atrial
isometric exercise stress test
isometric heart contraction
isometrics
isoproterenol infusion
isorhythmic AV (atrioventricular)
  dissociation
isotonic exercise
isotonic heart contraction
isotope (see *contrast medium*)
isotropic lung scan
isovolumetric contraction
isovolumetric period
isovolumic contraction time
isovolumic period
isovolumic relaxation
ISS (Injury Severity Score)
isthmic coarctation, congenital
isthmus
  aortic
  stenotic
isthmus aneurysm
isthmus of aorta
isthmus of Vieussens
Isuprel drip
ITA (internal thoracic artery) graft
ITC balloon catheter
IUGR (intrauterine growth retardation)
IV (interventricular) septum
I.V. or IV (intravenous)
I.V. bolus
I.V. drip
I.V. TKO (to keep open)
Ivalon prosthesis
IVB (intraventricular block)
IVC (inferior vena cava)
IVC filter
  percutaneous
  prophylactic
Ivemark syndrome

IVFA (intravenous fluorescein
   angiography)
IVH (intraventricular hemorrhage)
IVOX (intravascular oxygenator)
   artificial lung
IVP (intravenous pyelogram)
IVR (idioventricular rhythm)

IVS (interventricular septum)
IVSD (interventricular septal defect)
IVST (interventricular septal thickness)
IVUS (intravascular ultrasound)
Ivy bleeding time
Ixodes dammini

J, j

J (joule)
JA (jet area)
Jaccoud arthritis
Jaccoud sign
jacket, Medtronic cardiac cooling
Jackman orthogonal catheter
Jackson bronchoscope
Jackson-Olympus bronchoscope
Jackson sign
Jacobson-Potts clamp
Jaffé rate reaction, creatinine estimated using
Jahnke anastomosis clamp
Jako anterior commissure scope
James atrionodal bypass tract
James bundles or fibers
James intranodal bypass tract
Janeway lesion in infective endocarditis
Janeway skin lesion in bacterial endocarditis
Jannetta dissector
Janus syndrome
Jarvik-7 (and 8) artificial heart
Jarvik 7-70 total artificial heart
Jatene arterial switch procedure
Jatene-Macchi prosthetic valve

Jatene operation for transposition of great arteries
Javid carotid artery clamp
Javid endarterectomy shunt
Jelco intravenous catheter
Jelco needle
jeopardize
jeopardy, myocardial
Jerome Kay technique
Jervell and Lange-Nielsen syndrome
jet
    central
    high-velocity
    regurgitant
jet area (JA)
jet length (JL)
jet lesion
jet nebulizer
Jeune syndrome
Jeune-Tommasi syndrome
jeweler's forceps
Jewel pulse generator
J guide, Teflon
J guide wire
JL (jet length)
JL4 (Judkins left 4) catheter
JL5 (Judkins left 5) catheter

J loop technique on catheterization
Jobst compression stockings
Jobst garment
Jobst stockings
Jobst-Stride (or Stridette) support
  stockings
Johns Hopkins coarctation clamp
Johns Hopkins forceps
Johnson thoracic forceps
joint
  costochondral
  costotransverse
  costovertebral
  interchondral
  manubriosternal
  secondary cartilaginous
  sternal
  sternoclavicular
  sternocostal
  xiphisternal
joint hyperextendability
joint of thorax
Jonas modification of Norwood
  procedure
Jones criteria for acute rheumatic
  fever
Jones IMA forceps
Jones thoracic clamp
J orthogonal electrode
joule (pl. joules) (J)
joule shocks
J (junction) point on EKG tracing
J tip wire
J-tipped exchange guide wire
J-shaped lead
J-shaped tube
J-tipped spring guide wire
judicious vasodilation
Judkins 4 diagnostic catheter
Judkins cardiac catheterization
Judkins coronary angiography
Judkins coronary arteriography

Judkins coronary catheter
Judkins femoral catheterization
Judkins left 4 coronary catheter (JL4)
Judkins right 4 coronary catheter
  (JR4)
Judkins selective coronary
  arteriography
Judkins USCI catheter
jugular bulb, internal
jugular pulse tracing
jugular triangle, internal
jugular vein
  anterior
  external
jugular vein distention (JVD)
jugular veins filled from above
jugular veins filled from below
jugular venous distention (JVD)
jugular venous excursions
jugular venous impulse
jugular venous pressure (JVP)
jugular venous pressure collapse
jugular venous pulsation (pulse)
jugulovenous distention (JVD)
Julian thoracic forceps
jump vein graft
jump-graft
Junct (junctional)
junction
  aortic sinotubular
  atriocaval
  atrioventricular
  cardiophrenic
  caval-atrial
  chondrosternal
  costochondral
  iliocaval
  J
  mucocutaneous
  saphenofemoral
  sinotubular
  sternoclavicular

junctional bradycardia
junctional defect
junctional escape beats, atrio-
    ventricular
junctional extrasystole
junctional focus
junctional (nodal) rhythm
junctional impulse
junctional premature complex
junctional premature contraction,
    atrioventricular (AV)
junctional tachycardia
junction between AV node and bundle
    of His
June grass
Jürgensen sign
juvenile laryngoscope
juvenile sulfatidosis
juxta-anastomotic stenoses

juxta-apical impulse
juxta-arterial ventricular septal defect
juxtacapillary J receptors
juxtacrural
juxtaductal
juxtaductal coarctation of aorta
juxtaglomerular cell tumor
juxtaposed leftward
juxtaposed rightward
juxtaposition
juxtarenal aortic aneurysm
juxtarenal aortic atherosclerosis
juxtarenal cava
juxtatricuspid ventricular septal defect
JVD (jugulovenous or jugular venous
    distention)
JVP (jugular venous pressure)
J wave on EKG
J wire

K, k

K (vitamin) antagonist therapy
Kabuki make-up syndrome
kaliuretic effect of licorice
kallikrein-kinin system
Kalos pacemaker
Kangaroo pump
Kantrowitz vascular scissors
Kaplan-Meier life-table
Kaposi sarcoma
  endobronchial
  epicardial
  intrathoracic
  myocardial infiltration by
  pulmonary
Kaposi-Besnier-Libman-Sacks
  syndrome
Kapp-Beck-Thomson clamp
Karmody venous scissors
karolysis
Karp aortic punch forceps
Karplus sign of pleural effusion
Kartagener syndrome
Kartagener triad
Kartchner carotid artery clamp
karyorrhexis
Kasabach-Merritt phenomenon
Kasabach-Merritt syndrome

Kast syndrome
Kaster mitral valve prosthesis
Katayama snails
Katayama syndrome
Kattus treadmill exercise protocol
Katz-Wachtel phenomenon or sign
Kawai bioptome
Kawasaki disease or syndrome
Kawashima technique
Kaye-Damus-Stansel operation
Kayexalate enema
Kay-Lambert clamp
Kay-Shiley disk valve prosthesis
Kay-Shiley mitral valve
Kay-Suzuki disk prosthetic valve
Kay tricuspid valvuloplasty
KDA profile
Kearns-Sayre syndrome
keeled chest
keel, laryngeal
keel-like ridge
Keith bundle of fibers in heart
Keith-Flack sinoatrial node
Keith-Wagener-Barker classification of
  arteriolosclerosis, based on retinal
  changes, group 1-4
Kell blood antibody type

Kell blood group
Kellock sign of pleural effusion
Kelly forceps, curved
Kelly hemostat
Kelly retractor
Kelvin Sensor pacemaker
Kemp-Elliot-Gorlin syndrome
Kempner rice diet
Kendall Sequential Compression
    Device
Kennedy area-length method
Kennedy method for calculating
    ejection fraction
Kensey atherectomy catheter
Kensey catheter
Kent atrioventricular bundle in the
    heart
Kent bundle
Kent fibers
Kerckring nodule
Kerley A, B, or C lines
Kerrison rongeur
Keshan disease
ketamine, intramuscular
kick, atrial (AK)
Kidd blood antibody type
kidney arteriovenous fistula
kidney, Ask-Upmark
kidney transplantation
Killip classification (I through IV) of
    heart disease
Killip classification of pump failure
Killip-Kimball classification of heart
    failure
Killip wire to give heart shock during
    cardiac arrest
kilopound
Kim-Ray Greenfield caval filter
Kim-Ray Greenfield inferior vena
    caval filter
Kindt carotid artery clamp

kinetocardiogram
King bioptome
King cardiac device
King-Mills procedure
King multipurpose coronary graft
    catheter
King syndrome
Kingella infection
kinked innominate artery
kinking
    carotid artery
    innominate artery
kinking carotid artery
kinking of blood vessel
kinking of catheter
kinking of graft
kinking of patch
kinking of vessels secondary to shift
    of intrathoracic structures
kinocardiography
Kinsey atherectomy catheter
Kirklin atrial retractor
Kirklin fence
kissing atherectomy technique
kissing balloon technique
Klauder syndrome
Klebsiella pneumoniae
Klebsiella rhinoscleromatis
Klein-Waardenburg syndrome
Klippel-Feil sequence
Klippel-Feil syndrome
Klippel-Trénaunay syndrome
Klippel-Trénaunay-Weber syndrome
knee-chest position
knife
    Bailey-Glover-O'Neill commis-
        surotomy
    Bard-Parker
    Beaver
    Brock commissurotomy
    cautery

knife *(cont.)*
  commissurotomy
  Derra commissurotomy
  intimectomy
  Lebsche sternal
knitted Dacron graft
knitted double velour Dacron patch
  graft
knitted tantalum
knob
  aortic
  blurring of aortic
knock, pericardial
knots, half-hitch
knuckle sign
Kobert test for hemoglobin
Kocher grasping forceps
Kocher hemostats
Kocher maneuver
Koch reaction
Koch sinoatrial node
Koch triangle, apex of
Koch reaction
Koch sinoatrial node
KoGENate blood factor VIII product
Kohn, pores of
Kommerell diverticulum
Konno bioptome
Konno operation for aortic stenosis
Konno procedure for patch enlarge-
  ment of ascending aorta
Kontron balloon catheter

Kontron intra-aortic balloon
"koo sur koo" (coup sur coup)
Korányi-Grocco sign
Korányi-Grocco triangle
Korányi sign of pleural effusion
Korotkoff heart sound in blood
  pressure
Korotkoff method in Doppler
  cerebrovascular examination
Korotkoff sounds
Korotkoff test for collateral circulation
Kouchoukos method
Krayenbuehl vessel hook
Krehl, tendon of
Kronecker puncture
Krovetz and Gessner equation
Kugel anastomosis
Kugel artery
Kugel collaterals
Kugelberg-Welander syndrome
Kurtz-Sprague-White syndrome
Kussmaul breathing
Kussmaul-Maier disease
Kussmaul-Maier variant
Kussmaul respiration
Kussmaul syndrome
Kussmaul venous sign
Kveim test
KVO (keep vein open) rate
kyphoscoliotic heart disease
kyphosis, loss of thoracic

L, l

LA (left atrium)
LAA (left atrial appendage)
LAA (left auricular appendage)
LA/AR (left atrium/aortic root) ratio
LABA (laser-assisted balloon angioplasty)
Labbé syndrome
labeling, radioactive
labile blood pressure
labile hypertension
laboratory
    cardiac catheterization
    EP (electrophysiology)
labored breathing
labored respirations
LACD (left apexcardiogram,
calibrated displacement)
lactate dehydrogenase (LDH)
lactate, elevated plasma
lactic acid accumulation
lactic dehydrogenase
lacunae, bluish nail
lacunar infarct
LAD (left anterior descending)
coronary artery
LAD (left axis deviation)
LAD saphenous vein graft angioplasty

LAD wraps around the apex
Ladder diagram
LAE (left atrial enlargement)
Laënnec pearls
Laënnec sign
LAFB (left anterior fascicular block)
Lahey bag
Lahey thoracic forceps
LAID (left anterior internal diameter)
LAIS excimer laser for coronary
angioplasty
lake, lipid
Laks method
LAMA (laser-assisted microvascular
anastomosis)
LAMB (lentigines, atrial myxoma,
blue nevi) syndrome
Lambda pacemaker
Lambert aortic clamp
Lambert-Eaton syndrome
Lambert-Kay vascular clamp
Lambl excrescences
lamellar body density (LBD) count
lamina
    elastic
    internal elastic
lamina propria

laminated clot
laminar flow
laminated intraluminal thrombus
laminography, cardiac
Landis-Gibbon test
Lancisi muscle
Lancisi sign
landmark, bony
Landolfi sign
Landouzy-Dejerine dystrophy
Langerhans cell granulomatosis
Langhans giant cells
LAO (left anterior oblique)
LAO position
LAO projection
LAP (left atrial pressure)
laparotomy, median xiphopubic
Laplace effect
Laplace law
Laplace mechanism
large-bore slotted aspirating needle
large-caliber tube
large-cell carcinoma
large defibrillating patch
large obtuse marginal branch
large patch lead
large Q waves
large thymus shadow obscuring
　　cardiac silhouette
large vein pulsation
large venous tributaries
laryngeal cartilage
laryngeal edema
laryngeal epilepsy
laryngeal fistulectomy
laryngeal fracture
laryngeal keel
laryngeal nerve, recurrent
laryngeal nodule
laryngeal rales
laryngeal vertigo
laryngeal vestibule

laryngeal web
laryngectomy, radical
laryngis, pachyderma
laryngismus stridulus
laryngitis
　　acute
　　catarrhal
　　Haemophilus influenzae
　　hypertrophic
laryngitis sicca
laryngogram, contrast
laryngopharyngectomy
laryngoplegia
laryngoscope
　　juvenile
　　pediatric
laryngospasm
laryngostomy
laryngotracheal bronchitis
laryngotracheal fistulectomy
laryngotracheitis
larynx, artificial
laser
　　ARC (argon beam electro-
　　　　coagulator)
　　argon
　　CO_2 (carbon dioxide)
　　erbium:YAG
　　excimer
　　helium-neon
　　Ho:YAG (holmium:yttrium
　　　　aluminum garnet)
　　holmium
　　infrared-pulsed
　　ion
　　Lastec System angioplasty
　　microsecond pulsed flashlamp
　　　　pumped dye
　　Nd:YAG (neodymium:yttrium-
　　　　aluminum-garnet)
　　XeCl
laser ablation

laser angioplasty
laser-assisted balloon angioplasty
(LABA)
laser-assisted microvascular
anastomosis (LAMA)
laser balloon angioplasty (LBA)
laser desiccation of thrombus
Laserdish electrode
Laserdish pacing lead
Laserflo blood perfusion monitor
(BPM)
laser-light vaporization of intimal
plaque material
laser photocoagulation, intraoperative
(for ventricular tachycardia)
laser photocoagulation of capillary
malformation (CM)
Laserprobe-PLR Plus
laser recanalization
laser thermal coronary angioplasty
LASH (left anterior-superior hemiblock)
Laslett-Short syndrome
Lastac System angioplasty laser
late asthmatic response
late diastolic murmur
late false aneurysm
late graft occlusion
late inspiratory crackles
late-onset asthma
late phase
late potential activity, ventricular
late potentials (after-potentials)
lateral basal bronchi
lateral bronchi
lateral costotransverse ligament
lateral decubitus position
lateral leaflet obliteration
lateral precordial leads
lateral precordium
lateral thoracic vein periphlebitis
lateral thrombus

lateral webs
late systolic bulge
late systolic click
late systolic honk
late systolic impulse
late systolic murmur (LSM)
late systolic posterior displacement on
echocardiogram
late systolic retraction
late systolic whoop
latissimus dorsi muscle
Laubry-Pezzi syndrome
Laurence-Moon-Biedl-Bardet
syndrome
lavage
bronchoalveolar (BAL)
bronchopulmonary
bronchoscopy
continuous pericardial
pleural
saline
tracheal bronchial
tracheobronchial
law
Einthoven
Laplace
Starling
laxa, cutis
layer
bright
circumferential echodense
echodense
echo-free
hypoechoic
inner bright
musculofascial
parietal
platysma
sonolucent
subcuticular
visceral
lazy leukocyte syndrome

LBA (laser balloon angioplasty)
LBBB (left bundle branch block)
LBCD (left border of cardiac dullness)
LCA (left coronary artery)
LCF or LCX (left circumflex)
coronary artery
LCL (Levinthal-Coles-Lillie) bodies
LD or LDH (lactate dehydrogenase)
LD_1 or LDH_1 isoenzyme
LD_2 or LDH_2 isoenzyme
LDH_1, LDH_2, flipped
LDH_1 or LDH_2 isoenzyme
LDH_1/LDH_2 ratio
LDL (low-density lipoprotein)
lead (see also *electrode*)
Accufix bipolar
Accufix pacemaker
Accufix pacing
active fixation
anterior precordial
anterolateral
anteroseptal
atrial
atrial J
augmented bipolar limb
augmented limb: aVR, aVL, aVF
barb-tip
bifurcated J-shaped tined atrial
pacing and defibrillation
bipolar
bipolar endocardial
bipolar limb
bipolar precordial
braided
break in insulation of
Cadence TVL nonthoracotomy
CapSure
Cardifix EZ pacing
cathodal
chest
CM5

lead *(cont.)*
cobra-head epicardial
Cordis pacing
coronary sinus
CPI Sweet Tip
CPI ventricular
deep limb
DF (defibrillation, Telectronics
endocardial)
dislodgement of
EKG
electrode
Encor pacing
endocardial
Endotak C
Enguard pacing and defibrillation
EnGuard PFX
ensiform cartilage: V_E
epicardial lead
epicardial pacemaker
esophageal: E_{15}, E_{24}, E_{50}, etc.
finned pacemaker
fishhook
Frank XYZ orthogonal
grounding
Hombach placement of
impedance
infected
inferior
inferior precordial
inferolateral
J-shaped
Laserdish pacing
lateral
lateral precordial
left precordial
Lewis
limb
Mason-Likar placement of EKG
monitor
myocardial screw-in rate-sensing
nonthoracotomy

lead *(cont.)*
  I ("one") (right arm, left arm)
  orthogonal Frank XYZ EKG
  Oscor pacing
  pacemaker
  pacing
  pacing/sensing
  passive fixation
  precordial: V_1 through V_9
  rate-sensing
  reversed arm
  right precordial: V_{3R}, V_{4R}, etc.
  right ventricular endocardial
    sensing lead
  right-sided chest
  scalar
  screw-in
  screw-on
  screw-on epicardial pacemaker
  screw-on epimyocardial
  screw-tipped
  sew-on
  shock(ing)
  silicone
  SRT (segmented ring tripolar)
  standard (bipolar): I, II, III
  standard limb
  steroid-eluting
  steroid-eluting active fixation
  superior vena cava
  sutureless electrode
  Telectronic pacing
  Telectronics endocardial
    defibrillation (DF)
  temporary pacemaker
  third interspace: $3V_1$, $3V_2$, etc.
  III ("three") (left arm, left leg)
  three-turn epicardial
  tined
  tined atrial J pacing/defibrillation
  Transvene
  transvenous ventricular sensing

lead *(cont.)*
  tripolar tined endocardial
  II ("two") (right arm, left leg)
  two-turn epicardial
  unipolar
  unipolar limb
  unipolar precordial
  urethane
  vector
  ventricular
  V_1 through V_6
  Wilson central terminal on EKG
  XYZ Frank EKG
lead configuration
  bidirectional
  unidirectional
lead dislodgement
lead electrode malfunction
lead fracture
lead impedance
lead insulation break
lead malfunction
lead migration
lead placement, chronic
lead resistance
lead reversal
lead system, Transvene
lead threshold
leaflet, leaflets
  anterior mitral (AML)
  anterior mitral valve
  anterior motion of posterior mitral
    valve
  anterior tricuspid (ATL)
  aortic valve
  apposition
  arching of mitral valve
  ballooning of
  billowing mitral (BML)
  bowing of mitral valve
  calcified
  cleft

leaflet *(cont.)*
 coaptation of
 commissural
 conjoined
 degenerated
 doming of
 doughnut-shaped prolapsing
 flail mitral
 floating
 fluttering of valvular
 fused
 hammocking of
 incompetent
 mitral valve
 mural
 myxomatous valve
 nodularity of
 noncalcified mitral
 noncoronary
 paradoxical motion of
 poorly mobile
 posterior
 posterior mitral (PML)
 posterior mitral valve
 posterior tricuspid (PTL)
 prolapse of
 prolapsed
 pseudomitral
 redundant aortic
 redundant mitral valve
 sail-like anterior
 septal
 thickened
 tricuspid valve
 valve
leaflet cleft
leaflet fusion
leaflet incompetence
leaflet motion
leaflet prolapse
 anterior
 posterior

leaflet tip
leak, leakage
 air
 aortic paravalvular
 baffle
 blood
 capillary
 chyle
 current
 generalized capillary
 interatrial baffle
 mitral
 paraprosthetic
 paravalvar
 paravalvular
 periprosthetic
 perivalvular
leaking vein
leaky valve
leather valve cutter
leather venous valvulotome
Lebsche sternal knife
LeCompte maneuver
LeCompte modification of arterial
 switch operation
Lectron II electrode gel
ledge, eccentric
Lee bronchus clamp
Lee microvascular clamp
Lees artery forceps
Lee-White whole blood clotting time
 method
left accessory pathways
left anterior chest wall
left anterior descending (LAD) artery,
 superdominant
left anterior descending coronary
 artery takeoff
left anterior fascicular heart block
left anterior hemiblock
left anterior oblique projection
left atrial active emptying fraction

left atrial active emptying volume
left atrial appendage
left atrial cannulation
left atrial chamber
left atrial contraction
left atrial diameter
left atrial end-diastolic pressure
left atrial enlargement
left atrial maximal volume
left atrial myxoma
left atrial pressure (LAP)
left atrial tension
left atrial thrombosis
left atrial vent
left atrium, giant
left auricle
left auricular appendage (LAA)
left axis deviation
left border of heart
left bundle branch block (LBBB)
left bundle branch hemiblock
left circumflex (LCX) coronary artery
left common femoral artery
left coronary artery arising from
    pulmonary artery
left coronary artery, dominant
left coronary cusp
left coronary plexus (of heart)
left fibrous trigone
left fifth intercostal space
left free-wall pathway
left-handedness, ventricular
left heart catheter
left heart failure
left heart pressure
left iliac system
left internal mammary artery (LIMA)
    graft
left Judkins catheter
left lower lobe
left lower lobe collapse
left lower parasternal heave

left lung collapsed
left lung retracted under a laparotomy
    pad
left main coronary artery (LMCA)
left main stem bronchus
left paramedian incision
left pleural apical hematoma cap
left pleural cap
left posterior fascicular heart block
left posterior hemiblock
left posterolateral thoracotomy
left precordial Q waves
left pulmonary artery
left pulmonary cusp
left semilunar valve
left-sided heart failure
left sinoatrial node, vestigial
left sternal border
left subcostal approach
left-to-right shunt of blood
left-to-right ventricular shunt
left upper lobe, emphysematous
    expansion of
left ventricle
    double-inlet
    hypoplastic
    morphologic
left ventricle hypoplasia
left ventricular afterload
left ventricular assist device (LVAD)
    Novacor
    Thermocardiosystems
left ventricular bypass pump
left ventricular cavity pressure
left ventricular chamber
left ventricular contractility, deranged
left ventricular dysfunction, exercise-
    induced
left ventricular ejection fraction by
    acoustic quantification
left ventricular ejection time,
    increased

left ventricular end-diastolic pressure
(LVEDP)
left ventricular end-diastolic volume
left ventricular end-systolic volume
left ventricular filling
left ventricular heave, sustained
left ventricular hypertrophy (LVH)
left ventricular hypoplasia
left ventricular impulse, prolonged
left ventricular lift
left ventricular loading
left ventricular maximal volume
left ventricular outflow tract
obstruction (LVOTO)
left ventricular papillary muscle
left ventricular patch placed over
diaphragmatic surface of the left
ventricle
left ventricular preload
left ventricular preponderance
left ventricular pressure
left ventricular regional wall motion
abnormality
left ventricular segmental contraction
left ventricular stenotic pulmonary
artery
left ventricular stroke work (LVSW)
left ventricular stroke work index
(LVSWI)
left ventricular systolic pump function
left ventricular systolic time interval
ratio
left ventricular thrombosis
left ventricular thrust
left ventricular vent
left ventriculogram, -graphy
left vocal cord
leg claudication
leg edema
leg fatigue
leg pain at rest

leg, postphlebitic
Legend pacemaker
Legionella pneumophila infection
legionnaires' disease
Lehman ventriculography catheter
leiomyomatosis of heart
leiomyosarcoma of the heart
leiomyosarcoma, right atrial extension
of uterine
Leios pacemaker
Leitner syndrome
Lejeune thoracic forceps
Leland-Jones vascular clamp
Lemmon intimal dissector
Lemmon sternal approximator
Lemmon sternal spreader
Lenègre acquired complete heart block
Lenègre disease or syndrome
length
basic cycle (BCL)
basic drive (BDL)
basic drive cycle (BDCL)
chordal
drive cycle
paced cycle (PCL)
sinus cycle
VA block cycle
wave
lentigines, multiple
lentiginosis
cardiomyopathic
diffuse
lentis, ectopia
LEOPARD (lentigenes, electrocardiographic abnormalities, ocular
hypertelorism, pulmonary valve
stenosis, abnormalities of genitalia,
retardation of growth, and deaf-
ness) syndrome
Leptos pacemaker
leptospirosis

Leriche syndrome
Lermans-Means scratch
Lermans-Means systolic grating sound
lesion
  acanthotic
  accessible
  acquired
  angulated
  aortic arch
  atherosclerotic
  bifurcation
  Blumenthal
  Bracht-Wachter
  calcified
  circular cherry-red
  coin
  complex
  concentric
  constrictive
  coronary artery
  critical
  cryosurgical
  culprit
  de novo
  diffuse
  discrete
  eccentric
  eccentric restenosis
  endobronchial
  extrinsic
  flow-compromising
  flow-limiting
  focal
  friable
  hemodynamically significant
  high-grade
  high-grade obstructive
  hourglass-shaped
  hyperplastic
  intrinsic stenotic
  Janeway

lesion *(cont.)*
  jet
  lesions
  mixed
  multifocal
  multiverrucous friable
  noninfective endocardial
  occlusive
  occult
  ostial
  oval cherry-red raised
  partial
  regurgitant
  rheumatic
  secondary
  segmental
  serial
  space-occupying
  spherical
  stenotic
  subtotal
  tandem
  target
  telangiectatic
  tight
  total
  tubular
  type A, B, or C
  ulcerated
  unstable
  valvular regurgitant
  vegetative
lesser saphenous vein
lesser saphenous vein in situ bypass
less-than-full pause
lethal arrhythmias
lethal consequences
lethal midline granuloma
lethal myocardial injury
lethal tachyarrhythmia
lethargy

Letterer-Siwe disease
leukanakmesis
leukemia
  eosinophilic
  granulocytic
leukocyte-depleted terminal blood
  cardioplegic solution
leukocyte-poor red blood cells
leukocytes, polymorphonuclear
leukocytic infiltration of submucosa
leukocytic trapping of bacteria
leukocytoblastic vasculitis
leukocytosis
  intravascular polymorphonuclear
  polymorphonuclear
leukopenia, drug-induced
leukoplakia
leuko-poor red blood cells
Leukos pacemaker
Leukotrap RC (red cell) storage
  system
leukotrienes
Lev acquired complete heart block
Lev classification of complete AV
  block
Lev disease or syndrome
LeVeen plaque-cracker
level
  air-fluid
  beta thromboglobulin plasma
  beta$_2$-microglobulin
  complement
  cotinine
  elevated serum lactate
  fluid
  IgE
  interferon gamma
  peak and trough (of drug)
  ring shadows with air-fluid
  serum phosphorus
  subtherapeutic

level *(cont.)*
  theophylline
  thiocyanate blood
  threshold
level of first division of main stem
  bronchus
Levine-Harvey classification of heart
  murmur
Levine sign or test
Levinthal-Coles-Lillie (LCL) bodies
levocardia
levophase follow-through
levoposition
levorotatory
levotransposition (L-transposition)
levoversion
Lewis and Pickering test for
  peripheral circulation
Lewis angle
Lewis lead
Lewis upper limb cardiovascular
  disease
LGL (Lown-Ganong-Levine)
LGL variant syndrome
Lian-Siguier-Welti venous thrombosis
  syndrome
liberation of thromboplastic material
  into circulation
Libman-Sacks endocarditis disease
Libman-Sacks syndrome
licorice ingestion, chronic excessive
licorice ingestion-related hypertension
licorice, kaliuretic effect of
LICS (left intercostal space)
Liddle aorta clamp
Liddle syndrome
Lido-Pen Auto-Injector
lidocaine, aerosolized
lidocaine drip
lidocaine neurotoxicity
lidocaine spray, topical

Liebermann-Burchard reaction,
  Schultz modification of (for
  cholesterol)
Liebermann-Burchard test
Liebow and Carrington classification
  for pulmonary eosinophilia
lifelong smoker
Life-Pack 5 cardiac monitor
life-saver or doughnut of Teflon felt
lifestyle changes
lifestyle, sedentary
life-table
  Kaplan-Meier
  Mantel-Haenszel
life-threatening hemorrhage
life-threatening pneumothorax
life-threatening respiratory distress
life-threatening ventricular arrhythmias
lift
  aneurysmal
  ectopic
  late systolic parasternal
  left ventricular
  parasternal
  parasternal systolic
  pulmonary artery
  right ventricular
  sternal
  substernal
  sustained right ventricular
ligament
  conus
  Cooper
  costoxiphoid
  inferior pulmonary
  intra-articular
  lateral costotransverse
  Poupart
  pulmonary
  radiate
  sternopericardial
  superior costotransverse

ligament of Treitz
ligamentum arteriosum
ligamentum teres cardiopexy
ligate
ligation
  intrapericardial
  PDA (patent ductus arteriosus)
  selective vascular
ligation of communicating veins
ligation of perforators
ligature
  popliteal veins
  rubber band
  silk
  suture
  tape
light chain, myosin
lightheaded
lightheadedness
Lilienthal rib spreader
Lillehei-Cruz-Kaster prosthesis
Lillehei-Hardy-Hunter operation
Lillehei-Kaster mitral valve
  prosthesis
Lillehei-Kaster pivoting-disk
  prosthetic valve
Lillehei valve forceps
LIMA (left internal mammary artery)
  graft
limb asymmetry
limb-girdle dystrophy
limb, Gore-Tex
limb of bifurcation graft
limb salvage
limb-shaking TIA (transient ischemic
  attack)
limb-threatening ischemia
limb-threatening thrombosis
limbus fossa ovalis
limbus of Vieussens
limited respiratory chest excursion
limulus amebocyte lysate assay

Lincoln-Metzenbaum scissors
Lindesmith operation
Lindholm tracheal tube
line
    A (arterial)
    Aldrich-Mees
    anterior axillary
    aortic
    arterial
    axillary
    central venous
    central venous pressure (CVP)
    commissural
    Correra
    demarcation
    Eberth
    Ellis
    Ellis-Garland
    intravenous
    isoelectric
    Kerley A, B, C
    Linton
    lower lung
    Mees
    midaxillary
    midclavicular (MCL)
    midscapular
    midsternal
    monitoring
    peripheral intravenous infusion
    posterior axillary
    radial arterial
    subpleural curvilinear
    suture
    transcutaneous drive
    triple-lumen
    venous
    Z
    Zahn
linea alba
linear artifact
linear scar in lungs

linear shadow
linear tear
linea semicircularis
lingula involvement
lingula, right middle lobe
lingular artery
lingular bronchus
    inferior
    superior
lingular orifice
Linton line
Linx exchange guide wire
LINX-EZ cardiac device
Liotta-BioImplant LPB prosthetic
    valve
Liotta TAH (total artificial heart)
lipemia retinalis
lipid
    plasma
    serum levels of
lipid deposits
lipid-laden plaque
lipid lake
lipid-lowering therapy
lipid-rich material
lipid zone
lipofuscin
lipofuscinosis
    ceroid
    neuronal ceroid
lipoid material
lipoid pneumonia or pneumonitis
lipoma, cardiac
lipomatous hypertrophy of the
    interatrial septum
lipopolysaccharide
lipoprotein
    high-density (HDL)
    intermediate density (IDL)
    low-density (LDL)
    plasma
    very-low-density (VLDL)

lipoprotein lipase deficiency
lipoprotein plasminogen inhibition
lipoproteins
liposarcoma of the heart
liquefactive emphysema
LITE (low-intensity treadmill
    exercise) protocol
liters per minute per meter squared
    (L/min./m$_2$)
lithium pacemaker
Litten diaphragm phenomenon
Littleford-Spector introducer
Littman defibrillation pad
Litwak cannula
Litwak left atrial-aortic bypass
Litwak mitral valve scissors
livedo reticularis-digital infarct
livedo vasculitis
liver cirrhosis
liver function
liver-jugular sign
liverlike lung
livid
Livierato abdomino-cardiac sign
Livierato ortho-cardiac sign
Livierato reflex
L-loop heart
L-looping
L-loop ventricular situs
L-malposition of aorta
LMCA (left main coronary artery)
L/min./m^2 (liters per minute per
    meter squared)
loading dose
loading wire cut at tip and
    withdrawn, leaving two nylon
    strands holding device
loads
    combination flow and pressure
    predominantly flow
    pure pressure

lobar bronchus (pl. bronchi)
lobar cavitation
lobar consolidation
lobar emphysema, congenital
lobar lung atrophy
lobar pneumonia
lobe
    azygos
    left lower
    left middle
    left upper
    right lower
    right middle
    right upper
    sequestered (lung)
lobe collapse, left lower
lobectomy
    en masse
    right middle
    SIS (simultaneous individual
        stapling)
lobe of azygos vein
lobulated filling defect
lobulated saccular appearance
lobules
local blood oximetry
localization, CT-directed hook wire
localized mass effect
localized obstructive emphysema
localized stabbing pain
location, precordial impulse
locked lung syndrome
lock washer configuration
loculated collections of old clotted
    blood
loculated fluid collection
Loeffler (Löffler)
Loeffler disease
Loeffler endocarditis
Loeffler endomyocardial syndrome
Loeffler eosinophilia

Loeffler fibroblastic endocarditis
Loeffler parietal fibroplastic endocarditis
Loeffler syndrome
Loeffler variant
Loehr-Kindberg syndrome
Löffler (Loeffler)
Löfgren syndrome
log, episode
long ACE fixed-wire balloon catheter
long-acting bronchodilator
long-acting drugs
long axial oblique view
long-axis parasternal view
long-axis view
long chain acyl-CoA dehydrogenase
Longdwel Teflon catheter
longitudinal aortotomy
longitudinal arteriography
longitudinal arteriotomy
longitudinal incision
longitudinally
longitudinal muscles
longitudinal narrowing
long Péan clamp
long Q-T interval
long Q-T syndrome
long segment narrowing
Long Skinny over-the-wire balloon
  catheter
long thoracic nerve
loop
  capillary
  counterclockwise superiorly
    oriented frontal QRS
  endarterectomy
  flow-volume
  Gerdy interauricular
  J (on catheterization)
  P (on vectorcardiography)
  QRS
  reentrant

loop *(cont.)*
  rubber vessel
  silastic
  subclavian
  T (on vectorcardiography)
  vector
  ventricular
  vessel
  Vieussens
loop diuretics
loose cough
Lo-Por tracheal tube
Lo-Por vascular graft prosthesis
Lo-Profile and Lo-Profile II balloon
  catheter
Lo-Profile steerable dilatation catheter
loss of AV synchrony
loss of capture of pacemaker
loss of lung elasticity
loss of postural tone
loss of sensing of pacemaker
loss of thoracic kyphosis
loud friction rub
loud murmur (high-grade)
loud pulmonic component of second
  heart sound
loud pulmonic second sound
Louis, sternal angle of
Lovén reflex
low-amplitude P wave
low cardiac output syndrome
low-cholesterol diet
low-density lipoprotein (LDL)
low-dose heparin prophylaxis
lower left sternal border
lower lobe lung mass
lower lung line
lower rate interval
lower respiratory tract disease
Lower rings (Richard Lower)
Lower-Shumway cardiac orthotopic
  transplant technique

lower sternal pulsation
Lower tubercle (Richard Lower)
low-fat diet
low-flow syndrome
low-frequency diastolic murmur
low-frequency positive-pressure
    ventilation
low-grade fever
low-intensity systolic click
low-level treadmill
low moderate rejection
Lown and Graboys classification of
    ventricular arrhythmias
Lown classification of ventricular pre-
    mature beats
Lown-Ganong-Levine syndrome
    (LGL)
Lown modified grading system for
    ventricular arrhythmia
low-output heart failure
low-output syndrome
low oxygen saturation
low-pitched rhonchi
low-pitched, rumbling apical
    diastolic murmur
low-pressure cardiac tamponade
low-profile bioprosthesis
low-renin essential hypertension
    syndrome
low-salt diet
low-salt syndrome
low septal right atrium
low-sodium diet
low-speed rotational angioplasty
    catheter
low wedge pressure
Lp(a) (apolipoprotein)
LPA (left pulmonary artery)
LPFB (left posterior fascicular block)
LPH (left posterior hemiblock)
LPS balloon catheter
LPS Peel-Away introducer

LPV (left pulmonary vein)
LQTS (long QT syndrome)
LRA (low right atrium)
LSB (lower sternal border)
LSCVP (left subclavian central
    venous pressure)
LSM (late systolic murmur)
L-transposition (levotransposition)
L-transposition of great arteries
Lucas-Champonnière disease
Lucchese mitral valve dilator
Ludovici angle
Ludwig angina
Ludwig angle
Luer fitting
luer-locked
Luer-Lok ports
Luer-Lok syringe
lues myocarditis
luetic aortic aneurysm
luetic aortitis
luetic arteritis
Lukens collector
Lukens trap
Lumaguide catheter
lumbotomy
lumen, lumens, lumina
    aortic
    arterial
    bronchial
    cloverleaf-shaped
    crescentic
    D-shaped vessel
    double-barrel
    eccentrically placed
    elliptical
    false
    slit-shaped vessel
    slitlike
    star-shaped vessel
    true
    vascular

lumen diameter, minimal
lumen-intimal interface
lumenogram
luminal area
luminal caliber
luminal configuration, scalloped
luminal contour, irregular hazy
luminal cross-sectional area
luminal diameter
luminal dimension
luminal encroachment
luminal irregularity
luminal narrowing
luminal plaquing
luminal silhouette
luminal stenosis
luminal thrombosis
lump in the throat
lumpy appearance of lung
lung
    acquired unilateral hyperlucent
    air-conditioner
    airless
    aluminosis of
    arc welder's
    artificial
    bauxite
    bird breeder's
    bird fancier's
    bird handler's
    black
    brown
    bubbly
    budgerigar-fancier's
    cardiac
    cheese handler's
    cheese washer's
    coal miner's
    coal worker's
    coffee worker's
    collapsed
    consolidated

lung *(cont.)*
    cork handler's
    cork worker's
    corundum smelter's
    dark and mottled
    drowned
    dynamic
    empty collapsed
    eosinophilic
    farmer's
    fibroid
    fish-meal worker's
    fresh
    furrier's
    gangrene of
    grain handler's
    hardened
    harvester's
    hen worker's
    honeycomb
    humidifier
    hyperlucent
    hypogenetic
    light pink
    liverlike
    malt worker's
    maple bark-stripper's
    mason's
    meat wrapper's
    miller's
    miner's
    mottled gray
    mushroom worker's
    pigeon-breeder's
    pigeon-fancier's
    premature infant's
    pump
    rheumatoid
    septic
    shock
    silicotic
    silo-filler's

lung *(cont.)*
   silver finisher's
   silver polisher's
   static
   stiff noncompliant
   stretched
   subsegment of
   thatched roof worker's
   thresher's
   tropical eosinophilic
   underventilated
   unilateral hyperlucent
   vanishing
   wedge resection of
   welder's
   wet
   white
lung abscess
   nonputrid
   putrid
lung agenesis
lung allograft
lung apex (pl. apices)
lung architecture
lung biopsy
lung calculus
lung carcinoma
lung cirrhosis
lung collapse
   massive
   postoperative acute massive
lung compliance, decreased
lung consolidation
lung disease
   idiopathic eosinophilic
   interstitial
lunger disease
lunger pulmonary adenomatosis
lung expansion
lung fever
lung field, collapsed
lung fissure

lung hemangioma
lung hepatization
lung hypoplasia
lung infiltrates (infiltration)
lung inflammation
lung injury, penetrating
lung lobule
lung mass
lung mass with mediastinal invasion
lung necrosis
lung overinflation
lung parenchyma consolidation
lung periphery
lung reexpansion
lung resection
lung scan, perfusion and ventilation
lungs clear to A & P (auscultation
   and percussion)
lung segment, infarcted
lung sounds, adventitious
lung stiffness
lung transplantation
lung volume
   diminished
   end-expiratory
lung volume determination
   FRC (functional residual capacity)
   RV (residual volume)
   TLC (total lung capacity)
   VC (vital capacity)
lung washout
lungworm
lunula (pl. lunulae)
lupus erythematosus
   neonatal
   systemic
lupus-like syndrome
Luschka muscle
lusoria, dysphagia
Lutembacher complex
Lutembacher syndrome
Lutheran blood group

Lutz-Splendore-Almeida disease
Lutz-Splendore-Almeida paracoccidi-
oidomycosis
luxury perfusion
LV (left ventricular) function
pressure
LV (left ventricular) function wall
motion
LVAD (left ventricular assist device),
HeartMate
LVAS (left ventricular assist
system), Novacor
LVd (left ventricular diastolic dimen-
sion)
LVD (left ventricular dysfunction)
LVEDD (left ventricular end-
diastolic dimension)
LVEDI (left ventricular end-diastolic
volume index)
LVEDP (left ventricular end
diastolic pressure)
LVEF (left ventricular ejection
fraction)
LVESD (left ventricular end-systolic
dimension)
LVESVI (left ventricular end-
systolic volume index)
LVET (left ventricular ejection time)
LVFS (left ventricular functional
shortening)
LVFW (left ventricular free wall)
LVG (left ventriculogram)
LVH (left ventricular hypertrophy)
LVH with strain
LVID (left ventricular internal
diameter or dimension)
LVIDd (left ventricular internal
dimension at end-diastole)
LVIDD (left ventricular internal dias-
tolic dimension)
LVIDs (left ventricular internal
dimension at end-systole)

LVIV (left ventricular inflow
volume)
LVM (left ventricular mass)
LVMI (left ventricular mass index)
LVOT (left ventricular outflow tract)
LVOTO (left ventricular outflow tract
obstruction)
LVOV (left ventricular outflow
volume)
LVP (left ventricular pressure)
LVP1 and LVP2 (left ventricular
pressure on apex cardiogram)
LVPW (left ventricular posterior wall)
LVS (left ventricular support) system
LVs (left ventricular systolic)
dimension
LVS (left ventricular systolic)
pressure
LVSW (left ventricular stroke work)
LVSWI (left ventricular stroke work
index)
LVW (left ventricular wall)
Lyme carditis
Lyme disease
lymphadenopathy
hilar
mediastinal
paratracheal
lymph and emulsified fat
lymphangiectasis, pulmonary cystic
lymphangioma, cardiac
lymphangioma circumscriptum
lymphangioma diffusum
lymphangioma of the heart
lymphangitic pulmonary spread
lymphapheresis
lymphatic channels
lymphatic drainage of heart
lymphatic drainage of lungs
lymphatic duct
lymphatic malformation (LM)
lymphatic system

lymphatic vessels
lymphaticovenous malformation
  (LVM)
lymphatics, prominent septal
lymph capillaries
lymphedema
  acquired
  hereditary
  Meige
  Nonne-Milroy
  praecox
lymph node
  axillary
  brachiocephalic
  bronchopulmonary
  diaphragmatic
  hilar
  intercostal
  medial supraclavicular
  mediastinal
  parasternal
  peribronchial
  posterior mediastinal
  supraclavicular
  tracheobronchial
lymph node enlargement, hilar
lymph node metastases

lymph node syndrome, mucocutaneous
lymphocytes
  B (bone-marrow)
  circulating
  immunoblastoid
  T (thymus-dependent)
lymphocytic infiltrate
lymphocytic interstitial pneumonitis
lymphocytic splenomegaly, postcardiotomy
lymphogenous dissemination
lymphogenous metastasis
lymphography
lymphoid alveolitis
lymphoid interstitial pneumonia
lymphoma, multifocal
lymphoreticular malignant disease
lymphosarcoma of heart
lymph vessels of thymus
lyophilized allergen extract
lyophilized DPT (house dust mites)
lysis of clot
lysophospholipid
lysosomal enzymes
lysosomal storage disorders
lysosomes, myocytic
lytic intervention

M, m

m (meter)
m (murmur)
mA (milliampere)
MAC (minimal alveolar concentration)
MAC (mitral annular calcium)
MAC (monitored anesthesia care)
MAC (*Mycobacterium avium* complex)
MacCallum patch
machinery (or machinery-like) murmur
Macleod syndrome
macroangiopathy
macrocytic anemia
Macrodex
macrofistulous AV (arteriovenous)
  communications
macrophage reaction
macroreentrant tachycardia
macroreentry
MAD2 nebulizer
Maddahi method of calculating right
  ventricular ejection fraction
Maestro pacemaker
Maffucci syndrome
magna
  anastomotica
  arteria
  radicularis

magnesium plasma concentration
magnesium, serum
magnet application over pulse
  generator
magnet, doughnut
magnetic field gradient
magnetic moment
magnetic resonance angiography
  (MRA)
magnetic resonance imaging
  gated
  velocity-encoded
magnetic resonance signal
magnetic resonance spectroscopy
  (MRS)
magnetic resonance spin incoherence
magnetic resonance, tagging cine
magnification
  high-resolution
  signal
magnet mode
magnet rate
magnet response
magnitude
magnum guide wire
Magovern-Cromie ball-cage prosthetic
  valve

Mahaim and James fibers
Mahaim bundles (in the heart)
Mahaim fibers (in the heart)
Mahler sign
mahogany flush
MAI (*Mycobacterium avium-intra-cellulare*)
MAI infection
main bronchus
main pulmonary artery
main stem bronchial cartilage
main stem bronchus
main stem carina
maintenance dose
Majocchi disease
Majocchi purpura annularis telangiectodes
Mal de Meleda syndrome
maladie de Roger (Roger disease)
malaise
malaligned atrioventricular septal defects
malar flush
malarial pneumonitis
maldevelopment
maldistribution of ventilation and perfusion
malformation
    adenomatoid
    arteriovenous (AVM)
    coronary artery
    cystic adenomatoid
    Ebstein
    endocardial cushion
    fast-flow
    septal
    slow-flow
    valve
malformed phlebectasias in the calf
malfunction, lead electrode
malignant airway obstruction

malignant arrhythmia
malignant endocarditis
malignant hemangioendothelioma
malignant hypertension
malignant lymphoma of the heart
malignant melanoma metastatic to heart
malignant mesothelioma
malignant pheochromocytoma
malignant pleural implants
malignant teratoma of the heart
malignant vasovagal syncope
malignant ventricular arrhythmias
malignant ventricular dysrhythmias
malignant ventricular tachyarrhythmias
Malin anemia
Malin syndrome
malleable ribbon retractors
Mallinckrodt angiographic catheter
Mallory-Weiss tear in the mucosa at the cardioesophageal junction
malperfused
malperfusion
malposition of the heart
malt worker's lung
mammary souffle murmur
mammary-coronary artery bypass
mandibular advancement device, Herbst
maneuver, maneuvers
    Adson
    costoclavicular
    de-airing
    Heineke-Mikulicz
    hyperabduction
    Kocher
    Müller (Mueller) cardiac auscultation
    Osler
    Rivero-Carvallo
    scalene

maneuver *(cont.)*
  squatting
  transabdominal left lateral
  retroperitoneal
  Valsalva
manganese pneumonitis
manifest
manifold, Morse
Mannkopf sign
mannosidosis
manometer
  Riva-Rocci
  strain gauge
manometer-tipped cardiac catheters
Mansfield Atri-Pace catheter
Mansfield balloon
Mansfield catheter
Mansfield orthogonal electrode
  catheter
Mansfield Scientific dilatation balloon
  catheter
Manson schistosomiasis-pulmonary
  artery obstruction syndrome
Mantel-Haenszel life-table
mantle
  anechoic
  hypoechoic
Mantoux test
manual compression of lungs
manual pressure over carotid sinus
manual resuscitation bag
manual subtraction films
manubriosternal joint
manubriosternal syndrome
manubrium
MAO (monoamine oxidase)
MAO inhibitor
MA-1 ventilator
MAP (mean arterial pressure)
map, acceleration
map-guided partial endocardial
  ventriculotomy

maple bark disease
maple bark stripper's disease
maple bark stripper's lung
maple bark worker's suberosis
mapping
  activation-sequence
  body surface
  body surface potential
  catheter
  Doppler color flow
  electrophysiologic
  endocardial activation
  endocardial catheter
  epicardial
  ice
  intramural
  pace
  phase-shift velocity
  precordial
  retrograde atrial activation
  sinus rhythm
mapping probe, hand-held
Marable syndrome
marantic clot
marantic infective endocarditis
marantic thrombus
marasmus
Marathon guiding catheter
Marchiafava-Micheli paroxysmal
  nocturnal hemoglobinuria
Marchiafava-Micheli syndrome
marching paresthesia
Marfan syndrome
marfanoid hypermobility syndrome
margin
  cardiac
  costal
  obtuse
marginal artery, Drummond
marginal branch
marginal candidate
marginal circumflex bypass

marginal rales
marginal vein
Marie-Bamberger syndrome
markedly accentuated pulmonic
    component
marked respiratory distress
marked wheezes
marker
    gold
    immunologic
    radioactive string
    unreliable
marker-channel diagram
marker channel of pacemaker
markings
    bronchovascular
    coarse bronchovascular
    increased pulmonary vascular
    pulmonary vascular
    vascular
Maroteaux-Lamy syndrome
Marquette Holter monitor
Marquette 3-channel laser holder
marrow, sternal
Marshall, vein of
marsupialization of laryngeal cyst
Martin-Gruber anastomosis
Martorell aortic arch syndrome
Martorell-Fabre syndrome
Martorell hypertensive ulcer
Mary Allen Engle ventricle
MAS (Morgagni-Adams-Stokes)
    syndrome
mask
    BLB
    meter
    nonrebreather
    particle
    rebreathing
    ventilation
mask anesthesia

masking
mask ventilation
Mason-Likar 12-lead ECG system
mason's lung
Mason vascular clamp
mass
    airless
    cavitary
    cavitary lung
    cordlike
    doughy
    echogenic
    firm
    fixed
    fluid-filled
    freely movable
    friable
    hilar
    ill-defined
    indurated
    inflammatory polypoid
    interbronchial
    intracardiac
    intracavity
    intraventricular
    left ventricular (LVM)
    lower lobe lung
    lung
    movable
    mushy
    nonpulsatile
    nonpulsatile abdominal
    paracardiac
    polypoid calcified irregular
    pulsatile
    pulsatile abdominal
    right ventricular (RVM)
    rubbery
    saccular
    solid
    solitary

mass *(cont.)*
    spherical
    stony
    ventricular
    woody
mass effect
mass ligation in lung resection
massage
    carotid sinus
    external cardiac
    heart
    manual
    open cardiac
    vapor
    vigorous manual cardiac
massive aortic regurgitation
massive ascites
massive blood transfusion
massive edema
massive effusion
massive embolism (embolization)
massive exsanguinating hemorrhage
massive gastrointestinal bleeding
massive heart attack
massive infiltration
massive left hemothorax
massive lung collapse
Masson body in pulmonary alveoli
mast cell inhibitors
mast cell mediator
MAST (Medical Anti-Shock Trousers)
Master syndrome
Master two-step exercise stress test
    for coronary insufficiency
MAT (multifocal atrial tachycardia)
Matas aneurysmoplasty
matched V/Q defect
match test
material
    atheromatous
    contrast

material *(cont.)*
    lipoid
    PAS-positive proteinaceous
maternal hypotension syndrome
maternal rubella syndrome
Matson-Alexander rib elevator
Matson rib elevator
Matson stripper
matter, pulverized plaque particulate
Mattox aorta clamp
mattress suture
mattress-type suture
Maugeri syndrome
Maxair Autohaler
maxillary sinusitis
maximal capacity for work
maximal exercise test
maximal inspiratory effort
maximal intensity
    point of
    site of
maximal volume (of left atrium)
maximal voluntary ventilation (MVV)
maximum blood pressure
maximum diameter to minimum
    diameter ratio
maximum electrical activity
maximum midexpiratory flow
maximum predicted heart rate
    (MPHR)
maximum velocity of the jet
Maxon suture
May-Hegglin anomaly
Mayo curved scissors
Mayo exercise treadmill protocol
Mayo-Gibbon heart-lung machine
Mayo-Gibbon pump oxygenator
Mayo Hegar needle holder
Mayo hemostat
Mayo ligature carrier
Mayo Péan forceps

Mayo straight scissors
Mayo vein stripper
maze operation in atrial fibrillation
maze procedure, Cox
Mb (myoglobin)
MB band or fraction
MBF (myocardial blood flow)
MBIH catheter
MB isoenzyme of CK (CK-MB)
McArdle syndrome
MCAT (myocardial contrast appearance time)
McDowall oculovagal reflex
MCE (myocardial contrast echocardiography)
MCFSR (mean circumferential fiber shortening rate)
McGinn-White sign
McGoon coronary perfusion catheter
McGoon method of avoiding heart block
McGoon ratio
McHenry treadmill exercise protocol
mCi (millicurie)
McIntosh double-lumen catheter
MCL (midclavicular line)
McLeod blood phenotype
MCLS (mucocutaneous lymph node syndrome), acute febrile
MCS (middle coronary sinus)
MDI (metered dose inhaler)
MDR-TB (multidrug-resistant tuberculosis)
meadow fescue
Meadows syndrome
Meadox biograft
Meadox Microvel arterial graft
Meadox woven velour prosthesis
mean aortic pressure
mean arterial pressure (MAP)
mean atrial pressure

mean blood pressure
mean cardiac vector
mean circulatory filling pressure
mean circumferential fiber shortening rate (MCFSR)
mean corpuscular red cell volume
mean electrical axis of heart
mean left atrial pressure
mean maximal expiratory flow (MMEF)
mean mitral valve gradient
mean pulmonary artery (MPA) pressure
mean pulmonary capillary pressure (MPCP)
mean pulmonary transit time
mean rate of circumferential shortening
mean right atrial pressure
mean vectors
mean venous pulsation
Means-Lermans scratch
measles, German
measure, prophylactic
measurement
  cardiac output
  occlusion
  ventilometric
meat wrapper's lung
mechanical augmentation
mechanical circulatory support
mechanical cough
mechanical counterpulsation
mechanical dottering effect
mechanical insufflation
mechanical obstruction of respiratory tract
mechanical respiratory assist
mechanical stress
mechanical valve
mechanical ventilation
mechanical ventilatory support

mechanism
  compensatory
  Frank Starling
  heart rate reserve
  Laplace
  reserve
  sensing
  Starling
  triggering
  ventricular escape
Medcor pacemaker
MEDDARS analysis system for
  cardiac catheterization
media (pl. of medium)
  fibrotic and scarred
  tunica
media-adventitia interface
medial arteriosclerosis
medial basal bronchi
medial bronchi
medial calcified sclerosis
medial extension
medial fibroplasia
medial hyperplasia
medial incision
medialis, ramus
medial necrosis, cystic
medial papillary muscle
medial plantar artery
medial rotation of viscera to the right
  of midline
medial supraclavicular lymph nodes
medial surface of lung
median arcuate ligament of diaphragm
median sternotomy
  primary
  secondary
median sternotomy approach (incision)
medianus, ramus
median xiphopubic laparotomy
mediastinal adenopathy
mediastinal border

mediastinal emphysema
mediastinal fat
mediastinal fistula
mediastinal flutter
mediastinal hernia
mediastinal idiopathic fibrosis
mediastinal infection
mediastinal invasion
mediastinalis, pleura
mediastinal lymph nodes
mediastinal lymphadenopathy
mediastinal neoplasm
mediastinal node
mediastinal part of medial surface
  of lung
mediastinal pleura
mediastinal pleurisy
mediastinal prominence
mediastinal shift
mediastinal structures
mediastinal surface of lung
mediastinal tracheostomy
mediastinal tumor
mediastinal widening
mediastinitis
  fibrous
  indurative
  sclerosing
  silicotic
mediastinodiaphragmatic pleural
  reflection
mediastinopericarditis
mediastinoscope, -scopy
mediastinotomy
mediastinum
  anterior
  deviated
  inferior
  middle
  posterior
  superior
  widened

mediastinum displacement
mediator, mast cell
medical cardiac tamponade
medications (see also *contrast medium*
   and *drug-related terms*)
Abbokinase (urokinase)
Abbokinase Open-Cath (urokinase)
abcirximab antiplatelet agent
ablukast sodium
acadesine
Accupril (quinapril)
Accurbron (theophylline)
ACE (angiotensin-converting
   enzyme) inhibitor
acecainide (Napa)
Aceon (perindopril erbumine)
acetazolamide
acetylcholine chloride
acetylcysteine sodium
acrivastine
Actifed Plus
actisomide
Activase (alteplase)
actodigin
Adalat (also Adalat CC, Adalat
   Oros) (nifedipine)
adaprolol maleate
Adenocard (adenosine)
adenosine
Adizem-XL (diltiazem hydro-
   chloride)
ADR-529
Adrenalin Chloride (epinephrine)
adrenaline (also epinephrine)
AeroBid; AeroBid-M (flunisolide)
AeroChamber aerosol holding
   chamber
Aerolate III; Aerolate Jr.; Aerolate
   Sr. (theophylline)
Aeropent (aerosolized pentamidine
   isethionate)

medications *(cont.)*
   aerosolized pentamidine isethionate
      (Aeropent)
   Aerotrol inhalation aerosol device
   Airet (albuterol sulfate)
   Alatone (spironolactone)
   Alazide (spironolactone, HCTZ)
   Albunex
   albuterol (also salbutamol)
   albuterol sulfate
   Alconefrin (phenylephrine)
   Aldactazide (spironolactone,
      HCTZ)
   Aldactone (spironolactone)
   Aldoclor (chlorothiazide; methyl
      dopa)
   Aldomet (methyldopa)
   Aldomet Ester (methyldopate)
   Aldoril (HCTZ, methyldopa)
   Alec (dipalmitoylphosphatidyl-
      choline; phosphatidylglycerol)
   alfuzosin
   alipamide
   Alodopa (HCTZ; methyldopa)
   alprostadil
   alseroxylon
   Altace (ramipril)
   alteplase (Activase)
   althiazide (also altizide)
   Alupent (metaproterenol sulfate)
   ambuphylline
   ambuside
   Amicar (aminocaproic acid)
   amikacin
   amiloride
   aminocaproic acid
   aminophylline
   aminosalicylate sodium
   aminosalicylic acid
   amiodarone
   amiquinsin

medications *(cont.)*
amlodipine besylate
amlodipine maleate
ammonia N 13
ammonia spirit, aromatic
Amodopa (methyldopa)
amoxicillin
ampicillin
amrinone lactate
amyl nitrite
anaritide acetate
anazolene sodium
Ancef (cefazolin sodium)
ancrod
angiotensin amide (also angiotensinamide)
angiotensin-converting enzyme (ACE) inhibitors
anisindione
anisoylated plasminogen streptokinase activator complex (APSAC)
anistreplase
ansamycin (LM427)
antazoline phosphate
Antrizine (meclizine)
Apresazide (hydralazine; HCTZ)
Apresoline (hydralazine)
Apresoline-Esidrix (hydralazine; HCTZ)
aprindine
aprotinin
Aprozide (HCTZ; hydralazine)
APSAC (anisoylated plasminogen streptokinase activator complex)
AquaMephyton (phytonadione)
Aquaphyllin (theophylline)
Aquatensen (methyclothiazide)
Aramine (metaraminol bitartrate)
arbutamine
ardeparin sodium

medications *(cont.)*
Arfonad (trimethaphan camsylate)
argipressin tannate
Arkin Z
artilide fumarate
Arvin (ancrod)
A-64077
Asmalix (theophylline)
aspirin
Astelin (azelastine)
astemizole
Astenose
AsthmaHaler (epinephrine bitartrate)
AsthmaNefrin (racepinephrine)
atenolol
atiprosin maleate
atorvastatin calcium
Atromid-S (clofibrate)
atropine
atropine sulfate
Atrovent (ipratropium bromide)
Atrovent inhaler (ipratropium bromide)
Augmentin (amoxicillin trihydrate; clavulanate potassium)
Axid Pulvules (nizatidine)
azaclorzine
azanator maleate
azatadine maleate
azathioprine
azelastine
Azmacort inhaler (triamcinolone acetonide)
azolimine
azosemide
bacitracin
bamethan sulfate
bamifylline
barmastine
batroxobin

medications *(cont.)*
Baypress (nitrendipine)
BCG vaccine (bacillus Calmette-
Guérin)
beclomethasone dipropionate
Beclovent (beclomethasone
dipropionate)
Beconase AZ (beclomethasone
dipropionate)
belfosdil
bemarinone
bemitradine
bemoradan
benazepril
benazeprilat
bendacalol mesylate
bendroflumethiazide
benzathine penicillin G
benzonatate
benzoylpas calcium
benzthiazide
bepridil
beractant
beraprost sodium
Berotec (fenoterol hydrobromide)
beta blocker
Beta-2 (isoetharine)
beta-adrenergic blocking agent
Betachron E-R (propranolol)
Betadine (povidone-iodine)
betahistine
Betapace (sotalol hydrochloride)
betaxolol
bethanidine sulfate
bevantolol
bicarb (sodium bicarbonate)
Bicillin C-R; Bicillin L-A
(penicillin G benzathine)
biclodil
Bidil (hydralazine isosorbide)
bidisomide

medications *(cont.)*
bile acid sequestrant
Bio-Tab (doxycycline hyclate)
bisoprolol fumarate
bitolterol mesylate
Blocadren (timolol maleate)
Bonine (meclizine)
Bredinin
Brethaire (terbutaline sulfate)
Brethine (terbutaline sulfate)
Bretschneider-HTK cardioplegic
solution
bretylium tosylate
Bretylol (bretylium tosylate)
Brevibloc (esmolol)
Bricanyl (terbutaline sulfate)
brocrinat
bromhexine
bromindione
bromodiphenhydramine
brompheniramine maleate
Bronkometer (isoetharine mesylate)
Bronkosol (isoetharine)
bucainide maleate
bucindolol
Buckberg solution
bucromarone
bucrylate
bumetanide
Bumex (bumetanide)
bunaprolast
bupicomide
butamirate citrate
butaprost
buterizine
buthiazide
butopamine
butoprozine
butorphanol
butorphanol tartrate
caffeine

medications *(cont.)*
Calan; Calan SR (verapamil)
Calciparine (heparin calcium)
calcium chloride
Cam-ap-es (HCTZ; reserpine; hydralazine)
candoxatril
candoxatrilat
Capastat Sulfate (capreomycin sulfate)
capobenate sodium
capobenic acid
Capoten (captopril)
Capozide (captopril; HCTZ)
capreomycin sulfate
captopril
carbazeran
carbenicillin disodium
carbinoxamine maleate
carbocysteine
carbon dioxide (CO_2)
carbuterol
Cardene; I.V.; QD; SR (nicardipine)
Cardi-Omega 3 (omega-3 fatty acids; multiple vitamins and minerals)
cardiac glycoside
Cardilate (erythrityl tetranitrate)
Cardioquin (quinidine polygalacturonate)
Cardizem; CD; SR (diltiazem)
Cardura (doxazosin mesylate)
Carfin (warfarin sodium)
carsatrin succinate
Cartrol (carteolol)
carvedilol
Carwin
Catapres (clonidine)
Ceclor (cefaclor)
Cedax (ceftibutin)

medications *(cont.)*
Cedilanid-D (deslanoside)
CeeNu (lomustine)
Cefobid (cefoperazone sodium)
Cefotan (cefotetan disodium)
cefotaxime sodium
cefuroxime
celiprolol
Cerespan (papaverine)
ceronapril
Cetacaine spray (benzocaine)
cetiedil citrate
cetirizine
Chealamide (edetate disodium)
chlophedianol
chloral hydrate
chlorcyclizine
chlorothiazide sodium
chlorpheniramine maleate
chlorpheniramine polistirex
chlorpromazine
chlorthalidone
cholestyramine resin
Choloxin (dextrothyroxin sodium)
Cholybar (cholestyramine resin)
chromonar
CI-930
Cibadrex
ciclafrine
cicletanine
cifenline succinate
cilazapril
cinalikast
cinepazet maleate
cinnarizine
Cipralan (cifenline succinate)
Cipro (ciprofloxacin)
ciprofloxacin
ciprostene calcium
cisplatinum
Claforan (cefotaxime sodium)

medications *(cont.)*
Claritin (loratadine)
Claritin D (loratadine; pseudoephedrine)
clazolimine
clemastine fumarate
clindamycin
clindamycin palmitate
clindamycin phosphate
clofazimine
clofibrate
clofilium phosphate
clonidine
clonitrate
clopamide
clorexolone
clorprenaline
closiramine aceturate
cocaine flakes
codeine phosphate
codeine polistirex
codeine sulfate
codoxime
coenzyme Q10
Colestid (colestipol)
colestipol
colestolone
colfosceril palmitate
colterol mesylate
Combipres (clonidine)
CoQ10; Co-Q10 (coenzyme Q10)
Cordarone (amiodarone)
Corgard (nadolol)
Corsevin M (monoclonal
antibodies)
Corzide (nadolol)
Coumadin (warfarin sodium)
coumarin
Cozaar (losartan)
crilvastatin
cromitrile sodium
cromolyn sodium

medications *(cont.)*
curare
Cyclan (cyclandelate)
cyclandelate
cycliramine maleate
cyclizine
cyclopenthiazide
Cyclo-Prostin (epoprostenol)
cycloserine
Cyclospasmol (cyclandelate)
cyclosporine
cyclothiazide
dalteparin sodium
dapiprazole
Daranide (dichlorphenamide)
darodipine
Dazamide (acetazolamide)
DDAVP (desmopressin acetate)
debrisoquin sulfate
Decabid (indecainide)
Decadron (dexamethasone)
Decadron Phosphate Respihaler;
Turbinaire (dexamethasone
sodium phosphate)
Delaprem (hexoprenaline sulfate)
delapril
Demadex (torsemide)
Demi-Regroton (chlorthalidone;
reserpine)
Demser (metyrosine)
Deponit (nitroglycerin)
deslanoside
desmopressin acetate
dexbrompheniramine maleate
dexchlorpheniramine maleate
dexpropranolol
dexrazoxane
dextromethorphan hydrobromide
dextromethorphan polistirex
dextrothyroxine
Diamox (acetazolamide)
diapamide

medications *(cont.)*
  diazoxide
  dicirenone
  dicumarol
  diethylcarbamazine citrate
  Digibind (digoxin immune Fab)
  Digidote (digoxin immune Fab)
  digitalis
  digitoxin
  digoxin
  digoxin immune Fab
  Dilacor XR (diltiazem)
  Dilatrate-SR (isosorbide dinitrate)
  dilevalol
  diltiazem
  diltiazem malate
  dimefline
  dimethindene maleate
  diphenhydramine citrate
  diphenhydramine
  diphenylpyraline
  dipyridamole
  disaccharide tripeptide glycerol
    dipalmitoyl
  disobutamide
  disopyramide phosphate
  Disotate (edetate disodium)
  ditekiren
  Diucardin (hydroflumethiazide)
  Diupres-250; -500 (chlorothiazide;
    reserpine)
  Diurese (trichlormethiazide)
  Diurigen (chlorthiazide)
  Diuril (chlorthiazide)
  Diutensen-R (methychlothiazide;
    reserpine)
  dobutamine
  dobutamine lactobionate
  dobutamine tartrate
  Dobutrex (dobutamine)
  docetaxel
  dofetilide

medications *(cont.)*
  domiodol
  donetidine
  dopamine
  dopamine drip
  Dopastat (dopamine)
  dopexamine
  dorastine
  dornase alfa
  doxapram
  doxaprost
  doxazosin mesylate
  doxofylline
  Doxy 100; 200 (doxycycline
    hyclate)
  Doxychel Hyclate (doxycycline
    hyclate)
  doxycycline
  doxycycline calcium
  doxycycline fosfatex
  doxycycline hyclate
  doxylamine succinate
  draflazine
  drobuline
  droprenilamine
  Duo-Medihaler (isoproterenol)
  Duotrate; Duotrate 45 (penta-
    erythritol tetranitrate)
  Duricef (cefadroxil monohydrate)
  Dyazide (HCTZ; triamterene)
  Dyclone (dyclonine)
  Dyflex-200 (dyphylline)
  Dyflex-G (dyphylline; guaifenesin)
  Dyline-GG (dyphylline;
    guaifenesin)
  DynaCirc (isradipine)
  dyphylline
  Dyrenium (triamterene)
  ebastine
  Ecotrin (aspirin)
  ECS cardioplegic solution
  Edecrin (ethacrynic acid)

medications *(cont.)*
Edecrin Sodium (ethacrynic sodium)
edifolone acetate
E.E.S. (erythromycin ethylsuccinate)
efegatran sulfate
eicosapentaenoic acid (EPA)
Eldisine (vindesine sulfate)
Elixomin (theophylline)
Elixophyllin (theophylline)
Elixophyllin-GG (theophylline;
guaifenesin)
Elixophyllin-KI (theophylline;
potassium iodide)
emilium tosylate
eminase
E-Mycin (erythromycin)
enalapril maleate
enalaprilat
enalkiren
encainide
endralazine mesylate
Endrate (edetate disodium)
Enduron (methyclothiazide)
Enduronyl; Enduronyl Forte
(methyclothiazide; deserpine)
enflurane
enofelast
enoximone
enprofylline
EPA (eicosapentaenoic acid)
ephedrine
ephedrine sulfate
epinephrine bitartrate
epithiazide
epoprostenol and prostacyclin
epoprostenol sodium
eprosartan
epsilon-aminocaproic acid (EACA)
erythromycin ethylsuccinate
erythromycin stearate
Esidrix (HCTZ)

medications *(cont.)*
Esimil (HCTZ; guanethidine
monosulfate)
esmolol
ethacrynate sodium
ethacrynic acid
ethambutol
ethamivan
Ethaquin (ethaverine)
Ethatab (ethaverine)
ethaverine
Ethavex-100 (ethaverine)
ethionamide
Ethmozine (moricizine)
ethyl dibunate
ethylenediaminetetraacetic acid
(EDTA)
ethylnorepinephrine
etintidine
etozolin
Euro-Collins cooling solution
Exna (benzthiazide)
Exosurf; Exosurf Neonatal
(colfosceril palmitate)
Ezide (HCTZ)
felodipine
felypressin
Fenesin (guaifenesin)
fenoldopam mesylate
fenoterol
fenprinast
fenquizone
fenspiride
fentanyl citrate
fish oil
FK-506
flavodilol maleate
flecainide acetate
Flolan (epoprostenol)
Flonase (fluticasone)
flordipine
flosequinan

medications *(cont.)*
Flovent (fluticasone)
flucytosine
flunarizine
flunisolide
Fluosol
fluvastatin sodium
Fortaz (ceftazidime)
fosinopril sodium
fosinoprilat
fostedil
furosemide
Gastrocrom (cromolyn sodium)
gelsolin, recombinant human
gemfibrozil
Gemzar (gemcitabine)
Genabid (papaverine)
GenESA System (arbutamine)
gentamicin
Gey fixative solution
globulin, aerosolized pooled
    immune
globulin, immune
guaifenesin
guaithylline
guanabenz acetate
guanacline sulfate
guanadrel sulfate
guancydine
guanethidine monosulfate
guanethidine sulfate
guanfacine
guanine monophosphate
guanisoquin sulfate
guanoclor sulfate
guanoctine
guanoxabenz
guanoxan sulfate
guanoxyfen sulfate
halothane
Hank balanced salt solution
HCTZ (hydrochlorothiazide)

medications *(cont.)*
Hep-Lock; Hep-Lock u/P (heparin
    sodium)
heparin calcium
heparin sodium
hexobendine
hexoprenaline sulfate
hirudin
Hirulog (hirudin)
Hismanal (astemizole)
HMG CoA reductase inhibitor
hoquizil
Human Surf (surfactant, human
    amniotic fluid derived)
hyaluronidase
Hycodan (hydrocodone bitartrate;
    homatropine methylbromide)
Hycomine (hydrocodone bitartrate;
    phenylpropanolamine)
Hydralazide (hydralazine)
hydralazine
hydralazine polistirex
Hydrap-ES (HCTZ; reserpine;
    hydralazine)
Hydra-Zide (HCTZ; hydralazine)
Hydrazide (HCTZ; hydralazine)
Hydrex (benzthiazide)
hydrochlorothiazide (HCTZ)
hydrocodone bitartrate
hydrocodone polistirex
HydroDIURIL (HCTZ)
hydroflumethiazide
Hydro-Fluserpine #2 (hydroflume-
    thiazide; reserpine)
Hydromet (hydrocodone bitartrate;
    homatropine methylbromide)
Hydromox (quinethazone)
Hydropane (hydrocodone bitartrate;
    homatropine hydrobromide)
Hydro-Par (HCTZ)
Hydrophed (theophylline)
Hydropres (HCTZ; reserpine)

medications *(cont.)*
Hydro-Serp (HCTZ; reserpine)
Hydroserpine (HCTZ; reserpine)
Hydrosine (HCTZ; reserpine)
hydroxyamphetamine hydrobromide
Hygroton (chlorthalidone)
Hylorel (guanadrel sulfate)
HyperGAM+CF
Hypermune RSV (respiratory syncytial virus immune globulin, human)
Hyperstat (diazoxide)
Hytrin (terazosin)
ibopamine
ibutilide fumarate
icatibant acetate
icotidine
imazodan
Imdur (isosorbide mononitrate)
imipenem
Immther (disaccharide tripeptide glycerol dipalmitoyl)
indacrinone
indandione
indapamide
indecainide
Inderal; Inderal LA (propranolol)
Inderide LA (propranolol; HCTZ)
Indocin I.V. (indomethacin sodium trihydrate)
indolapril
indolidan
indomethacin sodium trihydrate
indoramin
indorenate
Infasurf
INH (isoniazid)
Inhibace (cilazapril)
Innovace (enalapril maleate)
Inocor (amrinone lactate)

medications *(cont.)*
inositol niacinate
inotropic agent
Intal (cromolyn sodium)
Integrelin
interleukin-1 receptor (IL-1R)
interleukin-4 receptor (IL-4R)
interleukin-6 (IL-6)
Intropin (dopamine)
Inversine (mecamylamine)
Iophylline (theophylline; iodinated glycerol)
ipazilide fumarate
Ipran (propanolol)
ipratropium bromide
iproxamine
isamoxole
ISDN (isosorbide dinitrate)
Ismelin (guanethidine monosulfate)
Ismo (isosorbide mononitrate)
Ismotic (isosorbide)
Iso-Bid (isosorbide dinitrate)
isoetharine
isoetharine mesylate
isomazole
ISON (isosorbide dinitrate)
isoniazid
Isoprinosine (inosine pranobex)
isoproterenol
isoproterenol sulfate
Isoptin; Isoptin SR (verapamil)
Isordil Tembid; Titradose (isosorbide dinitrate)
isosorbide dinitrate (ISDN)
isosorbide mononitrate
Isotrate Timecelles (isosorbide dinitrate)
Isovex (ethaverine)
isoxsuprine
isradipine
Isuprel Mistometer; Glossets (isoproterenol)

medications *(cont.)*
itazigrel
Kabikinase (streptokinase)
kanamycin sulfate
Kay Ciel (potassium chloride)
Kayexalate enema
Kaylixir (potassium gluconate;
   alcohol)
Kaysine (adenosine phosphate)
KCl (potassium chloride)
K-Dur 10; 20 (potassium chloride)
Keflex Pulvules (cephalexin mono-
   hydrate)
Kefzol (cefazolin sodium)
Kerledex (betaxolol; chlorthalidone)
Kerlone (betaxolol)
ketotifen fumarate
KIE (ephedrine; potassium iodide)
K-Lor (potassium chloride)
Klor-Con (potassium chloride)
Klor-Con/EF (potassium bicarbon-
   ate; potassium citrate)
Klorvess (potassium chloride)
K-Lyte DS (potassium bicarbonate;
   potassium citrate)
K-Lyte/Cl (potassium chloride)
K-Norm (potassium chloride)
Konakion (phytonadione)
Konyne 80 (factor IX complex,
   human)
Kredex (carvedilol)
K-Tab (potassium chloride)
labetalol
lacidipine
Laniazid; Laniazid C.T. (isoniazid)
Lanophyllin (theophylline)
Lanoxicaps (digoxin)
Lanoxin (digoxin)
Lasix (furosemide)
leniquinsin
Lescol (fluvastatin sodium)

medications *(cont.)*
leukocyte protease inhibitor,
   secretory
Levatol (penbutolol sulfate)
levcromakalim
levdobutamine lactobionate
levocarnitine
levonordefrin
Levophed Bitartrate; drip
   (norepinephrine)
levopropoxyphene napsylate
libenzapril
lidocaine
lidoflazine
LidoPen auto-injector (lidocaine)
lifarizine
lignocaine
Lipo-Nicin (niacin; niacinamide;
   multiple vitamins)
Liquaemin Sodium (heparin sodium)
lisinopril
Livostin (levocarbastine
lixazinone sulfate
lobeline
lodoxamide ethyl
lodoxamide tromethamine
lofexidine
Logiparin (low molecular weight
   heparin)
Loniten (minoxidil)
loop diuretic
Lopid; Lopid-SR (gemfibrozil)
Lopressor (metoprolol tartrate)
Lopressor HCT (metoprolol
   tartrate; HCTZ)
lorajmine
loratadine
lorcainide
Lorelco (probucol)
losartan potassium
losulazine

medications *(cont.)*
Lotensin (benazepril)
Lotensin HCT (benazepril; HCTZ)
lovastatin
Lovenox (enoxaparin sodium)
Lozol (indapamide)
Lugol fixative solution
Luramide (furosemide)
LuVax (monoclonal antibodies)
lyapolate sodium
lypressin
Macstim (macrophage colony
    stimulating factor)
mannitol
Marax; Marax-DF (theophylline;
    ephedrine sulfate; hydroxyzine)
Marpres (HCTZ; reserpine;
    hydralazine
Matulane (procarbazine)
Maxair Autohaler (pirbuterol
    acetate)
Maxzide (triamterene; HCTZ)
MDL-17043
mebutamate
mecamylamine
Medihaler-Epi (epinephrine
    bitartrate)
Medihaler-Iso (isoproterenol sulfate)
medium chain triglycerides (MCT)
medorinone
Medrol Dosepak (methylpredniso-
    lone)
medroxalol
mefenidil fumarate
mefruside
Melrose solution
meobentine sulfate
mephentermine sulfate
Mephyton (phytonadione)
Mepig (mucoid exopolysaccharide
    Pseudomonas hyperimmune
    globulin)

medications *(cont.)*
mesuprine
Metahydrin (trichlormethiazide)
Metaprel (metaproterenol sulfate)
metaproterenol polistirex
metaproterenol sulfate
metaraminol bitartrate
Metatensin (trichlormethiazide;
    reserpine)
methacholine chloride
methalthiazide
methicillin sodium
methimazole
methoxamine
methyclothiazide
methyldopa
methyldopate
methylprednisolone
metiamide
metizoline
metolazone
metoprolol fumarate
metoprolol succinate
metyrosine
Mevacor (lovastatin)
mexiletine
Mexitil (mexiletine
Micro-K; Micro-K 10 Extencaps;
    Micro-K LS (potassium chloride)
Midamor (amiloride)
midazolam
midazolam maleate
midodrine
milrinone lactate
Minipress; Minipress XL (prazosin)
Minitran (nitroglycerin)
Minizide (prazosin; polythiazide)
minoxidil
mioflazine
Miradon (anisindione)
mixed respiratory vaccine (MRV)
mixidine

medications *(cont.)*
mizorbine
Modalim
modecainide
Moderil (rescinnamine)
Moduretic (amiloride; HCTZ)
molsidomine
Monsel's hemostatic solution
Monocid (cefonicid sodium)
Monoket (isosorbide mononitrate)
Monopril (fosinopril sodium)
Mono-Vacc Test
moricizine
morphine sulfate
morpholinethyl-mycophenolic acid
morrhuate sodium
moxazocine
MRV (mixed respiratory vaccine)
MS (morphine sulfate)
mucoid exopolysaccharide *Pseudomonas* hyperimmune globulin
Mucomyst (acetylcysteine sodium)
Mudrane (aminophylline; ephedrine; potassium iodide; phenobarbital)
Mustargen (mechlorethamine
mustine hydrochloride
Mutamycin (mitomycin)
muzolimine
Myambutol (ethambutol)
Myidyl (triprolidine)
Mykrox (metolazone)
Myloral
MZB (mizorbine)
nadolol
nafamostat mesylate
nafronyl oxalate
Napa (acecainide)
NAPA (N-acetylprocainamide)
Napamide (disopyramide phosphate)
Naqua (trichlormethiazide)
Nasalcrom (cromolyn sodium)

medications *(cont.)*
Naturetin ((bendroflumethiazide)
Navelbine (vinorelbine tartrate)
nebivolol
nedocromil calcium
nedocromil sodium
Nephron (racepinephrine)
Neptazane (methazolamide)
niacin
niacinamide hydroiodide
nicardipine
nicergoline
Nicobid (niacin)
Nicoderm (nicotine)
Nicolar (niacin)
nicorandil
Nicorette; Nicorette DS chewing gum
nicotinic acid
nicotinyl alcohol
Nicotrol (nicotine)
nifedipine
nimodipine
Nimotop (nimodipine)
nisbuterol mesylate
nisoldipine
nitrendipine
Nitro-Bid; Plateau Caps (nitroglycerin)
Nitrocine Timecaps (nitroglycerin)
Nitrodisc (nitroglycerin)
Nitro-Dur; Nitro-Dur II (nitroglycerin)
Nitrogard (nitroglycerin)
nitroglycerin (NTG)
nitroglycerin spray
Nitroglyn (nitroglycerin)
Nitrol ointment; paste; patch (nitroglycerin)
Nitrolingual (nitroglycerin)
Nitrong (nitroglycerin)
Nitropress (sodium nitroprusside)

medications *(cont.)*
nitroprusside
Nitrostat (nitroglycerin)
noberastine
norepinephrine bitartrate
Norisodrine Aerotrol (isoproterenol)
Norisodrine with Calcium Iodide
    (isoproterenol sulfate; calcium
    iodide; alcohol)
Normiflo (low molecular weight
    heparin)
Normodyne (labetalol)
Normozide (labetalol; HCTZ)
Norpace; Norpace CR (disopyra-
    mide phosphate)
Norvasc (amlodipine)
noscapine
novel plasminogen activator (NPA)
NPA (novel plasminogen activator)
NTG (nitroglycerin)
NTS (nitroglycerin)
Nydrazid (isoniazid)
nylidrin
octodrine
ofornine
OKT3 monoclonal antibody
Oncovin (vincristine sulfate)
OPC-8212
OPC-18790
OPC-8212
Oretic (HCTZ)
Oretic Forte (HCTZ; deserpidine)
Orthoclone OKT3 (muromonab-
    CD3)
Osmitrol (mannitol)
Osmoglyn (glycerin)
ouabain
oxacillin sodium
oxagrelate
oxarbazole
oxatomide
oxfenicine

medications *(cont.)*
oxiramide
oxmetidine
oxmetidine mesylate
oxprenolol
oxtriphylline
oxygen
ozolinone
papaverine
Par Glycerol (iodinated glycerol)
pargyline
Pavabid HP; Plateau Caps
    (papaverine)
Pavacap Unicelles (papaverine)
Pavacen Cenules (papaverine)
Pavadur (papaverine)
Pavagen (papaverine)
Pava-Par (papaverine)
Pavarine Spancaps (papaverine)
Pavased (papaverine)
Pavasule (papaverine)
Pavatine (papaverine)
Paverolan Lanacaps (papaverine)
pazinaclone
pazoxide
PDE isoenzyme inhibitor
pelanserin
pelrinone
pemerid nitrate
penicillin V
pentaerythritol tetranitrate (PETN)
pentobarbital calcium
pentopril
pentoxifylline
pentrinitrol
Pentritol Tempules
Pentylan (pentaerythritol tetrani-
    trate)
perhexiline maleate
Periactin (cyproheptadine)
perindopril
perindopril erbumine

medications *(cont.)*
Peritrate; Peritrate SA (pentaerythritol tetranitrate)
Persantine (dipyridamole)
PETN (pentaerythritol tetranitrate)
PGE1 (prostaglandin E1; now
alprostadil)
Phenameth (promethazine)
phenindamine tartrate
phenindione
phenoxybenzamine
phenprocoumon
phentolamine mesylate
phenyl aminosalicylate
phenylephrine bitartrate
phenylephrine
Pherazine (promethazine)
Phyllocontin (aminophylline)
Physiotens (monoxidine)
picumeterol fumarate
Pima (potassium iodide)
pimagedine hydrochloride
pimobendan
pinacidil
Pindac (pinacidil)
pindolol
pipazethate
piperacillin sodium
piquizil
pirbuterol acetate
piretanide
piriprost potassium
pirmenol
pirolate
pirolazamide
piroximone
pivopril
Plasmalyte A cardioplegic solution
platelet concentrate
Platinol; Platinol-AQ (ciplastin)
Plendil (felodipine)

medications *(cont.)*
Pneumopent (pentamidine isethionate)
pobilukast edamine
Pockethaler
polythiazide
potassium chloride
potassium guaiacolsulfonate
potassium iodide
potassium-sparing diuretic
potassium-wasting diuretic
pranolium chloride
Pravachol (pravastatin sodium)
pravastatin sodium
prazosin
prednisolone
prednisone
prenylamine
Primacor IV (milrinone lactate)
Primatene Mist Suspension
primidolol
Prinivil (lisinopril)
prinoxodan
Prinzide (HCTZ; lisinopril)
Priscoline (tolazoline)
prizidilol
Pro-Air (procaterol)
Probeta (bisoprolol)
probucol
procainamide
Procan SR (procainamide)
Procardia; XL (nifedipine)
procaterol
Prograph (tacrolimus)
Prometa (metaproterenol sulfate)
Prometh (promethazine)
promethazine
Promine (procainamide)
Pronestyl; Pronestyl-SR
(procainamide)
propafenone

medications *(cont.)*
  propatyl nitrate
  propranolol
  propylhexedrine
  proscillaridin
  prostaglandin E1 (now alprostadil)
  ProStep (nicotine)
  Prostin VR Pediatric (alprostadil)
  protamine sulfate
  protein C
  Proventil (albuterol sulfate)
  Provocholine (methacholine
    chloride)
  proxorphan tartrate
  pseudoephedrine
  Pulmicort Turbuhaler (budesonide)
  Pulmocare nutritional supplement
  Pulmozyme (dornase alfa)
  pyrabrom
  pyrazinamide
  pyrinoline
  pyroxamine maleate
  Quadrinal
  quazinone
  quazodine
  quazolast
  Questran; Questran Light (chole-
    styramine resin)
  Quibron-T Dividose; Quibron-T/SR
    (theophylline)
  quinacrine
  Quinaglute Dura-Tabs (quinidine
    gluconate)
  Quinalan (quinidine gluconate)
  quinapril
  quinaprilat
  quinazosin
  quindonium bromide
  quinelorane
  quinethazone
  Quinidex Extentabs (quinidine
    sulfate)

medications *(cont.)*
  quinidine gluconate
  quinidine polygalacturonate
  quinidine sulfate
  Quinora (quinidine sulfate)
  quinpirole
  Quin-Release (quinidine gluconate)
  quinterenol sulfate
  quinuclium bromide
  racepinephrine
  ramipril
  ranolazine
  rapamycin (now sirolimus)
  Raudixin (*Rauwolfia serpentina*)
  Rauverid (*Rauwolfia serpentina*)
  rauwolfia derivative
  rauwolfia serpentina
  Rauzide (bendroflumethiazide;
    Rauwolfia serpentina)
  Reactine (cetirizine)
  recainam
  recainam tosylate
  recombinant tissue plasminogen
    activator (rt-PA)
  Recombinate (antihemophilic
    factor, recombinant)
  Regitine (phentolamine mesylate)
  Regroton (chlorthalidone; reserpine)
  Renese (polythiazide)
  Renese-R (polythiazide; reserpine)
  repirinast
  reproterol
  rescinnamine
  reserpine
  RespiGam (polyclonal antibodies)
  respiratory syncytial virus immune
    globulin, human
  R-Gen (iodinated glycerol)
  RheothRx Copolymer (poloxamer)
  Rhythmin (procainamide)
  ricin (blocked) conjugated murine
    monoclonal antibody

medications *(cont.)*
Ridaura (auranofin)
Rifadin (rifampin)
Rifamate (rifampin; isoniazid)
rifampin
rifampin, isoniazid and pyrazinamide
Rifater (rifampin, isoniazid and pyrazinamide)
Rimactane (rifampin)
Rimactane/INH (rifampin; isoniazid)
rimiterol hydrobromide
risotilide
ritolukast
rocastine
ropitoin
rotoxamine
RS 61443
rt-PA; rtPA (recombinant tissue plasminogen activator) (alteplase)
Rythmol (propafenone)
S-2 (racepinephrine)
Salazide; Salazide-Demi (hydroflumethiazide; reserpine)
salmeterol xinafoate
Saluron (hydroflumethiazide)
Salutensin; Salutensin-Demi (hydroflumethiazide; reserpine)
Sandimmune (cyclosporine)
saralasin acetate
Sclavo PPD Solution; Sclavo Test-PPD (tuberculin purified protein derivative)
Scleromate (morrhuate sodium)
sCR1 (soluble complement receptor I)
Sectral (acebutolol)
Seldane (terfenadine)
Seldane-D (terfenadine; pseudoephedrine)

medications *(cont.)*
Selecor (celiprolol)
sematilide
Ser-A-Gen (HCTZ; reserpine; hydralazine)
Ser-Ap-Es (HCTZ; reserpine; hydralazine)
Serevent (salmeterol xinafoate)
Seromycin Pulvules (cycloserine)
Serpalan (reserpine)
Serpazide (HCTZ; reserpine; hydralazine)
simvastatin
sirolimus
SK (streptokinase)
Slo-bid Gyrocaps (theophylline)
Slo-phyllin (theophylline)
Slo-phyllin GG (theophylline; guaifenesin)
Slow-K (potassium chloride)
sodium bicarbonate
sodium nitroprusside
Sodium Diuril (chlorothiazide)
Sodium Edecrin (ethacrynate sodium)
Sodium P.A.S. (aminosalicylate sodium)
Sofarin (warfarin sodium)
Solu-Medrol (methylprednisolone sodium succinate)
Sorbitrate; Sorbitrate SA (isosorbide dinitrate)
sotalol
soterenol
Sotradecol (sodium tetradecyl sulfate)
spirapril
spiraprilat
Spironazide (spironolactone; HCTZ)
spironolactone
spiroxasone

medications *(cont.)*
Spirozide (spironolactone; HCTZ)
SSKI (potassium iodide)
St. Thomas Hospital cardioplegic
solution
steroids
Stimate nasal spray (desmopressin
acetate)
Streptase (streptokinase)
streptokinase
streptomycin sulfate
sublingual nitroglycerin
sufotidine
sulfinalol
sulfonterol
suloctidil
suloxifen oxalate
sulukast
superoxide dismutase (SOD),
recombinant human
surface active extract of saline
lavage of bovine lungs
surfactant, human amniotic fluid
derived
surfactant TA, modified bovine
lung surfactant extract
surfomer
suricainide maleate
Survanta (beractant; modified
bovine surfactant extract)
Suscard Buccal (nitroglycerin)
suxemerid sulfate
tacrolimus
Tambocor (flecainide acetate)
Taxol (paclitaxel)
Taxotere (docetaxel)
tazifylline
tazolol
teludipine
temelastine
temocapril
Tenex (guanfacine)

medications *(cont.)*
Tenoretic (chlorthalidone; atenolol)
Tenormin (atenolol)
Tensilon (edrophonium chloride)
teprotide
terazosin
terbutaline sulfate
terfenadine
terlakiren
terodiline
Tessalon Perles (benzonatate)
tetracycline
tetrahydrozoline
tetrazolast meglumine
thalidomide
Tham (tromethamine)
Theochron (theophylline)
Theoclear; Theoclear L.A.
(theophylline)
Theo-Dur; Theo-Dur Sprinkle
(theophylline)
Theolair; Theolair-SR (theophylline)
Theo-Organidin (theophylline;
iodinated glycerol)
Theophyllin KI (theophylline;
potassium iodide)
theophylline (TH)
theophylline calcium salicylate
Theophylline Extended-Release
(theophylline)
Theo-Sav (theophylline)
Theospan-SR (theophylline)
Theostat 80 (theophylline)
Theo-24 (theophylline)
Theovent (theophylline)
Theo-X (theophylline)
thiazide diuretic
tiamenidine
tiaramide
tibenelast sodium
Tice BCG (BCG vaccine, Tice
strain)

medications *(cont.)*
Ticlid (ticlopidine)
ticlopidine
ticrynafen
Tilade (nedocromil sodium)
Tilarin (nedocromil sodium)
Timolide (timolol maleate; HCTZ)
tinabinol
Tine Test PPD (tuberculin purified
   protein derivative)
tinzaparin sodium
tiodazosin
tiotidine
tipentosin
tipropidil
tiqueside
tirilazad mesylate
tissue plasminogen activator (t-PA)
tobramycin
tocainide
tolamolol
tolazoline
tomelukast
Tonocard (tocainide)
topical lidocaine spray
Toprol XL (metoprolol succinate)
Tornalate (bitolterol mesylate)
torsemide
tosifen
t-PA; tPA (tissue plasminogen
   activator)
Trandate (labetalol)
tranilast
transcainide
Transderm-Nitro (nitroglycerin)
transdermal nitroglycerin
Trasylol (aprotinin injection)
Trecator-SC (ethionamide)
triamcinolone acetonide
triamterene
tribenoside
trichlormethiazide

medications *(cont.)*
Tridil (nitroglycerin)
triflocin
Tri-Hydroserpine (HCTZ;
   reserpine; hydralazine)
trimazosin
trimeprazine tartrate
trimethaphan camsylate
trimoxamine
tripamide
tripelennamine citrate
triprolidine
troleandomycin
tromethamine
Truphylline (aminophylline)
tuaminoheptane
tuberculin
Tuberculin Mono-Vacc Test
Tuberculin Tine Test, Old
Tubersol (tuberculin purified
   protein derivative
Unicard (dilevalol)
Uni-Dur (theophylline)
Uniphyl (theophylline)
Unipres (HCTZ; reserpine;
   hydralazine)
Ureaphil (urea)
urokinase
Vanceril (beclomethasone dipropionate)
vancomycin
Vaponefrin (racepinephrine)
Vaporole
Vascor (bepridil
Vaseretic (enalapril maleate;
   HCTZ)
Vasodilan (isoxsuprine)
vasopressin (VP)
vasopressin tannate
Vasotec (enalapril maleate)
Vasoxyl (methoxamine)
Velban (vinblastine sulfate)

medications *(cont.)*
Ventolin; Ventolin Rotacaps
 (albuterol sulfate)
VePesid (etoposide)
verapamil
Verelan (verapamil)
verlukast
verofylline
Versed (midazolam)
vesnarinone
Vibramycin (doxycycline monohydrate)
viprostol
Visken (pindolol)
vitamin B_{12} injections
Volmax (albuterol sulfate)
Voxsuprine (isoxsuprine)
warfarin potassium
warfarin sodium
Wyamine Sulfate (mephentermine
 sulfate)
Wytensin (guanabenz acetate)
xamoterol fumarate
xanoxate sodium
xanthinol niacinate
xenalipin
xipamide
Xylocaine IV for Cardiac Arrhythmias (lidocaine)
Zaditen (ketotifen)
zaltidine
zankiren
Zaroxolyn (metolazone)
Zebeta (bisoprolol fumarate)
Zestoretic (HCTZ; lisinopril)
Zestril (lisinopril)
Ziac (bisoprolol fumarate; HCTZ)
zileuton
zindotrine
Zinecard (dexrazoxane)
zinterol
Zixoryn (flumecinol)

medications *(cont.)*
Zocor (simvastatin)
zofenopril calcium
zofenoprilat arginine
zolertine
Medicon instruments for vascular and
 cardiac surgery
Medicon rib spreader
Medicon vascular and cardiac surgery
 instruments
Medigraphics analyzer
Medinvent stent
medionecrosis
 cystic
 Erdheim cystic
MediPort implanted vascular access
 device
Medi-Quet surgical tourniquet
Medi-Tech balloon catheter
Medi-Tech steerable system
Mediterranean anemia
medium crackles
Medrad contrast medium injector
Medrad guide wire
Medtel pacemaker
Medtronic aortic punch
Medtronic balloon catheter
Medtronic bipolar electrode
Medtronic cardiac cooling jacket
Medtronic Cardioverter
Medtronic demand pulse generator
Medtronic electrode
Medtronic endocardial defibrillation
 lead
Medtronic endocardial defibrillation-
 sensing/pacing lead
Medtronic External Tachyarrhythmia
 Control Device (ETCD)
Medtronic-Hall monocuspid tilting-
 disk valve
Medtronic-Hall prosthetic heart valve
Medtronic-Hall valve prosthesis

Medtronic-Hancock device
Medtronic Interactive Tachycardia
  Terminating System
Medtronic Minix
Medtronic pacemaker
Medtronic pacemaker generator
Medtronic patch leads
Medtronic PCD (programmable car-
  dioverter-defibrillator)
Medtronic prosthetic valve
Medtronic Radio-Frequency (RF)
  Receiver
Medtronic SPO pacemaker
Medtronic subcutaneous patch lead
Medtronic Symbios pacemaker
Medtronic temporary pacemaker
Medtronic Transvene electrode
medulla, adrenal
Meeker dissecting forceps
Meeker grasping forceps
Mee protocol
Mees lines
Mee technique
$MEF_{50\% \ VC}$ (mid-expiratory flow at
  50% vital capacity)
megahertz (MHz)
Meige lymphedema
Meigs capillaries
Meigs-Cass syndrome
Meigs syndrome
melanoma metastatic to heart,
  malignant
Melrose solution
Meltzer sign
membranacea, pars
membrane, membranes
  alveolar-capillary
  asphyxial
  basement
  Bichat
  diphtheritic
  Dorhas

membrane (cont.)
  fenestrated
  Gore-Tex surgical
  Henle
  Henle elastic
  Henle fenestrated
  hyaline
  pleuropericardial
  smooth glistening
  supramitral
  vernix
membrane oxygenator, SciMed
membrane potential
membranous bronchitis
membranous croup
membranous septum
membranous subvalvular aortic stenosis
membranous ventricular septal defect
MemoryTrace AT ambulatory cardiac
  monitor
Mendelson syndrome
Ménière syndrome
meningeal hemorrhage
meningitis, complicating
meningococcal endocarditis
meningococcal infection
meningococcal myocarditis
meningococcal pericarditis
meningococcus
meniscus (crescent) of contrast-saline
  mixture
meniscus of saline test for pneumoperitoneum
mercurial diuretics
mercury-in-Silastic strain gauge for
  blood flow determination
Meridian echocardiography
Mersilene braided nonabsorbable
  suture
Mersilene suture
"Mer-suh" (MRSA)
mesenchymal connective tissue

mesenchymal tissue migration
mesenteric angiography
mesenteric arterial thrombosis
mesenteric artery occlusion, acute
mesenteric artery, superior
mesenteric infarction
mesenteric venous thrombosis
mesh-wrapping of aortic aneurysm,
    subtotal
mesocardia
mesocaval anastomosis
mesothelioma, atrioventricular (AV)
    node
mesothelium, pleural
mesoversion of heart
Mester test for rheumatic disease
MET (measurement of oxygen
    consumption/kilogram/minute)
Meta MV pacemaker
Meta rate responsive pacemaker
metabolic aberration
metabolic acidemia
metabolic acidosis
metabolic alkalosis
metabolic cardiomyopathy
metabolic disorders affecting heart
    function
metabolic equivalents (mets)
metabolism
    glycosphingolipid
    myocardial
metaiodobenzylguanidine scintigraphy
metal fume fever
metal needle
metallic clips
metallic cough
metallic rales
metanephrine, urinary
metaplasia, squamous
metapneumonic empyema
metapneumonic pleurisy

metastasectomy, pulmonary
metastases to mediastinum
metastatic abscess
metastatic bronchogenic carcinoma
metastatic hypernephroma to heart
metastatic myocardial tumor
metasynchronous tumor
metazoal infestation
metazoal myocarditis
meter (m)
meter per second (m/sec) velocity
metered-dose aerosol
metered-dose inhaler (MDI)
meter mask
methacholine bronchial provocation
    test
methacholine challenge, inhaled
methacholine chloride challenge
methacholine chloride inhalation
methemoglobin reductase deficiency
methemoglobinemia
methimazole
method (see also *formula, operation,
    procedure, technique*)
    Anel
    Antyllus
    Barbero-Marcial
    Brasdor
    Brisbane
    Brisbane aortic valve and ascending
        aorta replacement
    Carpentier
    Danielson
    direct Fick
    Dodge area-length
    Douglas bag (for determining
        cardiac output)
    downstream sampling
    Ellman
    empty beating heart
    Fick

method *(cont.)*
  forward triangle
  GLH (Green Lane Hospital)
    insertion
  Graupner
  Hatle valve area
  Hetzel forward triangle
  indicator-dilution (for determining
    cardiac output)
  indocyanine green dye (cardiac
    output measurement)
  Kennedy ejection fraction
  Kouchoukos
  Laks
  Lee-White
  McGoon
  metrizamide contrast medium
  Narula
  Orsi-Grocco
  Pachon
  polarographic oxygen (for deter-
    mining cardiac output)
  Purmann
  pyramid ventricular volume
  Quick
  Sahli
  Scarpa
  Shimazaki area-length
  Stoney
  Strauss
  Theden
  thermodilution (cardiac output
    measurement)
  upstream sampling
  Valdes-Cruz
  van den Bergh
  Wardrop
  Westergren
methyl methacrylate repair of
  aneurysm
meticulous dissection

metrizoate acid contrast material
metrizamide contrast material
mets (metabolic equivalents)
Metzenbaum curved scissors
Metzenbaum straight scissors
Meyer vein stripper
MFAT (multifocal atrial tachycardia)
MHz (megahertz)
MI (mitral insufficiency)
MI (myocardial infarction)
MI (myocardial ischemia)
Michel aortic clamp
microaneurysm
microangiopathic anemia
microangiopathic hemolytic anemia
microangiopathy
  intraretinal (IRMA)
  thrombotic
microbubbles
  carbon dioxide
  hydrogen peroxide
  oxygen
  Renografin-76
microcavitation
microcirculation, pulmonary
microcytic anemia
microembolization, cholesterol
microfibrillar hemostat (INSTAT
  MCH)
microfibrillar protein fibrillin gene
microfilariae
microfistulous AV (arteriovenous)
  communications
microfistulous AV (arteriovenous)
  shunt
micro forceps
microglide
micrognathia
Micro-Guide catheter
microinfarct (of heart)
Microknit vascular graft prosthesis

Microlith P pacemaker
microlithiasis
  alveolar
  pulmonary alveolar
micromanometer-tip catheter
Micro Minix pacemaker
micronodular infiltrates
microscissors
microscope-aided pedal bypass
microsecond pulsed flashlamp pumped
  dye laser
microsphere, albumin
microsphere perfusion scintigraphy
Microthin P_2 pacemaker
Micro-Tracer portable EKG
microvascular anastomosis
microvascular circulation
microvascular clamp
microvasculature, pulmonary
Microvel double velour graft
Microvena nitinol wire
microvenoarteriolar fistula
microwave thermal balloon angioplasty
micturition syncope
midaortic arch
midaortic syndrome
midaxillary line
midcircumflex
midclavicular line (MCL)
mid-diastole
mid-diastolic mitral murmur
mid-distal
middle aortic syndrome
middle cardiac vein
middle lobe collapse
middle lobe of lung
middle lobe syndrome
middle mediastinum
mid-expiratory flow at 50% vital
  capacity ($MEF_{50\% VC}$)
mid-expiratory tidal flow
midgraft stenosis

mid-groove portion of lumina
mid-inspiratory flow at 50% vital
  capacity ($MIF_{50\% VC}$)
midlateral course
mid-left sternal border
midline hockey-stick incision
midline, infracolic
midline sternotomy
midline sternotomy incision
midlung zone
midmarginal branch of artery
midportion
midscapular line
midsternal area
midsternum
midsystole
midsystolic click–late systolic murmur
  syndrome
midsystolic closure of aortic valve
midsystolic murmur
midsystolic notching of velocity
  spectrum
midsystolic impulse
midsystolic retraction
mid-ventricular short-axis slice
midzone
$MIF_{50\% VC}$ (mid-inspiratory flow at
  50% vital capacity)
migraine equivalent
migraine, precordial
migrainous-like scintillations
migrating phlebitis
migration
  catheter
  lead
  mesenchymal tissue
  stent
migratory infiltrates, patchy
migratory patchy infiltration
migratory phlebitis
Mikros pacemaker
Mikro-tip angiocatheter

Mikro-tip micromanometer-tipped catheter
mild dyspnea
mild subcostal retractions
mild whole body hypothermia
miliary tuberculosis
milieu, therapeutic
milk leg syndrome
milk spot pericarditis
milking action of leg musculature
milky effusion
mill-house murmur
Millar catheter
Millar catheter-tip transducer
Millar micromanometer catheter
Millar MPC-500 catheter
Millar pigtail angiographic catheter
Miller-Dieker syndrome
miller's lung
Miller-Senn retractor
Miller septostomy catheter
milliampere (mA)
millicurie (mCi)
Millikan-Siekert syndrome
Milliknit Dacron prosthesis
Milliknit vascular graft prosthesis
millimeters of mercury (mm Hg)
milliseconds (ms, msec)
millivolt (mV)
Mills arteriotomy scissors
Mills valvotome; valvulotome
Miltex rib spreader
Milton angioedema disease
Milton edema
mimic, mimicked
mineralocorticoid excess
miner's asthma
miner's lung
minimal expiratory grunting
minimal lumen diameter
minimal luminal diameter (MLD)
minimal volume (of left atrium)

minimizes protrusion of device
minimum blood pressure
Mini-Profile dilatation catheter, USCI
minithoracotomy, right
Minix ST pacemaker
Minnesota classification of EKG
Minnesota criteria for high R waves
Minot–von Willebrand syndrome
minuscule
minute ventilation
minute ventilation sensor
minute vessels
minute volume
Mirage over-the-wire balloon catheter
MIRI (myocardial infarction recovery index)
mirror image
mirror-image brachiocephalic branching
mirror-image reversal of thoracic and abdominal viscera
mirror test for bronchial expectoration
MIS (minimally invasive surgery)
misery perfusion
missile trajectory
missile wound of heart
missing beat
mist tent
mite, house dust
mitigated (alleviate, relieve)
mitochondrial phosphorylation
mitral annular calcification
mitral annuloplasty
mitral annulus
mitral apparatus
mitral arcade
mitral atresia
mitral click syndrome
mitral click-murmur syndrome
mitral configuration of cardiac shadow on x-ray
mitral deceleration slope

mitral inflow velocities
mitral insufficiency
mitral leaflets, noncalcified
mitral leak
mitral orifice
mitral regurgitant murmur
mitral regurgitant signal area
mitral regurgitation
  congenital
  pansystolic
mitral regurgitation-chordal elongation
  syndrome
mitral ring calcification
mitral stenosis (see *stenosis*)
  congenital
  relative
  true
mitral valve
  Beall prosthetic
  billowing
  cleft
  hammock
  parachute
mitral valve abnormalities
mitral valve atresia
mitral valve calcification
mitral valve commissures
mitral valve configuration, fishmouth
mitral valve echogram
mitral valve leaflet tip
mitral valve myxomatous degeneration
mitral valve obstruction
mitral valve prolapse, holosystolic
mitral valve prolapse murmur
mitral valve prolapse syndrome
mitral valve regurgitation
mitral valve regurgitation without
  prolapse
mitral valve replacement
mitral valve septal separation
mitral valve stenosis (MVS)
Mitroflow pericardial prosthetic valve

Mitsubishi angioscope
Mitsubishi angioscopic catheter
mixed connective tissue disease
mixed grass pollen
mixed lesion
mixed restrictive-obstructive lung
  disease
mixed venous saturation
Mixter clamp
Mixter dissecting forceps
Mixter grasping forceps
Mixter right-angle clamp
MLD (minimal luminal diameter)
MM band
MMEF (mean maximal expiratory
  flow)
MM fraction
mm Hg (millimeters of mercury)
M-mode Doppler echocardiography
M-mode echocardiogram
M-mode echocardiogram in utero
M-mode echophonocardiography
M-mode transducer
MO (mitral orifice)
mobile pedunculated left atrial tumor
mobile thrombus
mobilization
Mobin-Uddin embolus trap
Mobin-Uddin umbrella filter
Mobin-Uddin vena caval filter
Mobitz classification (type I or II) of
  atrioventricular (AV) heart block
Mobitz I (and II) second-degree block
Mobitz type I on Wenckebach heart
  block
moccasin feet
modality
  alternative
  diagnostic
  pacing
  standard
  therapeutic

mode
A-mode (on echocardiogram)
AAI (noncompetitive atrial
    demand)
AAI rate-responsive
active
atrial triggered and ventricular
    inhibited
atrial-burst
atrioventricular dual-demand
B-mode (on ultrasound)
bipolar pacing
committed
DDD pacing
dual-demand pacing
DVI
fixed rate
full-to-empty VAD
inactive
inhibited pacing
M-mode (on echocardiogram)
noncommitted
pacing
semicommitted
sequential
stimulation
synchronous pacemaker
triggered pacing
underdrive
unipolar pacing
VVI (noncompetitive demand
    ventricular)
mode abandonment
model
figure-of-eight
leading circle
ring
moderate growth of normal
    respiratory flora
moderate respiratory acidemia
moderate respiratory distress
moderate wheezing

moderate whole body hypothermia
moderator band
modification
Bentall procedure, Cabrol II
Carpentier repair
Dor
Lecompte
Quaegebeur
slow-pathway
modified Bentall button technique
modified Blalock-Taussig shunt
modified Bruce protocol
modulation, respiratory
Moenckeberg ((Mönckeberg)
Mohr syndrome
moist atelectatic rales
moist mucous membranes
moist rales
MOL (middle of life)
molding, atheroma
Molina needle-catheter
moment, magnetic
Mönckeberg (Moenckeberg)
Mönckeberg arteriosclerosis
Mönckeberg calcification
Mönckeberg degeneration
Mönckeberg medial sclerosis
Monday fever syndrome
Mondor phlebitis disease
Mondor syndrome
Mondor thrombophlebitis
M1 (marginal branch #1)
M_1 heart sound (mitral valve closure)
Monge disease or syndrome
monilial endocarditis
monitor
Accucap CO_2/O_2
Accucom cardiac output
Accutorr
ambulatory Holter
Arrhythmia Net arrhythmia
CA (cardiac-apnea)

monitor *(cont.)*
  cardiac
  CardioDiary heart
  Commucor A+V Patient
  continuous Holter
  Dinamap blood pressure
  electrocardiograph
  Holter
  Ohmeda CO_2
  Polar Vantage XL heart rate
  VEST ambulatory function
monitor bed
monitored anesthesia care (MAC)
monitoring
  bedside
  continuous Holter
  continuous (of myocardial ischemia)
  cytoimmunologic
  hemodynamic
monitoring line
Monneret bradycardia
Monneret pulse
monoamine oxidase (MAO) inhibitor
monobacteriae
monoclonal antibody
  OKT3
  whole blood
monocrotic pulse
monocusp valve
monofilament absorbable suture
monofilament nylon suture
monofilament polypropylene sutures
Monolyth oxygenator
monomorphic premature ventricular
  contractions (PVCs)
monomorphic VT (ventricular tachycardia)
mononeuritis multiplex
mononuclear cell, pleomorphic
mononuclear infiltrate
monoparesis
monophasic contour of QRS complex

monophasic shock waveforms
monophasic waveforms, truncated
  exponential simultaneous
Monorail angioplasty catheter
Monorail balloon catheter
Monorail catheter system
Monostrut cardiac valve prosthesis
Monsel's hemostatic solution
moon facies
morbid event
morbidity and mortality
morbid thinking
morbus cordis
Morgagni-Adams-Stokes (MAS)
  attacks
Morgagni-Adams-Stokes syndrome
Morgagni, foramen of
moribund
morphine
morphologic left ventricle
Morquio syndrome
Morris aorta clamp
Morse manifold
Morse sternal spreader
mort d'amour syndrome
Morton Salt Substitute
mosaic-jet signals
Moschcowitz disease
Moschcowitz sign (of arterial occlusive disease)
Moschcowitz syndrome
Moschcowitz test for arteriosclerosis
Moschcowitz thrombotic thrombocytopenic purpura
moss-agate sputum
motion
  akinetic segmental wall
  anterior wall
  apical wall
  brisk wall
  catheter tip
  cusp

motion *(cont.)*
  discernible venous
  dyskinetic segmental wall
  dyskinetic wall
  forceful parasternal
  heaving precordial
  hyperkinetic segmental wall
  hypokinetic segmental wall
  hypokinetic wall
  inferior wall
  leaflet
  left ventricular regional wall
  palpable anterior
  paradoxical leaflet
  paradoxical (of chest wall)
  paradoxical septal
  posterior wall
  posterolateral wall
  regional hypokinetic wall
  regional wall
  rocking precordial
  segmental wall
  septal wall
  sustained anterior parasternal
  systolic anterior (SAM)
  trifid precordial motion
  ventricular wall
  visible anterior
motion artifact
motion cough
motor impairment
mottled density
mottled extremities
mottled gray lung
mottled thickening
mottling
Mounier-Kuhn syndrome
mountain sickness
  acute
  chronic
  chronic emphysematous

mountain sickness *(cont.)*
  chronic erythremic
  subacute
mouth-to-mouth respirations
movement
  basal (on x-ray)
  circus
  paradoxical
moyamoya ("puff of smoke")
moyamoya cerebrovascular disease
Moynahan syndrome
MPA (main pulmonary artery)
MPAP (mean pulmonary artery
  pressure)
M pattern on right atrial waveform
MPF catheter
MPHR (maximum predicted heart
  rate)
MPR (myocardial perfusion reserve)
MR (mitral regurgitation)
MRA (magnetic resonance
  angiography)
MRA gated inflow technique
MRI (magnetic resonance imaging)
MRI terms
  ECG-gated multislice technique
  ECG-gated spin-echo MR image
  echoplanar imaging
  FLASH (fast low-angle shot)
  free induction decay
  gradient-echo sequence imaging
  GRASS (gradient recalled acquisi-
    tion in steady state) cardiac MRI
  hydrogen density
  magnetic moment
  magnetic resonance signal
  multinuclear MRI
  multiphasic multislice technique
  paramagnetic substances
  proton density
  proton MRI

MRI terms *(cont.)*
  proton spectroscopy
  relaxation
  relaxation times
  resonant frequency
  short-axis plane
  spin density
  spin-echo imaging sequence
  surface coils
  TE (echo delay time)
  tesla
  T1 relaxation time
  T1-weighted image
  T2 relaxation time
  T2-weighted image
  TR (repetition time)
  transverse plane
  voxel
  XY plane
  ZY plane
MRS (magnetic resonance spectroscopy)
MRSA (pronounced "mer-suh")
  (methicillin-resistant
  Staphylococcus aureus)
ms (milliseconds)
MS (mitral stenosis)
MS (morphine sulfate)
MSA (multiple system atrophy)
  syndrome
msec (millisecond)
M-shaped pattern of mitral valve
MTEs (main timing events)
MTT (mean pulmonary transit time)
mucocele
mucociliary transport
mucocutaneous junction
mucocutaneous lymph node syndrome
mucoid degeneration, cardiac valve
mucoid impaction in bronchi
mucoid medial degeneration

mucoid plugging of airways
mucoid plugs
mucolipidosis
mucopolysaccharidoses (plural)
mucopolysaccharidosis cardiomyopathy
mucoproteins
mucopurulent bronchitis
mucopurulent exudate
mucopurulent secretions
mucopurulent sputum
mucosa
  bronchial
  endobronchial
  friable
mucosal inflammation
mucous membranes
  dry
  moist
mucous rales
mucoviscidosis
mucus
  bloody nasal
  inspissated
  tenacious
mucus hypersecretion
mucus plug or plugging
Mueller (Müller)
muffled breath sounds
muffled heart sounds
MUGA (multiple-gated acquisition)
MUGA blood pool radionuclide scan
MUGA scan, preoperative resting
mulibrey nanism
Müller (Mueller)
Müller catheter guide
Müller-Dammann pulmonary artery
  banding
Müller-Dammann technique
Müller maneuver (cardiac auscultation)
Müller sign (aortic regurgitation)

Mullins blade technique for dilatation
of patent foramen ovale
Mullins catheter introducer
Mullins cardiac device
Mullins modification of transseptal
catheterization
Mullins sheath
Mullins transseptal blade and balloon
atrial septostomy
Mullins transseptal catheter
Mullins transseptal sheath
multiadjustable fitting device
multicapture burst
multichannel ECG (EKG)
Multicor Gamma pacemaker
Multicor II pacemaker
multicrystal gamma camera
multidrug resistance
multidrug-resistant tuberculosis
(MDR-TB)
multidrug therapy
multifactorial
multifiber catheter
multifocal aggressive infiltrate
multifocal atrial tachycardia with
aberrancy
multifocal lesions
multifocal lymphoma
multifocal PVCs (premature ventricular contractions)
multifocal short stenoses
multiforme, erythema
multiform PVC
multiform ventricular complexes
multi-infarct dementia
multilaminar bodies
multilead electrode
multilesion angioplasty
Multilith pacemaker
Multi-Med triple-lumen infusion
catheter
multinuclear MRI

multinucleate giant cells
multiphasic multislice MRI technique
multiple blood transfusions
multiple chord, center line technique
in echocardiogram
multiple drug resistance
multiple endocrine neoplasia
multiple extrastimuli
multiple-gated acquisition (MUGA)
multiple lentigines
multiple logistic regression
multiple mural dilations
multiple organ failure
multiple-puncture tuberculin test
multiple sulfatase deficiency
multiple system atrophy (MSA)
syndrome
multiple-system disease
multiple unidentified respiratory flora
(MURF)
multiplex, mononeuritis
multiprogrammable pulse generator
multipurpose catheter
Multipurpose-SM catheter
multislice multiphase spin-echo
imaging technique
multislice spin-echo technique
multivalvular disease
multiverrucous friable lesions
multivessel angioplasty
multivessel disease
mural aneurysm
mural architecture
mural degeneration
mural endomyocardial fibrosis
mural infiltration
mural leaflet of mitral valve
mural thrombosis
mural thrombus (pl. thrombi)
mural thrombus formation
MURF (multiple unidentified respiratory flora)

mu rhythm (mu, twelfth Greek letter)
murmur (see also *sound*)
  accidental
  acquired heart
  amphoric
  anemic
  aneurysmal
  aortic diastolic
  aortic insufficiency
  aortic systolic
  apex
  apical
  apical diastolic
  arterial
  atrial systolic (ASM)
  atriosystolic
  attrition
  Austin Flint
  basal
  basal diastolic
  basal systolic
  basilar carotid
  bellows (blowing)
  blood
  blowing
  blowing pansystolic
  blubbery diastolic
  brachiocephalic systolic
  brain
  bronchial
  buzzing
  Cabot-Locke
  cardiac
  cardiopulmonary
  cardiorespiratory
  Carey Coombs (no hyphen)
  click
  coarse
  Cole-Cecil
  congenital heart
  continuous (CM)

murmur *(cont.)*
  continuous mammary souffle
  continuous rumbling
  cooing
  cooing-dove
  Coombs
  crescendo
  crescendo-decrescendo
  crescendo-decrescendo configuration
  crescendo presystolic
  Cruveilhier-Baumgarten
  decrescendo
  decrescendo holosystolic
  delayed diastolic (DDM)
  diamond-shaped
  diastolic (graded from 1 to 4)
  diastolic flow
  diastolic rumbling
  diffusely radiating
  diminuendo
  Docke
  Docke diastolic
  Duroziez
  dynamic
  early diastolic
  early systolic
  ejection
  ejection systolic (ESM)
  ejectionlike systolic
  endocardial
  even
  extracardiac
  extracardiac systolic arterial
  Flint
  Frantzel
  friction
  functional
  functional heart
  Gallavardin
  Gibson

murmur *(cont.)*
  goose honk
  grade 1/6 or I/VI
    2/6 or II/VI
    1-2/6 or I-II/VI
    1 to 6 or I to VI
  Graham Steell heart
  groaning
  grunting
  Hamman
  harsh
  heart
  hemic
  high
  high-frequency
  high-pitched
  high-pitched ejection
  Hodgkin-Key
  holodiastolic
  holosystolic
  holosystolic ejection
  honking
  Hope
  hourglass
  humming
  humming-top
  immediate diastolic (IDM)
  incidental
  innocent heart
  innocent systolic
  inorganic
  late apical systolic
  late diastolic
  late-peaking systolic
  late systolic (LSM)
  left ventricular outflow
  Levine Harvey grading system for
  loud (high-grade)
  low-frequency
  low-frequency diastolic
  low-pitched

murmur *(cont.)*
  low-pitched, rumbling apical
    diastolic
  machine-like
  machinery
  machinery-like
  mammary souffle
  mid-diastolic
  mid-diastolic flow
  mid-diastolic mitral
  midsystolic
  mid-to-late diastolic
  mill-house
  millwheel
  mitral
  mitral click
  mitral regurgitant
  mitral valve prolapse
  musical
  nun's venous hum
  obstructive
  organic
  outflow
  outflow midsystolic
  pansystolic (PSM)
  parasternal
  parasternal systolic
  pathologic
  pericardial
  peripheral pulmonic systolic
  plateau
  pleuropericardial
  prediastolic
  presystolic (PSM)
  presystolic Austin Flint
  presystolic crescendo
  protodiastolic
  prototypical holosystolic
  pulmonary outflow
  pulmonary trunk
  pulmonary valve flow

murmur *(cont.)*
  pulmonic radiating
  pulmonic systolic
  rasping
  regurgitant
  Roger
  rough
  rumbling
  rumbling diastolic
  Sansom rhythmical
  scratchy
  seagull
  seesaw (to-and-fro)
  Smith
  soft (low grade)
  squeaking
  Steell
  stenosal
  Still early systolic
  subclavicular
  supraclavicular
  supraclavicular systolic
  systolic (graded from 1 to 6)
  systolic ejection
  systolic mammary souffle
  to-and-fro (seesaw)
  Traube
  tricuspid
  tricuspid diastolic
  uneven
  unknown type
  valvular pulmonic stenosis
  variable
  vascular
  venous
  vibratory systolic
  waterwheel
  whooping
murmur abolished by digital pressure
murmur at the apex and left sternal
  border

murmur augmented by vigorous
  coughing
murmur grades: I to VI; 1 to 6
murmur increased during inspiration
murmur increased in intensity on
  Valsalva
murmur obliterated by digital pressure
murmur of long duration
murmur of short duration
murmur or gallop
murmur radiating into suprasternal
  notch
murmur radiating to apex of heart
murmur radiating to axilla
murmur radiating to base of neck
murmur radiating to neck
murmur radiating to sternal border
murmur, rub, or gallop
murmurs, clicks, or gallops
murmur transmitted to apex of heart
murmur transmitted to axilla
murmur transmitted to base of heart
murmur transmitted to carotids
murmur transmitted to neck
murmur with/without radiation
muscle, muscles
  accessory (of respiration)
  adductor magnus
  circular
  conal papillary
  electrically conditioned and driven
  skeletal
  fused papillary
  gastrocnemius
  intercostal
  Lancisi
  latissimus dorsi
  left ventricular
  longitudinal
  Luschka
  medial papillary

muscle *(cont.)*
  omohyoid
  papillary
  pectoralis major
  pectoralis minor
  peroneal
  plantaris
  platysma
  rhomboideus major
  sacrospinalis
  serratus anterior
  soleus
  sternocleidomastoid
  sternohyoid
  sternothyroid
  strap
  subaortic
  trapezius
  vastus medialis
  vocalis
muscle artifact
muscle cramps
muscle flap
muscle training, ventilatory
muscular atrioventricular septum
muscular bridging
muscular crus of diaphragm
muscular dystrophy
  Becker
  Duchenne
  Emery-Dreifuss
muscular subaortic stenosis
muscular venous pump
musculi pectinati
musculofascial layer
musculofascial pedicle
musculophrenic artery
musculophrenic branch
musculoskeletal pain
musculotendinous covering
mushroom picker's disease

mushroom worker's lung
mushroom worker's disease
mushy edema
mushy mass
musical murmur
musical rales
musical rhonchi
musical whoop
Musset sign (aortic aneurysm)
Mustard atrial baffle repair
Mustard baffle
Mustard correction of transposition of
  great vessels
mutation, fibrillin gene
mutism, akinetic
mV (millivolt)
MV (mitral valve)
MVA (mitral valve area)
MVD (mitral valve dysfunction)
MVO (maximum venous outflow)
MVO (mitral valve opening or orifice)
MVO_2 (myocardial oxygen consump-
  tion)
MVP (mitral valve prolapse)
MVP over-the-wire balloon catheter
MVR (mitral valve replacement)
MVS (mitral valve stenosis)
MVV (maximal voluntary ventilation)
MWT (maximum walking time)
myalgias and arthralgias
mycobacterial infection
mycobacteria, nontuberculous
mycobacteria susceptibility testing
mycobacterium, nonchromogenic
Mycobacterium abscessus
Mycobacterium avium complex
  (MAC)
Mycobacterium avium-intracellular
  (MAI) infection
Mycobacterium fortuitum
Mycobacterium gordonae

Mycobacterium kansasii
Mycobacterium simiae infection
Mycobacterium tuberculosis
Mycoplasma antibody titer
Mycoplasma pneumoniae infection
mycoplasmal pneumonia
mycosis
  fatal systemic
  Posadas
mycotic aneurysm of pulmonary
  artery
mycotic suprarenal aneurysm
mydriasis
myectomy
Myler catheter
myocardial blood flow (MBF)
myocardial blush
myocardial bridging
myocardial cell necrosis
myocardial contractile function
myocardial contractility
myocardial contraction
myocardial contracture
myocardial contrast appearance time
  (MCAT)
myocardial contusion
myocardial degeneration
myocardial depression
myocardial dysfunction
myocardial fibers degeneration
myocardial fibrosis
myocardial granulomatous disease,
  allergic
myocardial hibernation
myocardial hypoperfusion, resting
  regional
myocardial hypothermia
myocardial hypoxia
myocardial incompetency

myocardial infarction (see also
  infarction)
  anterior
  anterior wall
  anteroapical wall
  anterobasal
  anterolateral wall
  anteroseptal wall
  apical
  apical-lateral wall
  basal-lateral wall
  diaphragmatic wall
  esophageal spasm mimicking
  high lateral wall
  impending
  inferior (diaphragmatic)
  inferolateral wall
  inferoposterior wall
  intraoperative
  nontransmural
  perioperative
  posterior wall
  posterobasal wall
  posteroinferior
  posterolateral wall
  posteroseptal
  stuttering
  subendocardial
  transmural
  true posterior wall
  uncomplicated, non-Q-wave
  uncomplicated Q-wave
myocardial infiltration by Kaposi
  sarcoma
myocardial injury
  lethal
  nonlethal
myocardial insufficiency, Sternberg
myocardial irritability

myocardial ischemia, exercise-induced
  transient
myocardial lactate extraction
myocardial muscle
myocardial necrosis
myocardial oxygen consumption
myocardial oxygen demand
myocardial performance
myocardial perfusion
myocardial perfusion defect
myocardial perfusion imaging
myocardial perfusion imaging agent
  (see *contrast medium*)
myocardial perfusion scan
myocardial perfusion tomography
myocardial preservation
myocardial protection
myocardial recovery
myocardial reperfusion injury
myocardial revascularization
myocardial rupture
myocardial scan
myocardial screw-in rate-sensing lead
myocardial shortening, fractional
myocardial stiffness
myocardial straining
myocardial stunning
myocardial tagging
myocardial tissue viability
myocardial tumor, metastatic
myocardial uptake of thallium
myocardial work
myocardial-specific marker
myocardiopathy (see *cardiomyopathy*)
  dilated
  postpartum
  primary
  puerperium
  secondary

myocardiorrhaphy
myocarditic
myocarditis
  acute bacterial
  acute interstitial
  acute isolated
  acute rheumatic
  aseptic (of newborn)
  bacterial
  chronic
  chronic hypertrophic
  chronic interstitial
  chronic pernicious
  coxsackievirus
  diphtheritic
  eosinophilic
  fibroid
  fibrous
  Fiedler
  fragmentation
  fungal
  giant cell
  granulomatous
  Histoplasma
  hypersensitivity
  idiopathic
  infectious
  infective
  inflammatory
  influenzal
  interstitial
  isolated diffuse
  lues
  lymphocytic
  meningococcal
  metazoal
  neutrophilic
  nonspecific granulomatous
  parenchymatous

myocarditis *(cont.)*
  peripartum
  pernicious
  pneumococcal
  protozoal
  rheumatic
  rickettsial
  senile
  septic
  spirochetal
  staphylococcal
  subepicardial
  syphilitic
  toxic
  toxoplasmotic
  Trichinella
  tuberculoid
  tuberculous
  viral
myocardium
  ablation of
  asynergic
  calcification of
  dilated
  hibernating
  hypertrophied
  hypertrophy of
  ischemic reperfused
  ischemic viable
  jeopardized
  noninfarcted
  nonperfused
  perfused
  perfusion of
  reperfused
  rupture of
  stunned
  ventricular
  viable

myocardosis
myocellular area
myocyte necrosis
myocyte
  Anichkov (or Anitschkow)
  atrial
myocytic lysosomes
myocytolysis, focal (of the heart)
myoendocarditis
  acute
  subacute
myofibrillar area
myofibrillar intraventricular heart
  block
myofibril volume fraction
myoglobin (Mb) concentration, serum
myopathy
  myotubular
  nemaline
myopectoral inhibition of pacemaker
myopericarditis
myoplasty, sartorius
myopotential inhibition
myosin heavy chain
myosin light chain
myotonia atrophica cardiomyopathy
myotonia congenita
myotonic dystrophy
myotubular myopathy
myovascular
myriad
myxedema
myxoid degeneration
myxoma
  atrial
  biatrial
  cardiac
  familial (of the heart)
  heart

myxoma *(cont.)*
  left atrial
  pedunculated
  vascular
  ventricular
myxoma syndrome, with facial freckling
myxomatous degeneration of mitral
  valve

myxomatous degeneration of
  myocardium
myxomatous degeneration of valve
myxomatous proliferation in mitral
  valve prolapse
myxomatous proliferation of leaflets
  of mitral valve
myxomatous proliferation of spongiosa
myxomatous valve leaflet

N, n

Nabatoff vein stripper
N-acetylprocainamide (NAPA) level
nadir of lung function
nadir of QRS complex
nadir, protodiastolic
nail bed, clubbing of
nail bed color
nail bed cyanosis
nail-patella syndrome
nail-to-nailbed angle (clubbing)
Nakata index
NAME (nevi, atrial myxoma, myxoid
    neurofibroma, ephelides) syndrome
nanism, mulibrey
NAPA (N-acetylprocainamide) level
napkin-ring stenosis
Narcomatic flowmeter
narcosis, carbon dioxide
naris (pl. nares), anteverted
narrow anteroposterior diameter
narrow expiratory splitting
narrow inspiratory splitting
narrow QRS complex
narrowed pulse pressure
narrowed S_1 splitting
narrowed S_2 splitting

narrowing
    arterial
    atherosclerotic
    diffuse
    focal
    high-grade
    luminal
    residual luminal
    subcritical
narrowing in large airway
narrowing of bronchiolar passages
Narula method
nasal airway resistance
nasal antigen challenge
nasal CPAP (continuous positive
    airway pressure)
nasal flaring
nasogastric tube
nasopharyngeal temperature probe
nasotracheal suction
nasotracheal tube
Nathan pacemaker
National Heart, Lung, and Blood
    Registry guidelines
National Institutes of Health (NIH)
    catheter

native aortic valve, preservation of
native atherosclerosis
native coronary artery
native valve endocarditis
native ventricle
native vessel
natriuresis
natriuretic peptide, atrial
natural (intrinsic) heart rate
natural surfactant in the lungs
nature, evanescent
Naughton-Balke treadmill protocol,
  modified
Naughton cardiac exercise treadmill
  test
Naughton treadmill protocol, modified
navigating coronary structures
navigating heart structures
NBTE (nonbacterial thrombotic endocarditis)
Nd:YAG (neodymium:yttrium-
  aluminum-garnet) laser
near field
near-infrared spectroscopy
near-loss of consciousness
near-syncopal episode
near-syncope
nebulization therapy, continuous
  (CNT)
nebulize
nebulized bronchodilator
nebulized isoproterenol
nebulizer
  Acorn
  Aero Tech II
  air-powered
  DeVilbiss ultrasound
  Fisoneb
  hand-held
  high-frequency
  jet

nebulizer *(cont.)*
  MAD2
  Portasonic
  Pulmosonic
  Respirgard II
  Small Particle Aerosol
  Ultravent
  Varic ultrasound
  Wright
  ultrasonic (USN)
NEC (nonejection click)
Necator americanus infection
neck emphysema
neck, hyperextension
neck of the aneurysm
neck rotation
neck vein distention
neck veins
  distended
  elevated
  flat
  fullness of
neck vessel engorgement
necrosis
  acute tubular
  alveolar
  alveolar septa
  aorta idiopathic
  arteriolar
  caseous
  cheesy
  coagulation
  contraction band
  cystic medial
  embolic
  Erdheim cystic medial (of aorta)
  fibrinoid
  heart muscle
  hepatic
  hyaline
  ischemic

necrosis *(cont.)*
  lung
  myocardial
  myocyte
  perioperative myocardial
  skin (due to distal steal)
  subendocardial
  ventricular muscle
necrosis of lung
necrotic cells
necrotic debris
necrotic fibrinoid vegetation
necrotic flap
necrotizing angiitis
necrotizing arterial disease
necrotizing arteriolitis
necrotizing arteritis
necrotizing bronchitis
necrotizing emphysema
necrotizing granulomatous angiitis
  involving lungs
necrotizing pneumonia
necrotizing respiratory granulomatosis
necrotizing thrombosis
necrotizing vasculitis
needle
  Abrams
  Aldrete
  AMC
  aortic root perfusion
  aspirating
  Atraloc
  Becton Dickinson Teflon-sheathed
  Bengash-type
  beveled thin-walled
  Brockenbrough
  Brockenbrough transseptal
  BV-2
  cardioplegic
  Cope biopsy
  Cournand

needle *(cont.)*
  cutting
  DLP cardioplegic
  Dos Santos
  Jelco
  large-bore slotted aspirating
  metal
  Nordenstrom (Rotex II) biopsy
  olive-tipped
  percutaneous cutting
  pericardiocentesis
  pleural biopsy
  Potts
  Potts-Cournand
  Protect Point
  root
  Rotex II biopsy
  Seldinger
  slotted
  spinal
  swaged-on
  THI
  thoracentesis
  UMI
  venting aortic Bengash-type
needle biopsy, CT-scan directed
needle, sponge, and instrument counts
NEFA (non-esterified fatty acid)
  scintigraphy
negative chronotropic effect
negative deflection on EKG
needle holder
  Barraquer
  Berry sternal
  Castroviejo
  Crile-Wood
  Vital Cooley microvascular
  Vital Ryder microvascular
  Webster
needle hub
Nefertiti sniff position

negative image of pulmonary edema
negative pressure at the airway
  opening during expiration
negligible pressure gradient
Neisseria infection
Nelson scissors
Nelson thoracic trocar
nemaline myopathy
neoadjuvant therahemopostoperative
  bleeding
neoaorta
neoaortic valve
neodymium:yttrium-aluminum-garnet
  (Nd:YAG) laser
neointimal hyperplasia
neointimal proliferation
neonatal asphyxia
neonatal cystic pulmonary emphysema
neonatal lupus erythematosus
neonatal thyrotoxicosis
neonate
neonatorum, edema
neoplasia, multiple endocrine
neoplasm
  endobronchial
  mediastinal
  primary lung
neoplastic pericarditis
Neos M pacemaker
neostigmine test
nephritis
  arteriolar
  interstitial arteriosclerotic
  radiation
  vascular
nephritis repens
nephroblastoma
nephrosclerosis
nephrotic edema
Nernst equation in cardiac action
  potential (resting phase)

nerve
  Hering
  Kuntz
  long thoracic
  phrenic
  recurrent laryngeal
  supraclavicular
  vagus
nervous heart syndrome
nervous system, parasympathetic
NESC (nonejection systolic click)
neural crest origin, tumor of
neuralgia, glossopharyngeal
neurally mediated syncope
neurectomy, periaortic
neurocardiogenic syncope
neurocirculatory asthenia
neurofibroma of the heart
neurofibromatosis
neurogenic pulmonary edema
neurogenic sarcoma of the heart
neurologic signs, focal
neuromuscular blockade
neuronal ceroid lipofuscinosis
neuropathy, autonomic
neuroregulatory asthenia
neuroregulatory syncope
neurosis, postphlebitic
neurotoxicity, lidocaine
neurovascular bundle
neutral fat (triglyceride)
neutropenia
neutrophil alveolitis
neutrophil concentration
neutrophilia, absolute
nevus (pl. nevi)
nevus araneus
  senile
  spider
  stellar

New York Heart Association
(NYHA)
Newman-Keuls test
NH region of AV (atrioventricular)
node
NI-NR (no infection—no rejection)
niacin test for *Mycobacterium tuberculosis*
Nicaladoni-Branham sign
nicking, AV (arteriovenous)
Nicks procedure
nicotinic acid
nidus, thrombus
Niedner anastomosis clamp
night sweats
NIH (National Institutes of Health)
NIH cardiac device
NIH cardiomarker catheter
NIH left ventriculography catheter
NIH mitral valve forceps
Nikaidoh-Bex technique
Nikaidoh translocation of aorta
Nikolsky sign
nil blood loss
Nimbus Hemopump
nipple, blind
nipple sign, aortic
NIPS (noninvasive programmed
stimulation)
NIRS (near-infrared spectroscopy)
nitinol (nickel/titanium alloy) thermal
memory stent
nitrates, long-acting
nitrogen, blood urea (BUN)
nitrogen-13 ammonia radioactive
tracer
nitrogen washout
nitroglycerin (NTG)
sublingual (SL)
topical

nitroglycerin *(cont.)*
transdermal
translingual
transmucosal
nitroglycerin drip
nitroprusside
nitrous oxide
nl, Nml (normal)
NMR (nuclear magnetic resonance)
NMR spectroscopy
no CPR status
nocardial infection of the bronchi
nocardiosis
nocardiotic pericarditis
nociceptive
nocturia times two
nocturnal angina
nocturnal asthma
nocturnal cough
nocturnal polyuria
nocturnal worsening of asthma
nodal conduction
nodal contractions
nodal escape
nodal impulse
nodal premature contraction
nodal rhythm disorder
node, nodes (see also *nodules*,
nodulus)
aortic window
Aschoff
Aschoff-Tawara
atrioventricular (AV, AVN)
axillary lymph
cardiac
Flack sinoatrial
hilar
Keith-Flack sinoatrial
Koch sinoatrial
lymph

node *(cont.)*
  mediastinal lymph
  NH region of AV (atrioventricular)
  nonverrucous
  Osler
  pericardial lymph
  SA (sinoatrial)
  sentinel
  shotty lymph
  sick sinus
  singer's
  sinoatrial (SAN)
  sinoauricular
  sinus
  supraclavicular lymph
  Tawara atrioventricular
  vestigial left sinoatrial
no discernible findings
nodo-Hisian (nodohisian) bypass tract
nodosa
  chorditis
  panarteritis
  periarteritis
  polyarteritis
nodosum, erythema
nodoventricular bypass fiber
nodoventricular bypass tract
nodoventricular pathway
nodoventricular tachycardia
nodular aneurysm
nodular fibrosis
nodularity
  coarse
  valve leaflet
  vein
nodule, nodules (see also *node*,
  nodulus)
  Albini
  aortic valve
  Arantius
  Aschoff

nodule *(cont.)*
  Bianchi
  Cruveilhier
  hyalin
  Kerckring
  laryngeal
  Morgagni
  noncavitary
  ossific
  rheumatic
  rheumatoid
  silicotic
  singer's
  solitary lung
  solitary pulmonary
nodules of pulmonary trunk valves
nodulus Arantii (pl. noduli Arantii)
  (nodule of Arantius)
nodus arcus venae azygos
noise, respiratory
nonablative heating
nonaeruginosa pseudomonads
nonallergenic factors
nonallergic asthma
nonapneic snorer
nonarrhythmic
nonarrhythmogenic
nonasbestos pneumoconiosis
nonatopic
nonazotemic
nonbacterial endocarditis
nonbacterial thrombotic endocarditis
nonbacterial verrucous endocarditis
noncalcific subacute constrictive
  pericarditis
noncalcified mitral leaflets
noncardiac chest pain
noncardiac death
noncardiac dyspnea
noncardiac pulmonary edema
noncardiogenic pulmonary edema

noncardiogenic shock
noncaseating granuloma
noncaseating tubercles
noncavitary nodules
noncavitary prosthetic graft
nonchromogenic mycobacterium
noncircularity degree
noncoaxial catheter tip position
noncollagenous pneumoconiosis
noncompensatory pause
noncompliant plaque
noncontractile scar tissue
noncoronary cardiomyopathy
noncoronary cusp
noncoronary sinus
noncrushing vascular clamps
nondecremental
nondiaphoretic
nondistensible pericardium
nondominant vessel
nondrinker, nonsmoker
non-ejection click (NEC)
non-ejection systolic click (NESC)
non-everting suture
nonexpansional dyspnea
nonfilarial chylocele
nonfilling venous segment
nonforeshortened angiographic view
nonhypertension syndrome
nonimaging probe
nonimmune fetal hydrops
nonimmunocompromised host
nonimmunological fetal hydrops
noninducible tachycardia
noninfarcted segment
noninfectious reactions of lung
noninfective endocardial lesion
noninfective verrucous endocarditis
noninflammatory fluid accumulation
   in pleural cavity
noninvasive assessment

noninvasive technique
noninvasive testing
noninvasive vascular imaging
   technique
nonionic contrast material
nonlethal arrhythmias
nonlethal myocardial ischemic injury
non-lifestyle-limiting lower extremity
   claudication
nonlingular branches of upper lobe
   bronchus
Nonne-Milroy lymphedema
non-nodular fibrosis
non-nodular silicosis
nonobstructive cardiomyopathy
   (NOCM)
nonocclusive mesenteric arterial
   insufficiency
nonoperable disease
nonorthorhythmic
nonoxygenated blood
nonpalpable pulses
nonparoxysmal atrioventricular
   junctional tachycardia
nonparoxysmal automatic atrial
   tachycardia
nonparoxysmal AV (atrioventricular)
   nodal tachycardia
nonpenetrating trauma to heart
nonpleuritic precordial pain
nonpneumoconiotic
nonproductive cough
nonproductive dry cough
nonpulsatile abdominal mass
nonpulsatile mass
nonpurulent pericarditis
nonpurulent pulmonary secretions
nonpyogenic thrombosis
non-Q wave
non-Q-wave myocardial infarction
   (NQWMI)

nonrebreather mask
nonreversed saphenous vein graft
nonreversed translocated vein bypass
nonrheumatic aortic stenosis
nonrheumatic endocarditis
nonrheumatic valvular aortic stenosis
nonsegmental areas of opacification
nonselective beta blocker
nonshocked heart
non-small cell carcinoma of lung
non-small cell lung cancer (NSCLC)
nonsmoker, nondrinker
nonspecific changes
nonspecific granulomatous myocarditis
nonspecific inflammatory aortoarteritis
nonspecific irritants
nonspecific scooping (on EKG)
nonspecific ST and T wave changes
    (NSTTWC)
nonspecific ST segment changes
nonspecific ST segment and T wave
    changes
nonspecific T wave aberration
nonspecific T wave abnormality
nonspecific T wave changes
nonsteroidal anti-inflammatory drugs
    (NSAID)
nonstress test (NST)
nonsurvivor
nonsustained monomorphic ventricular
    tachycardia
nonsustained polymorphic ventricular
    tachycardia
nonthoracotomy cardioverter-
    defibrillator
nonthoracotomy endocardial lead
    systems
  CPI Endotak
  Medtronic Transvene
  Telectronics EnGuard systems
nonthoracotomy lead (NTL)

nontrabeculated atrium
nontransmural myocardial infarction
nontraumatic epidural hemorrhage
nontraumatizing catheter
nontuberculous mycobacteria
nonuniform rotational defect (NURD)
nonunion of operated sternum
nonvalved conduit
nonverrucous node
nonviable scar from myocardial
    infarction
Noonan AV (arteriovenous) fistula
    clamp
Noonan syndrome
NoProfile balloon catheter
Nordenstrom biopsy needle
no-reflow phenomenon
norepinephrine
normal (nl, Nml)
normal-appearing bronchi
normal flora
normal QRS axis
normal QRS complex
normal S_1 and S_2 (heart sounds)
normal sinus rhythm (NSR)
normalization of inverted T waves
normetanephrine
normocapnic
normochromic anemia
normocytic anemia
normokalemic reperfusion
normotensive
normothermia
normothermic cardiopulmonary
    bypass
normothermic fibrillating heart
normothermic temperature
normovolemia
normovolemic
normoxia
Northern blot analysis or test

Norwood operation for hypoplastic
   left-sided heart syndrome
   Fontan modification of
   Gill-Jonas modification of
   Jonas modification of
   Sade modification of
NOS (not otherwise specified)
NoSalt
nose cone
nosocomial infection
nosocomial infective endocarditis
nosocomial lung infection
nosocomial opportunistic infection
nosocomial pneumonia
nosocomial TB (tuberculosis) transmission
nostril symptoms
not a candidate for cardiac surgery
not a candidate for transplant surgery
notch
   anacrotic
   aortic
   dicrotic
   sternal
   suprasternal
notched aortic knob on chest x-ray
notched P wave
notching of pulmonic valve on
   echocardiogram
notching, rib
note
   drumlike percussion
   dull percussion
   flat percussion
   hyperresonant percussion
   percussion
   resonant percussion
   tympanitic percussion
no therapy zone
Nothnagel paresthesia
Nothnagel syndrome

not-so-sudden cardiac death
Novacor DIASYS cardiac device
Novacor implantable left ventricular
   assist device (LVAD)
Novacor LVAS (left ventricular assist
   system)
Novacor ventricular assist device
   (VAD)
Nova MR pacemaker
Nova II pacemaker
Novofil suture
no-wrap technique
noxious agent
noxious inhalants
noxious stimuli
NPC (nodal premature contraction)
NPJT (nonparoxysmal AV [atrioven-
   tricular] junctional tachycardia)
NPRJT (nonparoxysmal reciprocating
   junctional tachycardia)
NQWMI (non-Q-wave myocardial
   infarction)
NSAID (nonsteroidal anti-inflamma-
   tory drugs)
NSAID-precipitated asthma
NSCLO (non-small cell lung cancer)
NSR (normal sinus rhythm)
NSTTWC (nonspecific ST and
   T wave changes)
NTG (nitroglycerin)
N-13 ammonia uptake on PET scan
NTL (nonthoracotomy lead)
NTP (noninvasive temporary pace-
   maker)
Nu-Salt
nuchal rigidity
nuclear gated blood pool testing
nuclear magnetic resonance (NMR)
nuclear-tagged red blood cell bleeding
   study
null point

numb extremities
number of puffs of bronchodilator
number of puffs of corticosteroids
numbness
nummular sputum
nun's murmur (venous hum)
NURD (nonuniform rotational defect)
Nurolon suture
nutrient cardioplegia
nutrition heart syndrome
nutritional anemia

nutritional macrocytic anemia
Nycore angiography catheter
NYHA (New York Heart
  Association)
NYHA classification of angina
NYHA classification of congestive
  heart failure
NYHA classification of heart block
  (types I-IV)
nylon sutures
Nyquist limit

O, o

oat bran
oat cell carcinoma
oat-shaped cell
obesity, cardiopulmonary
obesity-related hypertension
objective symptoms
obligatory
obligatory admixture of systemic
    venous and pulmonary venous
    blood
oblique abdominal incision
oblique fissure of lung
oblique pericardial sinus
oblique sinus
oblique subcostal incision
oblique vein of left atrium
obliquity
obliterans
    arteriosclerosis
    bronchiolitis
    endarteritis
    thromboangiitis
obliterating phlebitis
obliteration, lateral leaflet
obliteration of the costophrenic angle
obliterative arteriolitis, pulmonary
obliterative arteriosclerosis

obliterative arteritis
obliterative bronchiolitis
obliterative cardiomyopathy
obliterative pericarditis
obliterative phlebitis
obscuration of hilum
obscure cardiomyopathy of Africa
obscured coronary anatomy
obstructed pulmonary artery
obstructing bronchogenic carcinoma
obstructing embolus
obstruction
    airway
    aortic arch
    aortic outflow
    aortoiliac
    bronchial
    chronic airways
    congenital left-sided outflow
    congenital subpulmonic
    cowl-shaped
    endobronchial
    fixed airway
    fixed coronary
    foreign body upper airway
    increased pulmonary
    intrathoracic airway

obstruction *(cont.)*
  intrathoracic upper airway
  intraventricular right ventricular
  irreversible airways
  malignant airway
  preocclusive
  pulmonary artery
  pulmonary outflow
  pulmonary vascular
  pulmonary venous
  respiratory tract, mechanical
  right ventricular outflow
  subpulmonic
  subvalvular aortic
  subvalvular diffuse muscular
  superior caval
  superior vena caval
  upper airway
  vascular
  venous
obstructive atelectasis
obstructive cardiomyopathy,
  hypertrophic
obstructive emphysema
obstructive hypertrophic cardiomyopathy
obstructive hypopnea
obstructive mitral valve murmur
obstructive murmur
obstructive pneumonia
obstructive pneumonitis
obstructive pulmonary disease (OPD)
obstructive pulmonary overinflation
obstructive rhinitis
obstructive shock
obstructive sleep apnea, idiopathic
obstructive small airways disease
obstructive thrombus within the lumen
obstructive ventilatory defect
obtunded infant, profoundly
obturating embolus

obturator
obtuse marginal (OM) coronary artery
obtuse marginal branch (OMB)
obtuse marginal bypass
obtuse marginal, first
obviate the morbidity
obviate the mortality
obviate the need for surgery
occipital vessels
occlude
occluded graft
occluder
  Clamshell
  Flo-Rester vessel
  Hunter-Sessions balloon
  radiolucent plastic
  Rashkind
  Rashkind double-disc
occluder button component folded and
  introduced into sheath
occluder delivered into left atrium
  under fluoroscopic control
occluder equals button
occluding spring emboli
occluding thrombus
occlusion
  acute mesenteric artery
  ASD transcatheter (with button
    device)
  balloon
  complete
  coronary
  coronary artery
  coronary orifices
  ductus arteriosus
  embolic
  graft
  intermittent
  late graft
  pressure-controlled intermittent
    coronary

occlusion *(cont.)*
  renal artery
  side branch
  snowplow
  subtotal
  tapering
  total
  vein graft
  vessel (atraumatic)
occlusion measurement
occlusion of internal carotid arteries
  above the clinoids
occlusive arterial thrombus
occlusive impedance phlebography
occlusive lesion
occult circulatory abnormalities
occult constrictive pericarditis
occult disease
occult hypertension
occult lesion
occult pericardial constriction
occupational asthma
occupational disease
occupational stress
Ochsner forceps
Ochsner graft
Ochsner retractor
octapolar catheter
ocular cardiac reflex syncope
ocular pneumoplethysmography
  (OPG)
oculoplethysmography/carotid
  phonoangiography (OPG/CPA)
oculopneumoplethysmography
ODAM defibrillator
Oehler symptoms
Oertel treatment
offending organism
offending pericardial fluid, evacuation
  of
OHD (organic heart disease)

ohm, ohms
Ohmeda 6200 CO_2 monitor
oil embolism
OKT3 monoclonal antibody
OKT3 prophylaxis
oligemia
oligemic
oligonucleotide probes
oliguria, postoperative
Oliver-Cardarelli sign
olive-tipped needle
Olympus angioscope
Olympus BF P-10 bronchoscope
Olympus BF 4B2 bronchoscope
Olympus BF 3C4 bronchoscope
Olympus bioptome
Olympus bronchoscope
OMB (obtuse marginal branch)
OMB1 (obtuse marginal branch #1)
Omed bulldog vascular clamp
Omega-NV balloon
omega-3 fatty acids
omentum
  gastrohepatic
  sigmoid
ominous chest discomfort
ominous findings
ominous prognosis
ominous sign
Omnicarbon prosthetic heart valve
Omnicarbon prosthetic valve
Omnicor pacemaker
Omniflex balloon catheter
Omni-Orthocor II pacemaker
Omniscience prosthetic heart valve
Omniscience single leaflet cardiac
  valve prosthesis
Omniscience tilting-disk valve
  prosthesis
Omniscience valve device
Omni-Stanicor pacemaker

Omni-Theta pacemaker
Omni tract retractor system
omohyoid muscle
Ondine curse
O'Neill clamp
one-second forced expiratory volume
    (FEV$_1$)
one-stage clotting test
one-stage prothrombin time test
onionskin configuration of collagenous
    fibers
onlay graft
onset
    acute
    early
    insidious
onset of atrial systole
opacification
    nonsegmental areas
    pedal artery
opacities, patchy alveolar
opacity
opalescent sputum
OPD (obstructive pulmonary disease)
open cardiac massage
open endarterectomy
opening
    amplitude of valve
    buttonhole
    slitlike
    valvular
opening pressure, airway
opening snap (OS)
    high-pitched
    palpable
open lung biopsy
open pneumothorax
open tuberculosis
open valvotomy
operation (see also *procedure,*
    method, technique)
    ablation of bundle of His

operation *(cont.)*
    aneurysmectomy
    annuloplasty
    aorticopulmonary window
    aortic-pulmonary shunt
    aortic root replacement
    aortic valve repair
    aortic valve replacement
    aortic valvuloplasty
    aortofemoral bypass
    aortopulmonary window
    arterial switch
    arteriotomy
    atherectomy
    atrial baffle
    atrial switch
    atrioventricular valve replacement
    AV (aortic valve) repair
    Babcock
    Baffe
    balloon atrial septostomy
    balloon mitral valvuloplasty
    balloon valvuloplasty
    banding of pulmonary artery
    Bentall inclusion technique
    bidirectional Glenn
    BIMA (bilateral internal mammary
        artery) reconstruction
    blade and balloon atrial septostomy
    Blalock-Hanlon atrial septectomy
    Blalock-Hanlon cardiac
    Blalock-Taussig anastomosis
    Blalock-Taussig cardiac
    Brockenbrough commissurotomy
    Brock transventricular closed
        valvotomy
    Brom repair (aortic stenosis)
    CABS (coronary artery bypass
        surgery)
    carotid endarterectomy
    Carpentier annuloplasty
    Carpentier tricuspid valvuloplasty

operation *(cont.)*
  catheter ablation of bundle of His
  catheter balloon valvuloplasty
    (CBV)
  coarctectomy
  commissurotomy
  commissurotomy of pulmonary
    valve
  Cooley anastomosis
  coronary atherectomy
  corridor
  costectomy
  cryosurgery
  cryosurgical interruption of AV
    (atrioventricular) bypass tract
  cryosurgical interruption of AV
    (atrioventricular) node
  Damus-Kaye-Stansel (DKS)
  David
  decortication of lung
  De Vega tricuspid annuloplasty
  directional coronary angioplasty
    (DCA)
  directional coronary atherectomy
    (DCA)
  division of accessory bundle of
    Kent
  Dor remodeling ventriculoplasty
  ELCA (excimer laser coronary
    angioplasty)
  electrode catheter ablation
  encircling endocardial ventricu-
    lotomy
  end-to-side portocaval anastomosis
  endocardial ablation
  endocardial resection
  endocardial to epicardial resection
  femorodistal bypass
  femoropopliteal bypass
  fenestrated Fontan
  first-stage Norwood

operation *(cont.)*
  Fontan-Kreutzer repair
  Fontan tricuspid atresia
  Glenn
  heart transplant
  heart-lung transplant
  Heller esophagocardiomyotomy
  hemi-Fontan
  Hunter
  infarctectomy
  inferior vena cava interruption
  infundibular resection
  internal saphenous vein grafting
  intra-atrial baffle
  Jatene arterial switch
  Jatene transposition of great
    arteries
  Kay tricuspid valvuloplasty
  Kaye-Damus-Stansel (KDS)
  King-Mills procedure
  Konno patch enlargement of aorta
  laser recanalization
  ligamentum teres cardiopexy
    fundoplication
  ligature of popliteal veins
  Lillehei-Hardy-Hunter
  Lindesmith
  Lower-Shumway heart transplant
  Matas aneurysmoplasty
  maze
  median sternotomy
  mitral valve replacement
  Müller-Dammann pulmonary artery
    banding
  Mullins blade and balloon
    septostomy
  Mullins transseptal atrial
    septostomy
  Mustard atrial baffle repair
  Mustard correction of transposition
    of great vessels

operation *(cont.)*
  Nicks
  Norwood hypoplastic left-sided
    heart
  Norwood univentricular heart
  open heart
  open mitral commissurotomy
  orthotopic cardiac transplant
  pacemaker implantation
  palliative
  palliative arterial switch
  Park blade and balloon atrial
    septostomy
  partial encircling endocardial
    ventriculotomy
  patent ductus arteriosus (PDA)
    ligation
  percutaneous aortic valvuloplasty
    (PAV)
  percutaneous balloon mitral
    valvuloplasty
  percutaneous coronary rotational
    atherectomy (PCRA)
  percutaneous mitral balloon
    valvotomy (PMBV)
  percutaneous transluminal
    angioplasty (PTA)
  percutaneous transluminal balloon
    dilatation (PTBD)
  percutaneous transluminal coronary
    angioplasty (PTCA)
  percutaneous transvenous mitral
    commissurotomy
  pericardial window
  pericardiectomy
  peripheral artery bypass
  peripheral laser angioplasty (PLA)
  phlebectomy
  photoablation, laser
  plastic
  plication repair of flail leaflet

operation *(cont.)*
  pneumonectomy
  postcardiotomy intra-aortic balloon
    pumping
  Potts anastomosis between
    descending aorta and left
    pulmonary artery
  Potts-Smith side-to-side anastomosis
  profunda Dacron patchplasty
  profundaplasty
  pulmonary artery banding
  pulmonary balloon valvuloplasty
  pulmonary valvotomy
  pulmonary valvuloplasty
  Rashkind balloon atrial septotomy
  Rashkind-Miller atrial septostomy
  Rastelli
  recanalization
  redirection of inferior vena cava
  Reed ventriculorrhaphy
  Ross
  Sade modification of Norwood
  sandwich patch closure
  Schede thoracoplasty
  selective subendocardial resection
  Senning atrial baffle repair
  Senning transposition
  septectomy
  septostomy
  SIMA (single internal mammary
    artery) reconstruction
  Simpson atherectomy
  Starnes
  stellectomy
  Sucquet-Hoyer anastomosis
  sympathectomy, regional cardiac
  synthetic patch angioplasty
  systemic to pulmonary artery
    anastomosis
  Takeuchi repair
  Tanner

operation *(cont.)*
thoracoabdominal aortic aneurysm
(TAAA) surgery
thromboendarterectomy
thrombolysis, intracoronary
transcatheter closure of atrial septal
defect
transmural resection
Trendelenburg excision of varicose
veins
triangular resection of leaflet
tricuspid valve annuloplasty
tunnel
unifocalization
valved venous transplant
valvotomy
valvuloplasty
valvulotomy
vein patch angioplasty
vein stripping
venotomy
ventricular endoaneurysmorrhaphy
ventricular exclusion
ventriculorrhaphy
ventriculotomy
Vineberg cardiac revascularization
Vineberg implantation of internal
mammary artery into
myocardium
Waterston anastomosis for
congenital pulmonary stenosis
Waterston extrapericardial
anastomosis
wedge-shaped sleeve aneurysm
resection
wrapping of abdominal aortic
aneurysm
opening snap (OS)
open lung biopsy
OPG/CPA (oculoplethysmography/
carotid phonoangiography)

ophthalmic retractor
opisthorchiasis
Opisthorchis infestation
Opitz disease
Opitz thrombophlebitic splenomegaly
O point of cardiac apex pulse
opportunistic infection
opportunistic organism
opposing pleural surfaces
Op-Site dressing
optic loupe
Optima MP pacemaker
Optima MPT Series III pacemaker
Optima MPI Series III pulse generator
Optima SPT pacemaker
Optiscope catheter
oral airway
oral anticoagulation
oral aspirin provocation
oral contraceptive-induced hypertension
oral drugs
oral steroid contraceptives are
contraindicated
orbit, artifacts due to body contour
orders or status
Do Not Attempt Resuscitation
(DNAR)
Do Not Resuscitate (DNR)
organic dust toxic syndrome
organic granulomatosis
organism
causative
offending
opportunistic
organs of respiration
orifice (see also *ostium*)
aortic
atriotomy
atrioventricular
cardiac

orifice *(cont.)*
  coronary
  coronary sinus
  double coronary
  hypoplastic tricuspid
  inferior vena cava
  lingular
  mitral
  narrowed
  pulmonary
  regurgitant
  segmental
  slitlike
  tricuspid
  valve
orifice-to-annulus ratio
origin, anomalous
origin of artery
origin of vessel
Orion pacemaker
Ormond syndrome
oroendotracheal tube
oropharynx
oropharyngeal airway
orotracheal direct vision intubation
orotracheal intubation
Orsi-Grocco method
ORT (orthodromic reciprocating
  tachycardia)
Orthoclone
Orthocor II pacemaker
orthodromic atrioventricular (AV)
  reciprocating tachycardia
orthodromic reciprocating tachycardia
  (ORT)
orthodromic tachycardia
orthogonal angiographic projection
orthogonal lead arrangement for EKG
orthogonal view on angiography
orthopnea
  three-pillow
  two-pillow

orthopnea position
orthopneic position
orthorhythmic
orthostasis
orthostatic blood pressure
orthostatic dyspnea
orthostatic hypotension, hyperadrenergic
orthostatic hypotension variant
orthostatic primary hypotension
orthostatic syncope
orthostatism, vasovagal
orthotopic cardiac transplantation
orthotopic heart transplantation
orthotopic total heart replacement
Ortner syndrome
OS (opening snap)
os, coronary sinus
Osborn wave (hypothermia)
Osborn wave on EKG
oscillation, pressure
oscillatory
oscillography
oscilloscope, Tektronix
Oscor active fixation leads
Oscor pacing lead
os infundibulum
O'Shaughnessy artery forceps
Osler (see *Weber-Osler-Rendu*
  syndrome)
Osler disease
Osler hereditary hemorrhagic telangi-
  ectasia
Osler-Libman-Sacks syndrome
Osler maneuver
Osler nodes in subacute bacterial
  endocarditis
Osler polycythemia vera
Osler sign
Osler triad
osmotic diuretics
osmotic edema

osmotic effect
osmotic pressure, plasma colloid
ossific nodule
osteoarthropathy, pulmonary
osteogenesis imperfecta syndrome
osteomyelitis of sternum
osteosarcoma of heart
osteosclerotic anemia
ostia
ostial cannulation
ostial lesion
ostial reimplantation, coronary
ostial revascularization, coronary
ostial stenosis
ostium (pl. ostia) (see also *orifice*)
  aortic
  artery
  atrioventricular
  coronary
  coronary sinus
ostium atrioventriculare commune
ostium primum defect
ostium secundum defect
outcome, portend a poor
outflow
  hypoplastic subpulmonic
  maximum venous (MVO)
  subpulmonic
outflow anastomosis
outflow disease progression
outflow midsystolic murmur
outflow tract
outflow tract prosthesis
outlet chamber, rudimentary
outlet, widened thoracic
out of synchrony
outpouching of portion of wall of
  artery
output
  adequate cardiac
  augmented cardiac
  cardiac (CO)

output *(cont.)*
  Dow method for cardiac
  Fick method for cardiac
  Gorlin method for cardiac
  Hetzel forward triangle method for
    cardiac
  inadequate cardiac
  low cardiac
  pulmonic
  reduced systemic cardiac
  Stewart-Hamilton technique for
    cardiac
  stroke
  systemic
  thermodilution cardiac
  ventricular
output amplitude
oval cherry-red raised lesion
ovalis, annulus
ovalocytosis, hereditary
ovarian carcinoma metastatic to heart
over-and-over stitch or suture
overdistention
overdistention of alveolar spaces in
  lungs
overdistention of lung tissue
overdistention, pulmonary
overdrive pacing
overdrive suppression
overexpansion, pulmonary
Overholt thoracic forceps
overinflation
  lung
  unilateral
overload, overloading
  acute hemodynamic
  cardiac
  chronic hemodynamic
  diastolic
  fluid
  pressure
  right ventricular

overload *(cont.)*
  systolic ventricular
  volume
overlying epicardial fat
over-read (noun)
over-responsive programming
overriding great artery
overriding great vessel
overriding of annulus
overriding of aorta
overriding of tricuspid valve
overriding ventricular septum of aorta
oversensing, pacemaker
over-the-wire balloon catheter
overventilation
  alveolar
  total
overwhelming sepsis
ovoid heart
Owren disease
Owren factor V deficiency
oxalosis
"ox heart" (cor bovinum)
oxidative phosphorylation
oxihemoglobin
oximeter
  American Optical
  ear
  finger
  Hewlett-Packard ear
  intracardiac
  Oxytrak pulse
  pulse
oximetry
  ear
  exercise
  finger
  pulse
  reflectance
Oxycel

oxygen (O_2)
  arterial blood gases on 100%
  heated humidified
  increased
  supplemental
oxygenated blood
oxygenated cardioplegic solution
oxygenated perfluorocarbon blood
  substitute
oxygenation, extracorporeal membrane
oxygenation of blood, inadequate
oxygenator
  Bentley
  bubble
  Capiox-E bypass system
  disk
  film
  membrane
  Monolyth
  pump
  rotating disk
  SciMed membrane
  screen
  Shiley
oxygen by mask
oxygen by nasal cannula
oxygen by nasal cathether
oxygen by nasal prong
oxygen by nonrebreather mask
oxygen-carrying capacity
oxygen capacity
oxygen consumption index
oxygen content
oxygen debt, severe
oxygen deficit
oxygen delivery
oxygen delivery index
oxygen-dependent emphysema
oxygen difference, arteriovenous

oxygen extraction index
oxygen extraction ratio
oxygen saturation
  aortic
  low
  PA (pulmonary artery)
  RA (right atrium)
oxygen stepup (or step-up)
oxygen tension gradient, alveolar-arterial

oxygen toxicity
oxygen unsaturation
oxygen utilization capacity
oxygen via nasal cannula
oxyhemoglobin dissociation curve
oxyhemoglobin saturation
Oxytrak pulse oximeter
ozena

P, p

P (posterior)
PA (pulmonary artery)
PA oxygen saturation
PA pressure
PAB (premature atrial beat)
PABP (pulmonary artery balloon
    pump)
PAC (premature atrial complex, or
    contraction)
paced beat
paced impulse
paced ventricular evoked response
    (PVER)
pacemaker (see also *generator*)
    AAI (atrial demand inhibited)
    AAIR
    AAT (atrial demand triggered)
    Accufix
    Acculith
    Activitrax
    Activitrax II single-chamber VVI
    Activitrax variable rate
    activity sensing
    Aequitron
    AFP
    AICD
    AID-B

pacemaker *(cont.)*
    antitachycardia
    AOO (atrial asynchronous)
    Arco
    Arcolithium
    artificial
    Arzco
    Astra
    ASVIP (atrial synchronous,
        ventricular inhibited)
    asynchronous (atrial or ventricular)
        mode
    atrial asynchronous
    atrial demand inhibited
    atrial demand triggered
    atrial synchronous ventricular
    atrial synchronous, ventricular-
        inhibited (ASVIP)
    atrial tracking
    atrial triggered, ventricular-
        inhibited
    Atricor
    atrioventricular junctional
    atrioventricular sequential
    Aurora dual-chamber
    Autima II dual-chamber cardiac
    automatic

357

pacemaker *(cont.)*
 AV (atrioventricular) junctional
 AV (atrioventricular) sequential
 Avius sequential
 Basix
 Biorate
 Biotronik
 bipolar
 burst
 Byrel SX
 Byrel-SX/Versatrax
 Cardio-Pace Medical Durapulse
 Chardack-Greatbatch implantable
  cardiac pulse generator
 Chorus
 Chorus dual-chamber
 Chorus II dual-chamber
 Chorus RM rate-responsive dual-
  chamber
 Chronocor IV external
 Circadia dual-chamber rate-adaptive
 Classix
 Command PS
 committed mode
 Cook
 Cordis
 Cordis Gemini
 Cordis Sequicor
 Cosmos 283 DDD
 Cosmos II DDD
 Cosmos pulse generator
 CPI (Cardiac Pacemakers, Inc.)
 CPI Astra
 CPI DDD
 CPI 910 ULTRA II
 cross-talk
 Cyberlith
 Cybertach automatic-burst atrial
 Cybertach 60
 Daig ESI-II or DSI-III screw-in
  lead
 Dash rate-adaptive

pacemaker *(cont.)*
 Dash single-chamber rate-adaptic
  cardiac
 DDD (fully automatic sequential)
 DDDR mode
 DDI mode
 Delta
 demand
 Devices, Ltd.
 diaphragmatic
 Diplos M
 downward displacement of
 Dromos
 dual-chamber
 Durapulse
 DVI (AV sequential)
 Ectocor
 ectopic atrial
 Ela
 Electrodyne
 Elema-Schonander
 Elevath
 Elgiloy
 Elite dual-chamber rate-responsive
 Encor
 endless loop, dual-chamber
 Enertrax
 Ergos O_2
 escape
 external transthoracic
 externally controlled noninvasive
  programmed stimulation
 Fast-Pass lead
 fixed-rate, asynchronous atrial
 fixed-rate, asynchronous ventricular
 fixed-rate permanent
 fully automatic, atrioventricular
  universal dual-channel
 Galaxy
 Gemini 415 DDD
 General Electric
 Genisis (*not* Genesis)

pacemaker *(cont.)*
Guardian
hermetically sealed standbys
implanted
Intermedics
Intermedics Quantum
internal
Intertach
intraperitoneal migration of
junctional
Kalos
Kelvin 500 Sensor
Lambda
latent
Legend
Leios
Leptos-01
Leukos
lithium
Maestro
Medcor
Medtel
Medtronic
Medtronic RF 5998
Medtronic SPO 502
Medtronic Symbios
Medtronic temporary
Meta MV
META rate responsive
Micro Minix
Microlith P
Midros
Minix
Minix ST
Microthin P2
Multicor Gamma
Multicor II
Multilith
multiprogrammable
myopectoral inhibition of
Nathan
natural

pacemaker *(cont.)*
Neos M
noncompetitive atrial demand
noncompetitive atrial synchronous
noncompetitive atrial triggered
noncompetitive demand ventricular
noncompetitive ventricular
synchronous
noncompetitive ventricular
triggered
noninvasive temporary (NTP)
Nova MR
Omnicor
Omni-Orthocor
Omni-Stanicor
Omni-Theta
Optima MP; MPT; SPT
Optima MPI Series III pulse
generator
Orion
Orthocor II
oversensing
Pacesetter
Pacesetter AFP
Pacesetter Synchrony
Pacesetter systems
PASAR (permanent scanning anti-
tachycardia)
PASAR tachycardia reversion
Pasys
PDx pacing and diagnostic
permanent
permanent rate-responsive
permanent rate-responsive dual-
chamber
permanent ventricular
Permathane Pacesetter lead
Phoenix single-chamber
Phymos 3D (foreign)
Pinnacle
PolyFlex lead
Prima

pacemaker *(cont.)*
  Prism-CL
  Programalith
  programmable
  Prolith
  Pulsar NI
  P wave triggered ventricular
  QT interval sensing
  QT sensing
  Quantum
  radiofrequency
  rate responsive
  Relay
  rescuing
  respiratory-dependent
  RS4
  runaway
  screw-in lead
  secondary
  Seecor
  Sensolog
  Sensor Kelvin
  Sequicor
  shifting
  Siemens-Elema
  Siemens-Pacesetter
  single-chamber
  sinus node
  Sorin
  Spectraflex
  Spectrax programmable Medtronic
  Spectrax SXT
  standby
  Stanicor
  Starr-Edwards
  supraventricular ectopic
  Swing DR1 DDDR
  Symbios
  synchronous mode
  Synergyst DDD
  tachycardia-terminating
  Tachylog

pacemaker *(cont.)*
  Telectronics
  temperature-sensing
  temporary
  temporary transvenous
  Thermos
  tined lead
  transcutaneous
  transthoracic
  transvenous
  Trios M
  Triumph VR
  troubleshooting of
  undersensing malfunction of
  Unilith
  unipolar
  universal
  variable rate
  VAT (atrial synchronous
    ventricular)
  VDD (atrial synchronous
    ventricular inhibited)
  Ventak AICD
  Ventricor
  ventricular
  ventricular asynchronous
  ventricular demand inhibited (VVI)
  ventricular demand triggered (VVT)
  Versatrax and Versatrax II
  Vicor
  Vista
  Vitatrax II
  Vitatron
  VOO (ventricular asynchronous)
  VVD mode
  VVI (ventricular demand inhibited)
  VVI/AAI
  VVIR mode
  VVT (ventricular demand
    triggered)
  wandering
  wandering atrial (WAP)

pacemaker *(cont.)*
Xyrel
Zitron
Zoll NTP (noninvasive temporary)
pacemaker adaptive rate
pacemaker afterpotential
pacemaker amplifier refractory period
pacemaker amplifier sensitivity
pacemaker artifact
pacemaker AV disable mechanism
pacemaker battery
pacemaker battery failure
pacemaker battery status
pacemaker burst pacing
pacemaker capability
pacemaker capture
   erratic
   lack of
pacemaker cell
pacemaker classifications
pacemaker code system
pacemaker complication
pacemaker crosstalk
pacemaker-defibrillator
pacemaker demand
pacemaker electrode
pacemaker escape interval
pacemaker failure
pacemaker generator pouch
pacemaker hysteresis
pacemaker implantation
pacemaker insertion
   transarterial
   transvenous
pacemaker introducer
pacemaker lead
pacemaker lead impedance
pacemaker loss of capture
pacemaker loss of sensing
pacemaker malfunction
pacemaker marker channel
pacemaker-mediated tachycardia

pacemaker mode (see *pacemaker*)
   AOO
   AAI
   DDD
   DDDR
   DDI
   DVI
   universal
   VOO
   VDD
   VVD
   VVI
   VVIR
   VVT
pacemaker oversensing
pacemaker pacing mode
pacemaker pocket
pacemaker potential
pacemaker programmability
pacemaker programmed settings
pacemaker rate
pacemaker reprogramming
pacemaker self-inhibition
pacemaker sensing
pacemaker sensitivity
pacemaker spike
pacemaker stimulus output amplitude
pacemaker syndrome
pacemaker system analyzer
pacemaker tester system
pacemaker threshold
pacemaker twiddler's syndrome
pacemaker undersensing
pace mapping
Paceport catheter
pacer-dependent
pacer spike
Pacesetter AFP pacemaker
Pacesetter cardiac pacemaker
Pacesetter introducer
Pacesetter Synchrony pacemaker
Pacesetter systems pacemaker

pace-termination
Pacewedge dual-pressure bipolar
  pacing catheter
Pachon method
Pachon test of collateral circulation in
  aneurysm
pachyderma laryngis
pachypleuritis
Pacifico venous cannula
pacing (see also *pacemaker*)
  activity sensor modulated atrial rate
  adaptive
  adaptive burst
  antitachycardia
  asynchronous
  asynchronous atrioventricular
    sequential
  atrial
  atrial overdrive
  atrial rate adaptive
  atrial synchronous ventricular
  autodecremental
  AV sequential
  backup bradycardia
  bipolar atrial
  burst
  burst-overdrive
  cardiac
  committed
  competitive
  constant rate atrial
  continuous rapid atrial
  coronary sinus
  coupled
  decremental
  demand
  double ventricular
  dual-chamber
  endocardial
  epicardial
  external
  external cardiac

pacing *(cont.)*
  extrastimulus
  fixed-rate
  incremental
  incremental atrial
  noncommitted
  overdrive
  paired
  permanent
  phrenic nerve
  physiologic
  prophylactic
  P synchronous
  P triggered ventricular
  ramp
  ramp atrial
  ramp overdrive
  rapid atrial
  rapid ventricular
  rate adaptive
  rate responsive (RRP)
  scan
  scanning
  semicommitted
  sequential
  single-chamber
  synchronous
  temporary cardiac
  temporary transvenous
  transcutaneous
  transesophageal
  transesophageal atrial
  transesophageal cardiac
  transthoracic cardiac
  transvenous
  triggered
  ultrafast train
  ultrarapid
  underdrive
  unipolar
  ventricular
  ventricular burst

pacing *(cont.)*
  ventricular cardiac
  ventricular demand
  ventricular overdrive
  ventricular triggered
  vibration based
  pacing analyzer
  pacing cable, alligator
  pacing-induced termination of
    arrhythmia
  pacing lead fracture
  pacing mode (see *pacemaker*)
  pacing/sensing lead
  pacing stimulus
  pacing system analyzer (PSA)
  pacing threshold
  pacing wire, pacing wires
  pacing wire fracture
pack, moist laparotomy (lap)
pack-a-day smoking history
packed red blood cells (PRBCs)
pack-years of cigarette smoking
$PaCO_2$) (arterial partial pressure of
  CO_2) (mm Hg)
pad, pads
  defibrillator
  epicardial fat
  insulating
  laparotomy (lap)
  Littmann defibrillation
  R2 defibrillator
  Telfa
PAD (pulmonary artery diastolic)
  pressure
PAD (pulsatile assist device)
paddle
  defibrillatory
  pediatric defibrillator
PA diastolic pressure
PADP-PAWP (pulmonary artery
  diastolic and wedge pressure)
  gradient

pad sign of aortic insufficiency
PAEDP (pulmonary artery end-
  diastolic pressure)
Page episodic hypertension with
  tachycardia
Page syndrome
Paget-Schroetter (Schrötter) syndrome
Paget-Schroetter venous thrombosis of
  axillary vein
Paget-von Schroetter syndrome
PAI (plasminogen activator inhibitor)
pain (see also *angina*)
  acme
  anginal chest
  anomalous
  atypical chest
  boring
  burning
  calf
  cardiaclike chest
  chest
  chest wall
  concomitant chest
  crushing
  crushing chest
  deep visceral
  dull
  esophageal
  evanescent chest
  excruciating
  exertional
  exertional chest
  exquisite
  focal
  heartburn type of
  hemicranial
  ischemic rest
  localized stabbing
  musculoskeletal
  noncardiac chest
  nonpleuritic precordial
  parasternal chest

pain *(cont.)*
  pericardial
  pinching chest
  pleuritic
  pleuritic chest
  postprandial
  pounding
  precordial chest
  pressure
  pulsating
  radiating (to left arm, shoulder)
  referred cardiac
  reproducible
  rest
  retrosternal chest
  sharp
  squeezing
  squeezing chest
  stabbing
  sternal border
  substernal chest
  suffocating chest
  thoracic
  throbbing
  unrelenting
  unremitting
  viselike
  waning
  waxing and waning
pain abolished by breath-holding
pain accompanied by abdominal
  fullness
pain accompanied by nausea
pain accompanied by palpitations
pain accompanied by sensation of gas
pain accompanied by shortness of
  breath
pain accompanied by sweating
pain accompanied by weakness
pain aggravated by coughing
pain aggravated by deep breathing

pain aggravated by deep inspiration
pain continued unabated
pain following heavy meal
pain indistinguishable from angina
pain induced with methacholine
pain in sternal articulations
painless edema
pain like "being crushed under a
  heavy load"
pain on drinking cold liquid
pain on exposure to cold
pain on strong emotion
pain on swallowing
pain precipitated by emotional upset
pain precipitated by exertion
pain precipitated by strong emotion
pain radiating to back
pain radiating to epigastrium
pain radiating to jaw
pain radiating to left arm
pain radiating to neck
pain radiating to right arm
pain radiating to throat
pain rapidly extinguished by
  withdrawal of stimulus
pain relieved by antacids
pain relieved by belching
pain relieved by bowel movement
pain relieved by carotid massage
pain relieved by cimetidine
pain relieved by eating
pain relieved by food intake
pain relieved by leaning forward
pain relieved by passage of flatus
pain relieved by rest
pain reproduced by palpation
pain reproducible with moderate
  exercise
pain unaffected by position
pain unrelated to meals
pain unrelieved by nitroglycerin

pain when angry
pain when excited
pain "like being caught in a vise"
pain "like someone sitting on my
  chest"
P-A interval
paired beats
palate, high arched
pale thrombus
palliation
palliative operative procedure
palliative surgery
palliative therapy
pallid breath-holding spells
Pallister-Hall syndrome
pallor
  circumoral
  elevation
pallor of extremity
pallor of lower extremities
palmar pulses, palpable
Palmaz balloon-expandable iliac stent
Palmaz-Schatz coronary stent
Palmaz-Schatz stent prototype
Palmaz vascular stent
Palmeri QRS score
palpability
palpable A wave
palpable anterior motion
palpable aortic ejection sound
palpable apical impulse
palpable ejection click
palpable opening snap
palpable palmar pulses
palpable peripheral pulse
palpable popliteal pulse
palpable presystolic bulge
palpable pulmonic ejection sound
palpable S_3 or S_4
palpable systolic pulsation
palpable thrill

palpation
  fist
  precordial
palpation reproduces the pain
palpatory
palpitation, palpitations
  flip-flop
  flopping
  fluttering
palsy, cranial nerve
PAM (pulmonary artery mean)
  pressure
PAN (periarteritis nodosa)
panacinar emphysema
panaortic
panarteritis nodosa
pancarditis
panchamber enlargement
pancreatitis, acute
pancuronium
panel, anergy
paninspiratory crackles
panlobular emphysema
pansinusitis
pansystolic mitral regurgitation
pansystolic murmur (PSM)
pantaloon embolus
pantyhose, support (see *stockings*)
panzerherz (dense pericardial
  calcification)
PaO_2 (arterial partial pressure of O_2)
  (mm Hg)
PAP (pulmonary artery pressure)
papaverine-soaked sponge
papillary fibroelastoma
papillary muscle
  anterior
  posterior
  septal
papillary muscle rupture
papillary muscle dysfunction

papillary muscle infarction
papilledema
papillomas
Pappenheimer bodies
PA pulse amplitude
PA systolic pressure
PAPVR (partial anomalous pulmonary
venous return)
para-arterial angiomatosis arteritis
paraaminosalicylic acid hypersensitivity
paracardiac mass
paracardiac-type total anomalous
venous return
paracentesis of pericardium
parachute deformity of mitral valve
parachute mitral valve
parachute technique for distal
anastomosis
paracicatricial emphysema
paracoccidioidomycosis
paracoronary right ventriculotomy
paracorporeal
paracostal
paradoxic respiratory splitting
paradoxic splitting
paradoxical bronchospasm
paradoxical embolism
paradoxical embolus
paradoxically
paradoxical motion
paradoxical motion of the chest wall
paradoxical movement
paradoxical pulse
paradoxical septal motion
paraganglioma, cardiac
Paragonimus westermani infection
parainfluenza virus
paralysis of diaphragm
paralysis
periodic
phrenic nerve

paralytic chest
paramagnetic substances
paramagnetism
paramedian position
paramediastinal glands
parameter, parameters
physiologic
clinical
ventricular function
parameter study
paramyotonia congenita
paranasal sinuses
paraneoplastic process
paraneoplastic syndrome
parapharyngeal abscess
paraprosthetic leakage
paraprosthetic-enteric fistula
pararenal aortic aneurysm
pararenal aortic atherosclerosis
paraseptal emphysema
paraseptal position
parasite (pulmonary)
Ascaris
Echinococcus multilocularis
(alveolaris)
Entamoeba
filaria
hookworm
liver fluke
lung fluke
Schistosoma haematobium
Schistosoma japonicum
Schistosoma mansoni
schistosomes
Strongyloides
tapeworms
Toxocara
Trichina
Trichuris
parasitic circulation in angio-
osteohypertrophic syndrome
parasitic infection, intestinal

parasitic infestation
parasitic pericarditis
paraspinal pleural stripe
parasternal bulge
parasternal chest pain
parasternal heave
parasternal incision
parasternal lift
parasternal long-axis view
parasternal lymph nodes
parasternal motion
    forceful
    sustained anterior
parasternal murmur
parasternal short-axis view
parasternal systolic lift
parasternal systolic murmur
parasternal view of heart
parasternal window
parasympathetic nervous system
parasystole
    atrial
    junctional
    ventricular
parathyroid hormone
parathyroidectomy
paratonia
paratracheal lymphadenopathy
paravalvar leak
paravalvular leak
paravertebral gutter
parchment heart syndrome
parchment right ventricle
Pardee T wave
parenchyma
    lung
    pulmonary
parenchymal hemorrhage
parenchymal infiltrates, pulmonary
parenchymal lung disease
parent vein

parenteral bronchodilators
parenteral fluids
parenteral steroids
paresis, vocal cord
paresthesia, paresthesias
    marching
    Nothnagel
    vasomotor
parietal band
parietal extension of infundibular
    septum
parietalis, pleura
parietal layer
parietal pericardium
parietal pleura
parietal pleurectomy
Parietaria judaica
parietoalveolar pneumonopathy
Park blade and balloon atrial
    septostomy
Park blade septostomy
Parkes Weber syndrome
Parks bidirectional Doppler flowmeter
paroxysmal atrial fibrillation
paroxysmal atrial tachycardia (PAT)
paroxysmal coughing
paroxysmal crisis, hypertensive
paroxysmal dyspnea
paroxysmal hyperpnea
paroxysmal hypertension
paroxysmal nocturnal dyspnea (PND)
paroxysmal nocturnal hemoglobinuria
    (PNH)
paroxysmal sneezing
paroxysmal supraventricular
    tachycardia (PSVT)
paroxysmal tachycardia
paroxysmal wheezing
paroxysmal wheezing dyspnea
paroxysms of cough
paroxysms of hypertension

parrot fever
pars membranacea
Parsonnet probe
partial anomalous pulmonary venous
return (PAPVR)
partial collapse of lung
partial dislodgement
partial encircling endocardial
ventriculotomy
partial exsanguination
partial graft preservation
partial lung collapse
partial occluding (or occlusion) clamp
partial pericardial absence
partial pressure of arterial CO_2
($PaCO_2$)
partial pressure of arterial O_2 (PaO_2)
partial rebreather
partial thromboplastin time test
partial volume effect, artifact due to
particle debris
particle masks
partition, atrial
parvovirus B19
parvovirus, human (HPV)
parvus et tardus, pulsus
parvus pulse
PAS (pulmonary artery systolic)
pressure
PAS-positive proteinaceous material
PASAR (permanent scanning antitachycardia) pacemaker
PASAR tachycardia reversion pacemaker
PASG (pneumatic antishock garment)
PASP/SASP (pulmonary to systemic
arterial systolic pressure) ratio
passage of clots
passages, narrowing of bronchiolar
passer
right-angle
Schnidt (*not* Schmidt)

passive clot
passive filling
passive fixation lead
passive hyperemia
passive hyperimmune therapy (PHT)
passively congested lung tissue
passive pneumonia
passive smoking exposure
passive vascular congestion
passive venous distention
Passovoy defect
Passovoy mild hemorrhagic diathesis
PASYS (single-chamber cardiac
pacing system)
PAT (paroxysmal atrial tachycardia)
with block
Patau syndrome (trisomy 13)
patch
autologous pericardial
Carrel
Dacron Sauvage
felt
Gore-Tex cardiovascular
Gore-Tex soft tissue
gusset-type
kinking of
MacCallum
outflow cardiac
pericardial
Teflon felt
Teflon intracardiac
transannular
transdermal nitroglycerin
vein
patch closure of septal defect
patch crinkling
patch electrode
anterior anodal
posterior cathodal
subcutaneous
patch electrodes placed outside the
pericardium

patch graft annuloplasty
patch graft aortoplasty
patch graft, Dacron onlay
patch graft of outflow tract
patching, transannular
patch lead, HV-1
patch lead placement, intrapericardial
patch placement, extrapericardial
patchplasty, profunda Dacron
patchy alveolar opacities
patchy atrophy of renal cortex
patchy consolidation
patchy infiltration, migratory
patchy migratory infiltrates
patchy zones of hemorrhagic exudate
patchy zones of purulent exudate
patency
   arterial
   coronary artery
   coronary bypass graft
   ductus arteriosus
   graft
   vein
patency and valvular reflux of deep
   veins
patency of balloon-dilated vessel
patency of ductus arteriosus, persistent
patency of ductus venosus, persistent
patency of the radial artery-to-cephalic
   vein anastomosis
patency of vein graft
patency of vessel
patent bifurcation
patent bronchus sign
patent ductus arteriosus (PDA)
patent ductus arteriosus closure
patent ductus arteriosus double
   umbrella closure
patent ductus arteriosus, silent
patent foramen ovale
patent graft
patent trifurcation

patent, widely
Pathfinder catheter
pathogenesis of bleeding syndrome
pathogenic coagulation process
pathognomonic symptoms
pathologic diagnosis
pathophysiologic changes in airways
   obstruction
pathophysiology
pathway
   ablation of accessory
   accessory (AP)
   accessory atrioventricular (AV)
   accessory conduction (ACP)
   anomalous
   anomalous atrioventricular
      conduction
   antegrade
   antegrade fast
   anterior internodal
   atrio-His; atrio-Hisian; atriohisian
   atrioventricular (AV)
   AV (atrioventricular) nodal
   Bachmann
   bystander
   concealed accessory
   concealed atrioventricular
   dual AV nodal
   Embden-Meyerhof
   Embden-Meyerhof-Parnas
   fast
   flow
   free-wall accessory
   internodal
   left accessory
   multiple accessory
   nodoventricular
   paranodal
   paraseptal accessory
   posterior septal
   preferential intranodal
   reentrant

pathway *(cont.)*
  retrograde
  septal
  slow
  slow AV nodal
  Thorel
  Wenckebach
patient-controlled analgesic (PCA)
  system
patient risk factors
Patrick-McGoon technique
pattern
  A fib (atrial fibrillation)
  bigeminal
  blood flow
  contractile
  DNA ploidy
  dP/dt upstroke
  early repolarization
  hemodynamic
  juvenile T wave
  left ventricular contraction
  left ventricular strain
  M (on right atrial waveform)
  M-shaped mitral valve
  P pulmonale
  pseudoinfarct
  pulmonary flow
  pulmonary vascular
  QR
  reticulogranular
  right ventricular strain
  RR' (RR prime)
  RSR' (RSR prime)
  S1Q3; S1Q3T3; S1S2S3
  speckled
  spectral
  strain
  tachypneic breathing
  trigeminal
  ventricular contraction

patulous
Paul-Bunnell test
Paul sign
pause, pauses
  asystolic
  compensatory
  full
  incomplete
  less-than-full
  noncompensatory
  postextrasystolic
  sinus
PAV (percutaneous aortic
  valvuloplasty)
PA Watch position-monitoring
  catheter
PAWP (pulmonary artery wedge
  pressure)
PBF (pulmonary blood flow)
PBLs (peripheral blood lymphocytes)
PBPC (peripheral blood progenitor
  cell)
PBPI (penile-brachial pressure index)
  to assess cardiac disease
PBVI (pulmonary blood volume
  index)
PBSC (peripheral blood stem cell)
  collections
PCA (patient-controlled analgesic)
  system
PCBS (percutaneous cardiopulmonary
  bypass support)
PCD (programmable cardioverter-
  defibrillator)
PCD ICD with biphasic shocks
PCD ICD "active can" model
  (Medtronic)
PCD pulse generator
PCD tiered therapy
P cell
P congenitale

PCG (phonocardiogram, -graphy)
PCICO (pressure-controlled intermit-
tent coronary occlusion)
PCL (paced cycle length)
pCO_2, PCO_2 (partial pressure of
carbon dioxide)
PCP (*Pneumocystic carinii* pneumonia)
prophylaxis
PCP (pulmonary capillary pressure)
PCr (phosphocreatine) analysis
PCRA (percutaneous coronary
rotational atherectomy)
PCS (proximal coronary sinus)
PCU (progressive care unit)
PCVD (pulmonary collagen vascular
disease)
PCWP (pulmonary capillary wedge
pressure)
PDA (patent ductus arteriosus) (on
echo report; congenital defect)
PDA (peripheral directional
atherectomy)
PDA (posterior descending artery)
PDE isoenzyme inhibitor
PDF (probability density function)
PDP (postural drainage and
percussion)
PDS suture
PDS Vicryl suture
PDT guide wire
PDx pacing and diagnostic pacemaker
PE (pericardial effusion)
PE (pulmonary embolism)
peacock sound
peak and trough drug levels
peak, carotid pulse
peak circumferential wall stress
peak dP/dt
peak early diastolic filling velocities
peaked P wave
peak exercise

peak expiratory flow (PEF)
peak expiratory flow rate (PEFR)
peak filling rate
peak flow
peak flow variability
peak flow velocity
peak-inflation pressures
peak late diastolic filling velocities
peak level of drug
peak of wave
peak regurgitant flow velocity
peak regurgitant wave pressure
peak systolic pressure
peak systolic velocity
peak tidal expiratory flow
peak-to-peak pressure gradient
peak velocity of blood flow on
Doppler echocardiogram
Péan clamp
Péan forceps
pearls, Laënnec
Pearson chi-squared test (calculation
used for artificial heart)
PEC (pulmonary ejection click)
P_ECO_2 (partial pressure of end-tidal
$PECO_2$)
pectoral ectopia cordis
pectoral electrode
pectoral fremitus
pectoralis fascia
pectoralis major muscle
pectoralis major syndrome
pectoralis minor muscle
pectoriloquy
aphonic
whispered
whispering
pectoris, angina (see *angina pectoris*)
pectus carinatum
pectus excavatum
pedal artery opacification

pedal edema
pedal pulses
  absent
  diminished
  intact
  palpable
pediatric biplane TEE (transesophageal
  echocardiography) probe
pediatric defibrillator paddles
pediatric laryngoscope
pedicle
  IMA (internal mammary artery)
  musculofascial
  phrenic
  vascular
pedicle flap
pedunculated myxoma
pedunculated thrombus
peel-away sheath
peeling back mechanism on electrophysiology study
PEEP (positive end-expiratory
  pressure)
PEF (peak expiratory flow)
PEI (postexercise index)
pelvic varices
Pemco prosthetic valve
Penaz methodology for monitoring
  blood pressure
pencil, electrocautery
Penderluft syndrome
penetrating aortic ulceration
penetrating atherosclerotic aortic ulcer
penetrating atherosclerotic ulceration
penetrating chest trauma
penetrating injury to aortic arch
penetrating injury to innominate artery
penetrating injury to superior vena
  cava
penetrating lung injury
penetrating trauma to heart

penetrating ulceration
penetrating wound of descending
  thoracic aorta
Penfield dissector
Penfield elevator
penicillin prophylaxis
penile-brachial pressure index (PBPI)
  to assess cardiac disease
Penn State total artificial heart (TAH)
Penn State ventricular assist device
  (VAD)
Pennington grasping forceps
Penrose drain
pentalogy, Fallot
penultimate
PEP (pre-ejection period)
PE Plus II balloon dilatation catheter
peptide, atrial natriuretic
Peptostreptococcus
perceived exertion scale, Borg
percent of predicted maximum heart
  rate
perceptual disturbances following
  open heart surgery
Percor DL balloon catheter
Percor DL-II (dual-lumen) intra-aortic
  balloon catheter
Percor-Stat-DL catheter
percussion, auscultation and
percussion note
  drumlike
  dull
  flat
  hyperresonant
  resonant
  tympanitic
percussion sound
percussion wave of carotid arterial
  pulse
percutaneous aortic balloon valvuloplasty

percutaneous aspiration of pericardial
   cyst
percutaneous balloon aortic valvotomy
percutaneous balloon pulmonary
   valvotomy
percutaneous cardiopulmonary bypass
   support (PCBS)
percutaneous cardiopulmonary
   support, temporary
percutaneous coronary rotational
   atherectomy (PCRA)
percutaneous cutting needle
percutaneous endomyocardial biopsy
percutaneous groin puncture
percutaneous inferior vena cava (IVC)
   filter
percutaneous insertion
percutaneous insertion via femoral
   vein
percutaneous intra-aortic balloon
   counterpulsation
percutaneous intracoronary angioscopy
percutaneous lead introducer
percutaneous patent ductus arteriosus
   closure
percutaneous pericardial biopsy
percutaneous pericardioscopy
percutaneous puncture technique
percutaneous radiofrequency catheter
   ablation
percutaneous retrograde atherectomy
percutaneous revascularization
percutaneous technique
percutaneous thoracoscopy
percutaneous transatrial mitral
   commissurotomy
percutaneous transcatheter ductal
   closure (PTDC)
percutaneous transluminal angioplasty
   (PTA)
percutaneous transluminal carotid
   angioplasty

percutaneous transluminal coronary
   angioplasty (PTCA)
percutaneous transluminal coronary
   balloon angioplasty
percutaneous transthoracic aspiration
percutaneous transtracheal aspiration
percutaneous umbrella closure of
   patent ductus arteriosus
percutaneously cannulated
percutaneously inserted
percutaneously introduced
perennial fever
perennial rhinitis
Perez sign
perfluorocarbon blood substitute,
   oxygenated
perforated aortic cusp
perforating arteries
perforation
   cardiac
   transseptal
perforator
   first septal
   ligation of
   septal
   stripping of
perforator vessel
performance (see *function*)
perfusate
perfuse
perfused
perfusion
   adequate coronary
   antegrade
   coronary
   diminished systemic
   extremity
   homogenous
   hypothermic
   isolated heat
   luxury
   misery

perfusion *(cont.)*
 myocardial
 peripheral
 pulsatile
 regional (by mixed venous blood)
 retrograde cardiac
 tissue
perfusion abnormality
perfusion and ventilation lung scan
perfusion catheter
perfusion defect
perfusionist, pump
perfusion lung scan
perfusion of myocardium
perfusion of underventilated lung
perfusion pressure
 diastolic
 transmyocardial
perialveolar fibrosis
perianeurysmal retroperitoneal fibrosis
periaortic fibrosis
periaortic inflammation and fibrosis
periaortic neurectomy
periarterial sympathectomy
periarteritis, disseminated necrotizing
periarteritis nodosa (PAN)
peribronchial alveolar spaces
peribronchial connective tissue
peribronchial cuffing
peribronchial distribution
peribronchial fibrosis
peribronchial lymph nodes
peribronchiolar hemorrhage
pericardectomy (pericardiectomy)
pericardiaca, pleura
pericardiacophrenic vein
pericardial absence
 congenital
 partial
pericardial baffle
pericardial basket

pericardial biopsy, percutaneous
pericardial cavity
pericardial chyle with tamponade
pericardial constriction, occult
pericardial cradle
pericardial cyst
pericardial diaphragmatic adhesions
pericardial disease
pericardial effusion
pericardial effusion with cardiac tamponade
pericardial flap
pericardial fluid
 evacuation of offending
 exudative
 transudative
pericardial fluid analysis
pericardial fluid aspiration
pericardial fold
pericardial fremitus
pericardial friction rub
pericardial hematoma
pericardial infusion
pericardial knock
pericardial lavage, continuous
pericardial pain
pericardial patch
pericardial reflection (on x-ray)
pericardial reserve volume
pericardial restraint
pericardial rub
pericardial sac
pericardial sinus (sinuses)
pericardial sling
pericardial space, free
pericardial tamponade
pericardial tap (tapping)
pericardial window operation
pericardiectomy (pericardectomy)
pericardiocentesis, diagnostic
pericardiocentesis needle

pericardiolysis
pericardioscopy, percutaneous
pericardiotomy syndrome
pericarditis
  actinomycotic
  acute
  acute benign
  acute fibrinous
  acute nonspecific
  acute rheumatic
  adhesive
  advanced tuberculous constrictive
  amebiasis
  amebic
  bacterial
  bread-and-butter
  calcific constrictive
  carcinomatous
  cholesterol
  chronic
  chronic constrictive
  chronic effusive
  constricting
  constrictive
  coxsackievirus
  drug-induced
  dry
  effusion-constrictive
  effusive-constricting
  enteroviral
  external
  fibrinous
  fibrous
  fungal
  gonococcal
  hemorrhagic
  idiopathic
  idiopathic benign
  infective
  inflammatory
  localized
  mediastinal

pericarditis *(cont.)*
  meningococcal
  milk spot
  neoplastic
  nocardiosis
  noncalcific subacute constrictive
  nonpurulent
  obliterating
  obliterative
  occult constrictive
  parasitic
  Pick chronic constrictive
  pneumococcal
  pneumopyopericardium
  postcardiotomy
  postinfarction
  postirradiation
  postoperative
  postoperative constricting
  purulent
  pyopericardium
  radiation-induced
  restrictive
  rheumatic
  rheumatoid
  serofibrinous
  serous
  staphylococcal
  Sternberg
  streptococcal
  subacute constrictive
  suppurative
  syphilitic
  traumatic
  tuberculous
  uremic
  viral
pericarditis calculosa
pericarditis episternocardiaca
pericarditis-liver pseudocirrhosis
  syndrome
pericarditis obliterans

pericarditis sicca
pericarditis villosa
pericarditis with effusion
pericardium
  adherent
  autologous
  bread-and-butter
  calcified
  congenitally absent
  diaphragmatic
  empyema
  fibrous
  inelastic
  inflamed
  nondistensible
  parietal
  pericardial
  serous
  shaggy
  soldier's patches of
  thickened
  visceral
pericardium calcareous deposits
pericardium exposed
pericardium fibrosum
pericardium opened in inverted T
  fashion
pericardium serosum
pericatheter thrombi
perichondritis
pericostal sutures
periendocarditis
  acute
  subacute
perigraft hematoma
perihilar area
perihilar density
perihilar edema
perihilar region
peri-infarction block
peri-infarction conduction defect

peri-infarction heart block
peri-infarction ischemia
peri-infarctional defect
perimedial dysplasia
perimembranous ventricular septal
  defect
perimuscular plexus
perinatal respiratory distress syndrome
period
  absolute refractory (ARP)
  accessory pathway effective
    refractory
  antegrade refractory
  atrial effective refractory
  atrial refractory
  diastolic filling
  effective refractory (ERP)
  ejection
  functional refractory (FRP)
  isoelectric
  isovolumetric
  isovolumic
  pacemaker amplifier refractory
  postventricular atrial refractory
    (PVARP)
  pre-ejection (PEP)
  presphygmic
  rapid filling (RFP)
  refractory
  relative refractory (RRP)
  retrograde refractory
  sphygmic
  symptom-free
  systolic ejection (SEP)
  ventricular effective refractory
    (VERP)
  ventricular refractory
  ventriculoatrial effective refractory
  vulnerable
  Wenckebach
periodic breathing

periodic chills
periodic dizziness
periodic edema
periodic paralysis
periodicity
    AV node Wenckebach
    circadian
period of isovolumic contraction
period of rapid ventricular filling
period of reduced ventricular filling
perioperative blood loss
perioperative complications
perioperative myocardial infarction
perioperative myocardial necrosis
perioperative plasmapheresis
perioperative stroke
perioral cyanosis
periorbital Doppler study
periorbital fullness
periosteal incision
periosteum
periostitis
peripancreatic arteries
peripartum cardiomyopathy
peripartum dilated cardiomyopathy
peripartum myocarditis
peripelvic collateral vessel
peripheral air-space disease
peripheral angiopathy
peripheral angioplasty
peripheral arterial cannula
peripheral blood flow
peripheral blood lymphocytes (PBLs)
peripheral blood progenitor cell
    (PBPC)
peripheral blood stem cell (PBSC)
    collections
peripheral cholesterol embolization
    syndrome
peripheral circulatory vasoconstriction
peripheral cutaneous vasoconstriction

peripheral cyanosis
peripheral directional atherectomy
    (PDA)
peripheral edema
peripheral embolus
peripheral infiltrates
peripheral intravenous infusion line
peripheral laser angioplasty (PLA)
peripherally inserted central catheter
    (PICC)
peripheral pulmonic stenosis
peripheral pulmonic systolic murmur
peripheral pulse (pulses)
peripheral pulse deficit
peripheral resistance
peripheral small airways study
peripheral vascular disease,
    arteriosclerotic
peripheral vascular resistance,
    decreased
peripheral vasodilators
peripheral veins, absent
peripheral venous cannula
peripheral venous reservoirs
peripheral vessels
periphery of the lung
periphlebitis
    breast
    lateral thoracic vein
    sclerosing
    sclerosing breast
    thoracoepigastric vein
peripheral pulmonary artery stenosis
periprosthetic leak (leakage)
perirenal hematoma
peritoneal dialysis, continuous ambu-
    latory
peritoneovenous shunt
periumbilical area tenderness
perivalvular dehiscence
perivalvular disruption

perivalvular leak
perivascular canal
perivascular cell
perivascular distribution
perivascular edema
perivascular fibrosis
perivascular space of Virchow-Robin
Perma-Hand suture
permanent disability
permanent idiopathic hypotension
permanent impairment
permanent lead introducer
permanent rate-responsive dual-
 chamber pacemaker
permanent rate-responsive pacemaker
permanent reciprocating atrioventricular junctional tachycardia
Permathane Pacesetter lead pacemaker
permeability of capillaries
permeability-type pulmonary edema
pernicious anemia
pernicious myocarditis
peroneal area
peroneal artery
peroneal muscles
peroneal-tibial trunk
peroneal vein
peroneal vessel
perpetuation of atelectasis
Persantine thallium scanning
Persantine thallium stress test
persistent bronchopleural fistula
persistent common atrioventricular
 canal
persistent fetal circulation
persistent marginal vein
persistent ostium primum
persistent ostium secundum
persistent patency of ductus arteriosus
persistent patency of ductus venosus
persistent splenomegaly

persistent truncus arteriosus
persistent upright T waves
personality type A
personality type B
perspiring
Perthes test for collateral circulation
 in varicose veins
pertussis
pertussoid eosinophilic pneumonia
pervenous catheter
PES (programmed electrical stimula-
 tion) interval
PET (positron emission tomography)
PET balloon, USCI
PET balloon with window and
 extended collection chamber
PET balloon Simpson atherectomy
 device
PET scan
petechia (pl. petechiae)
petechial hemorrhage
Petit sinus
PETN (pentaerythritol tetranitrate)
PFD (persistent fetal dispersion) of
 AV node
PFR (peak filling rate)
PF3 (platelet factor 3) syndrome
PFTs (pulmonary function tests)
Pfuhl-Jaffé sign
PFWT (pain-free walking time) on
 treadmill
PG (pulse generator)
PGE_1 (prostaglandin E_1)
pH interval
pH-stat strategy
phagocytized hemosiderin
phagocytosis
Phalen stress test
Phaneuf artery forceps
Phantom cardiac guide wire
pharmaceutical cardioversion

pharmacologic stress dual-isotope
   myocardial perfusion SPECT
pharmacologic stress echocardiography
pharmacologic stress technique
pharyngeal
pharyngitis
   acute
   catarrhal
   granular
   phlegmonous
   pneumococcal
   staphylococcal
   ulcerative
   viral
pharynx
phase (see also *period*)
   bradycardic agonal
   diastolic depolarization
   expiratory
   inspiration
   inspiratory
   plateau (in cardiac action
      potentials)
   prolonged expiratory
   prolonged inspiratory
   rapid early repolarization
   rapid filling
   rapid repolarization
   resting (of cardiac action potentials)
   upstroke (of cardiac action
      potentials)
phase angle
phase-shift velocity mapping
PHCA (profound hypothermic
   circulatory arrest)
P$_2$ heart sound (pulmonary valve
   closure)
phenomenon (pl. phenomena) (see
   also *sign, reaction*)
   aliasing
   anniversary
   Aschner

phenomenon *(cont.)*
   Ashman
   Austin Flint
   booster
   Bowditch staircase
   coronary steal
   Cushing
   dip
   dip and plateau
   Doppler
   embolic
   Friedreich
   Gaertner (Gärtner)
   Gallavardin
   gap conduction
   Goldblatt
   Hering
   Kasabach-Merritt
   Katz-Wachtle
   Litten diaphragm
   no-reflow
   Raynaud
   R-on-T
   Schellong-Strisower
   staircase
   steal
   stone heart
   tactile precordial
   treppe
   vasovagal
   Wenckebach
phenotype
   Cellano
   McLeod blood
phenylephrine
pheochromocytoma
   extra-adrenal
   intra-adrenal
   malignant
phlebectasia
   deep
   deep malformed

phlebectasia *(cont.)*
  diffuse
  superficial
phlebectomy
phlebitis
  adhesive
  anemic
  blue
  breast
  chest wall
  chlorotic
  migrating
  migratory
  obliterating
  obliterative
  plastic
  postvenography
  productive
  proliferative
  sclerosing breast
  septic
  superficial breast
  suppurative
phlebitis migrans
phlebodynia
phlebofibrosis
phlebogram, phlebography
  ascending
  ascending contrast
  direct puncture
  impedance
phleboid
phlebolith
phlebophlebostomy
phleboplasty
phleborheography
phleborrhagia
phleborrhaphy
phleborrhexis
phlebosclerosis
phlebosis
phlebostasis

phlebostenosis
phlebothrombosis
phlebotomy
  bloodless
  therapeutic
phlegm (see *sputum*)
phlegmasia
  cellulitic
  thrombotic
phlegmasia alba dolens puerperarum
phlegmasia cerulea dolens
phlegmonous pharyngitis
Phoenix single-chamber pacemaker
Phoenix total artificial heart
phonocardiogram (PCG)
phonocardiography, intracardiac
phonocardiographic
phonocatheter
phonomechanocardiography
phosphatase, histamine acid
phosphatidylinositol
phosphocreatine (PCr)
phosphodiesterase inhibitors
phosphofructokinase
phosphoinositides
phospholamban
phospholipids, desaturated
phosphorus level, serum
phosphorylase kinase deficiency
phosphorylation
  mitochondrial
  oxidative
photoablation, laser
photocoagulation
  intraoperative laser (of ventricular
    tachycardia)
  laser
photodisruption
photometer, HemoCue
photoplethysmography (PPG)
photoplethysmographic monitoring
phrenic artery

phrenic nerve pacing
phrenic nerve paralysis
phrenic pedicle
PHT (passive hyperimmune therapy)
phthinoid chest
phthisis, aneurysmal
PHTN (pulmonary hypertension)
Phylax implantable cardioverter-defibrillator (Biotronik)
Phymos 3D pacemaker
physical finding(s)
  cardinal
  salient
physiologic(al) anemia
physiologic fibrinolysis
physiologic pacing
physiologic regurgitation
physiologic shunt flow
physiologic solution
physiologic splitting of S$_2$
physiologic stress technique
physiologic third heart sound
physiotherapy, vigorous chest
PI (pulmonic insufficiency)
PIB (peri-infarction block)
PIBC (percutaneous intra-aortic balloon counterpulsation)
PIC (plasmin inhibitor complex)
PICA (posterior inferior communicating artery)
PICD (peri-infarction conduction defect)
Pick chronic constrictive pericarditis
Pick disease of heart
Pick syndrome
pickwickian syndrome
picture
  clinical
  hemodynamic
PIE (pulmonary infiltrates with eosinophilia)

PIE (pulmonary interstitial emphysema)
PIE (pulmonary infiltrate-eosinophilia) syndrome
Pierce-Donachy ventricular assist device (VAD)
pigeon breast
pigeon breeder's pneumonitis
pigeon breeder's syndrome
pigeon-breeder's lung
pigeon chest
pigeon-fancier's disease
pigeon-fancier's lung
piggy-back cardiac transplantation
pigmentation
pigmenti, incontinentia
pigtail catheter
PIH (pregnancy-induced hypertension)
Pilling Wolvek sternal approximator
piloerection
Pilotip catheter guide
PIMS (programmable implantable medication system)
pinching chest pain
pincushion distortion, radiographic
pink puffer
pink tetralogy of Fallot
pinked up extremity
Pinnacle pacemaker
Pins sign in pericarditis
PIP (peak inspiratory pressure)
pipestem arteries
piriform (pyriform) sinus
pistol-shot femoral and radial pulse
pistol-shot sound in aortic regurgitation
pitch
pitting edema
PJC (premature junctional contraction)
PJT (paroxysmal junctional tachycardia)
PLA (peripheral laser angioplasty)

PLA-I (platelet antigen)
placebo effect
placement
  annular
  intracoronary stent
  intrapericardial patch lead
  subannular
placental souffle
placental transfusion syndrome
planar exercise thallium-201
  scintigraphy
plane
  circular
  four-chamber
  frontal
  short-axis
  subadventitial
  subintimal cleavage
  transmedial
  transverse
  valve
  XY
  ZY
plane-type synovial joint
planimeter, -metry
planogram
plantar hyperplasia
plantar ischemia test for circulation
plantaris muscle
plaque, plaquing (noun)
  arterial
  arteriosclerotic
  atheromatous
  atherosclerotic
  calcified
  concentric atherosclerotic
  coral reef
  disrupted
  eccentric
  eccentric atherosclerotic
  echogenic

plaque (cont.)
  echolucent
  endocardial
  fatty
  fibrofatty yellow
  fibrotic
  fibrous
  fissured atheromatous
  Hollenhorst
  intraluminal
  lipid-laden
  luminal
  noncompliant
  obstructive
  pleural
  pulverized
  residual
  sessile
  stenotic
  talc
  ulcerated
plaque cleaving
plaque compression
plaque constituents
plaque-containing artery
plaque cracker, LeVeen
plaque disintegration by laser pulses
plaque erosion
plaque fracture (or fracturing)
plaque regression
plaque remodeling
plaque rupture
plaque splitting
plaque tearing
plaque vaporization
plaquing of arteries
Plasbumin
plasma
  fresh frozen
  platelet-rich
plasma aldosterone, circadian rhythm

plasma cell pneumonia, interstitial
plasma cells
plasma coagulation factors
plasma colloid osmotic pressure
plasma concentration
plasma expanders
plasma infusion, fresh frozen
plasma lactate, elevated
Plasmalyte A cardioplegic solution
plasmapheresis
Plasma-Plex
plasma renin activity
    inappropriately elevated
    suppressed
Plasma-Saver
Plasma TFE vascular graft
plasma thromboplastin component
    (PTC)
plasma viscosity
plasma volume expander (Hespan or
    hetastarch)
plasmapheresis, perioperative
Plasmatein
plasmin inhibitor complex (PIC)
plasminogen activator
    recombinant tissue-type
    tissue
    tissue-type
    urokinase-type
plasminogen activator inhibitor (PAI)
plasminogen deficiency
plasminogen streptokinase activator
    complex
Plasmodium falciparum infestation
plastic clot
plastic phlebitis
plastic pleurisy
plasty, sliding
plastysma layer
plate
    ground
    pusher

plateau
    elevated diastolic
    ventricular
plateau murmur
plateau phase in cardiac action
    potentials
plateau phenomenon, dip and
platelet
    blood
    HLA-type specific
    giant
platelet activating factor
platelet adhesiveness
platelet aggregation
platelet antiaggregant drugs
platelet count
platelet-derived growth factor
platelet factor 4
platelet-rich plasma
platelet-rich thrombus
platelet thrombosis or thrombus
platelet trapping
platelike atelectasis
platelike fibrous scar in lungs
platinum asthma
platysma
pledget, pledgets
    cotton
    oval
    Teflon felt
pledgeted Ethibond suture
pledgeted everting mattress sutures
pledgeted mattress suture
Plegisol cardioplegic solution
pleomorphic mononuclear cells
Plesch test
plethora of findings
plethoric appearance
plethysmogram, -graphy
    body box
    Doppler ultrasonic velocity detector
    segmental

plethysmogram *(cont.)*
  exercise strain gauge venous
    impedance (IPG)
  Medsonic
  strain-gauge
  venous
pleura (pl. pleurae)
  cervical
  congested
  costal
  diaphragmatic
  edematous
  inflamed
  mediastinal
  parietal
  pericardiac
  pulmonary
  roughened
  silicotic visceral
  visceral
  wrinkled
pleuracentesis
pleura costalis
pleuracotomy
pleura diaphragmatica
pleural adhesions, fibrous
pleural apical hematoma cap
pleural-based area of increased opacity
pleural biopsy
pleural biopsy needle
pleural cap, left
pleural carcinomatosis
pleural cavity
pleural crackle
pleural crepitation
pleural cupola (pl. cupolae)
pleural effusion
  chylous
  eosinophilic
  milky
pleural empyema
pleural exudate

pleural fibrosis, asbestos-induced
pleural fistula
pleural flap
pleural fluid, iridescent
pleural fremitus
pleural friction rub
pleuralgia
pleural implants, malignant
pleural margins
pleural mesothelium
pleural plaque
pleural poudrage
pleural pressure
pleural rales
pleural recesses
pleural reflection
pleural rub
  coarse
  creaking
  faint
  grating
  harsh
  loud
  scratchy
  shuffling
  soft
pleural sac
pleural shock
pleural sleeve
pleural space
pleural tap
pleural thickening, diffuse
pleural trauma
pleura mediastinalis
pleura parietalis
pleura pericardiaca
pleura pulmonalis
pleura visceralis
pleurectomy, parietal
Pleur-evac suction tube
pleurisy
  acute

pleurisy *(cont.)*
 acute fibrinous
 adhesive
 blocked
 cholesterol
 chronic
 chyliform
 chyloid
 chylous
 circumscribed
 costal
 diaphragmatic
 diffuse
 double
 dry
 encysted
 exudative
 fibrinopurulent
 fibrinous
 hemorrhagic
 ichorous
 indurative
 interlobar, interlobular
 mediastinal
 metapneumonic
 plastic
 pneumococcal
 primary
 proliferating
 pulmonary
 pulsating
 purulent
 sacculated
 secondary
 septic
 serofibrinous
 seropurulent
 serous
 single
 staphylococcal
 streptococcal
 suppurative

pleurisy *(cont.)*
 typhoid
 visceral
 wet
pleurisy with effusion
pleuritic chest pain
pleuritic exudate
pleuritic pain
pleuritic rub
pleuritis
pleurodesis
pleurodesis via talc poudrage
pleurodynia
pleuropericardial incision
pleuropericarditis
pleuropneumonia-like organisms
 (PPLO)
pleuropulmonary adhesions
plexectomy
plexiform fibrosis
plexogenic pulmonary arteriopathy
 (PPA)
plexus
 anterior coronary
 anterior pulmonary
 cardiac
 deep cardiac
 esophageal
 extradural vertebral
 great cardiac
 perimuscular
 pulmonary
 right coronary (of heart)
 superficial cardiac
 vascular
 vertebral venous
plexus aorticus
plexus cardiacus
plexus pulmonalis
plexus vascularis
plexus vasculosus
plexus venosus

plicated
plication
  annular
  annulus
  commissural
  inferior vena cava
  pulmonary artery
  vein
  vena cava
plication repair of flail leaflet
ploidy pattern, DNA
P loop (on vectorcardiography)
plop, tumor
PLR (peripheral laser recanalization)
PLT (primed lymphocyte test)
plucked chicken appearance
plug
  Alcock catheter
  mucus
  Teflon Bardic
plugging
  mucoid
  mucous
plug of tenacious bronchial exudate
plumb-line sign
plump vessel
PM (posterior mitral)
PMD (papillary muscle dysfunction)
PMI (point of maximum impulse)
PMI (point of maximal intensity)
  hyperdynamic
  hyperkinetic
PMI displaced downward
PMI displaced laterally
PMI displaced to left
P mitrale
PML (posterior mitral leaflet)
PMT AccuSpan tissue expander
PMV (percutaneous mitral balloon
  valvotomy)
PMV (percutaneous mitral balloon
  valvuloplasty)

PMV (prolapsed mitral valve)
PMVL (posterior mitral valve leaflet)
PNC (premature nodal contraction)
PND (paroxysmal nocturnal dyspnea)
pneumatic antishock garment (PASG)
pneumatic compression
pneumatic foot compression garment
pneumatic garments for shock
pneumatic HeartMate LVAD
pneumatic splint
pneumatocele, tension
pneumococcal bronchitis
pneumococcal empyema
pneumococcal myocarditis
pneumococcal pericarditis
pneumococcal pharyngitis
pneumococcal pleurisy
pneumococcal pneumonia
pneumococcus (pl. pneumococci)
pneumoconiosis
  bauxite
  coal worker's
  collagenous
  nonasbestos
  noncollagenous
  rheumatoid
  talc
pneumoconiosis siderotica
pneumoconstriction
Pneumocystis carinii pneumonia (PCP)
pneumocystis pneumonitis
pneumogram
pneumomediastinum, postoperative
pneumonectomy
  complete
  partial
pneumonectomy after contralateral
  lobectomy
pneumonia (see also *pneumonitis*)
  acute
  acute eosinophilic
  allergic

pneumonia *(cont.)*
aspiration
atypical interstitial
bacterial
bronchiolitis obliterans organizing
capillary
chronic
chronic eosinophilic
classic interstitial
community-acquired
consolidative
Cryptococcus neoformans
delayed resolution of
desquamative interstitial (DIP)
Eaton agent
endogenous lipoid
eosinophilic
Escherichia coli (*E. coli*)
exogenous
Friedländer
fungal
granulomatous
gray hepatization stage of
Haemophilus influenzae
hypersensitivity
hypostatic
incomplete resolution of
infantile
inhalation
interstitial
interstitial plasma cell
irradiation
Klebsiella pneumoniae
Legionella
lipoid
lobar
lobular
lymphoid interstitial
Mycoplasma (mycoplasmal)
necrotizing
nonbacterial
nosocomial

pneumonia *(cont.)*
obstructive
passive
pertussoid eosinophilic
pneumococcal
pneumococcus
Pneumocystis carinii (PCP)
postobstructive
postoperative
post-traumatic
primary atypical
Proteus
protozoal
Pseudomonas
red hepatization stage of
rheumatic
rickettsial
right-sided
segmental
staphylococcal
streptococcal
Streptococcus
subacute allergic
toxic
viral
pneumonia, aspiration, following:
alcoholic intoxication
anesthesia
CNS (central nervous system)
　　disease
convulsive disorders
disturbances of consciousness
excessive sedation
immersion
marked debility
vomiting
pneumonia, bacterial, causes of:
bacterial pathogens
Escherichia coli
Francisella tularensis
Friedländer bacillus
gram-negative bacilli

pneumonia, bacterial *(cont.)*
  Group A hemolytic streptococci
  Hemophilus influenzae
  Klebsiella pneumoniae
  Staphyloccus aureus
  Streptococcus pneumoniae
  tubercle bacillus
pneumonia-induced septic shock
pneumonia vaccine
pneumonia, viral, caused by:
  adenoviruses
  coxsackievirus (or Coxsackie virus)
  cytomegalovirus
  echovirus
  herpes simplex
  herpesvirus
  influenza
  parainfluenza viruses
  Reovirus
  respiratory syncytial virus
  rhinoviruses
  varicella
  viruses of childhood exanthems
pneumonic fever
pneumonitis (see also *pneumonia*)
  acid aspiration
  acute interstitial
  aspiration
  bacterial
  chemical
  cholesterol
  chronic
  congenital rubella
  cytomegalovirus
  early
  granulomatous
  hypersensitivity
  interstitial
  lipoid
  lymphocytic interstitial
  malarial
  manganese

pneumonitis *(cont.)*
  Mycoplasma (mycoplasmal)
  pneumocystis
  pigeon breeder's
  radiation
  staphylococcal
  trimellitic anhydritic
  uremic
  ventilation
pneumonocirrhosis
pneumonopathy
  alveolar
  eosinophilic
  parietoalveolar
pneumonopexy
pneumonophthisis
pneumonorrhaphy
pneumopericarditis
pneumopericardium, tension
pneumophila, Legionella
pneumopleuritis
pneumopyopericardium pericarditis
pneumotachograph
pneumothorax
  artificial
  blowing
  clicking
  closed
  congenital
  diagnostic
  extrapleural
  induced
  life-threatening
  open
  positive-pressure
  pressure
  simultaneous bilateral spontaneous
    (SBSP)
  spontaneous tension
  sucking
  tension
  therapeutic

pneumothorax *(cont.)*
  traumatic
  tuberculous
  uncomplicated
  valvular
pneuPAC ventilator/resuscitator
PNH (paroxysmal nocturnal
  hemoglobinuria)
pO_2, PO_2 (oxygen partial pressure or
  tension)
pocket (see also *pouch*)
  air
  endocardial
  infraclavicular
  pacemaker
  pacemaker tissue
  rectus sheath
  regurgitant
  subcutaneous pacemaker
  subpectoral
pockets of Zahn
poikilocyte
point
  A
  Arrhigi
  C
  coaptation
  commissural
  D
  de Mussey
  E
  Erb
  F
  J (junction)
  Mussey
  null
  O
point of maximal intensity (PMI)
point of maximum impulse (PMI)
Poiseuille layer (or space)
poisoning, cyanide
poker back

Poland sequence syndrome
polar anemia
polarcardiography
polarity
polarizing
Polar-Mate bipolar microcoagulator
polarographic oxygen method for
  determining cardiac output
Polar Vantage XL heart rate monitor
Polhemus-Schafer-Ivemark syndrome
pollen, mixed grass
pollinosis
polyaneurysmatic
polyangiitis overlap syndrome
polyarteritis nodosa
polychondritis, relapsing
polycystic kidney disease
polycythemia
  compensatory
  primary
  secondary
  spurious
  true
polycythemia vera
polycythemic
polydactyly
Polydek suture
PolyFlex lead pacemaker
polygelin colloid contrast medium
polygenic hypercholesterolemia
polymer fume fever
polymerase chain reaction (PCR)
polymeric endoluminal paving stent
polymicrobial infection
polymorphic ventricular tachycardia
polymorphic VT/VF (ventricular
  tachycardia/ventricular fibrillation)
polymorphonuclear leukocytes
polymorphonuclear lymphocytes
polymyositis
Polynesian bronchiectasis
polyolefin rubber diaphragm

polyp, cardiac
polypoid calcified irregular mass
polysomnography
polysplenia
Polystan perfusion cannula
Polystan venous return catheter
polytetrafluoroethylene (PTFE) fumes
polytetrafluoroethylene (PTFE) graft
polyunsaturated fats
polyurethane foam embolus
polyuria, nocturnal
polyvalvular dysplasia, congenital
Pompe disease
Ponfick shadow
Pontiac fever
pontine intracerebral hemorrhage
pool, circulating fibrinogen
pooling of blood in extremities
pooling, venous
poor compliance
poor drainage of bronchial secretions
poorly controlled hypertension
poor outcome, portend a
poor prognosis
poor R-wave progression
poor short-term prognosis
pop-off suture
popliteal artery aneurysmorrhaphy
popliteal artery entrapment syndrome
popliteal artery, infragenicular
popliteal artery occlusive disease
popliteal-blind peroneal graft
popliteal bypass
popliteal-distal bypass graft
popliteal fossa
popliteal in situ bypass
popliteal pulses, palpable
popliteal space
popliteal to distal in situ bypass
popliteal trifurcation
popliteal vein ligature
Poppen-Blalock carotid clamp

poppet
  ball
  barium-impregnated
  disk
  prosthetic heart valve
  prosthetic valve
popping sound
porcine heterograft
porcine valve prosthesis
porcine xenograft bioprosthesis
porcine xenograft, glutaraldehyde-
  preserved
pores of Kohn
porous electrode
porous tip electrode
porphyrins
port
  injection
  Quinton vascular access
  side-arm pressure
  vent
Port-A-Cath
portable heart-lung machine
portacaval anastomosis, end-to-side
portacaval shunt
portal hypertension
portal vein thrombosis
Portasonic nebulizer
portend, portends
portend a poor outcome
Porter syndrome
portion, conal
Portnoy ventricular cannula
port wine stain
Posadas disease
Posadas mycosis
Posadas-Wernicke coccidioidomycosis
Posadas-Wernicke disease
position
  anterior oblique
  catheter tip
  coaxial catheter tip

position *(cont.)*
45°
Fowler
infragenicular
infrapulmonary
knee-chest
lateral decubitus
left anterior oblique (LAO)
left lateral decubitus
Nefertiti sniff
noncoaxial catheter tip
orthopnea
orthopneic
paramedian
pulmonary capillary wedge
right anterior oblique (RAO)
semi-Fowler
semilateral
spiral
squatting
steep Trendelenburg
30°
Trendelenburg
wedge
position confirmed by fluoroscopy with
  aid of radiopaque marking on knot
position sensor, Hall-effect
positive deflection on EKG
positive end-expiratory pressure
  (PEEP)
positive inotropic effect
positive-pressure pneumothorax
positive-pressure ventilation
positive skin test
positive tilt test
Positrol cardiac device
Positrol II catheter
positron emission tomography (PET)
positron emitters
POSSIS epicardial pacing lead
postablation

postangioplasty mural thrombosis
postangioplasty stenosis
post-arrest hypoxic encephalopathy
postcapillaries
postcapillary venules
postcardiac injury syndrome
postcardiotomy delirium
postcardiotomy intra-aortic balloon
  pumping
postcardiotomy lymphocytic
  splenomegaly
postcardiotomy pericarditis
postcardiotomy psychosis syndrome
postcardiotomy shock
postcardiotomy syndrome
postcommissurotomy syndrome
postconversion electrocardiogram
postdeployment
postductal type of coarctation
posterior annulus, redundant scallop of
posterior-aorta transposition of great
  arteries
posterior axillary line
posterior basal bronchi
posterior border of lung
posterior bronchi
posterior cathodal patch electrode
posterior coronary plexus (of heart)
posterior cusp
posterior descending artery (PDA)
posterior descending branch
posterior fascicular block
posterior fossa compression syndrome
posterior fossa hypertension
posterior free wall
posterior inferior communicating
  artery (PICA)
posterior intercostal artery
posterior intercostal branch
posterior interventricular groove
posterior interventricular sulcus

posterior interventricular vein
posterior lumbar vessel
posterior leaflet prolapse
posterior mediastinal lymph nodes
posterior mediastinum
posterior mitral valve leaflet
posterior papillary muscle
posterior parietal peritoneal incision
posterior patch aortoplasty (Nicks
  procedure)
posterior pulmonary plexus
posterior rectus fascia exposed
posterior segment of lung
posterior semilunar valve
posterior table
posterior tibial pulse
posterior to the phrenic nerve
posterior ventricular branch
posterior wall myocardial infarction
posterior wall thickness
posterobasal wall myocardial infarction
posterolateral branch
posterolateral incision
posterolateral thoracotomy incision
posterolateral thoracotomy, left
posterolateral wall myocardial
  infarction
posteroseptal Kent bundle
postexercise tracing
postextrasystolic potentiation
postextubation stridor
posthemorrhagic anemia of newborn
postinfarction course
postinfarction failure
postinfarction ventricular aneurysm
postinfarction ventriculoseptal defect
postinfectious bronchiectasis
postinflammatory pulmonary fibrosis
postirradiation pericarditis
postirradiation vascular insufficiency
postischemic recovery

postmalignant arrhythmia
postmastectomy lymphedema
  syndrome
post-MI (myocardial infarction)
  syndrome
postmortem clot
postmortem thrombus
postmyocardial infarction syndrome
postmyocardiotomy infarction
postmyocarditis dilated cardiomyopathy
postnasal catarrh
postnasal discharge
postnasal drainage
postnasal drip
postobstructive pneumonia
postoperative acute cholecystitis
postoperative bronchopneumonia
postoperative cardiac function
postoperative choreiform movements
postoperative choreoathetosis
postoperative chylothorax
postoperative constricting pericarditis
postoperative mediastinal hemorrhage
postoperative oliguria
postoperative pericarditis
postoperative pneumomediastinum
postoperative pneumonia
postoperative pulmonary edema
postoperative renal failure
postoperative shock
postoperative transfusion
postpartum cardiomyopathy
postpartum myocardiopathy
postpartum thrombophlebitis
postperfusion lung syndrome
postperfusion pulmonary vasculitis
postperfusion syndrome
postpericardiotomy syndrome
postphlebitic incompetence
postphlebitic leg

postphlebitic neurosis
postphlebitic syndrome
postprandial angina
postprandial pain
postprandial syncope
postprimary tuberculosis
post-PTCA heparinization
post-PTCA residual stenosis
post-PVC sinus beat
postradiation fibrosis
postshock escape interval
postshock PA
postshock pacing
postshock pacing period
postshock pause
postshock PW
postshock VVI pacing
poststenotic dilatation
poststreptococcal inflammatory
    process
postthrombolytic coronary reocclusion
postthrombotic syndrome
post-tourniquet occlusion angiography
posttransfusion purpura
posttransfusion syndrome
posttransplantation lymphoproliferative
    disorder (PTLD)
posttransplant coronary artery disease
posttussive inspiratory rhonchi
posttussive rales
posttussive rhonchi
posttussive syncope
postural drainage
postural drainage and percussion
    (PDP)
postural drainage with clapping and
    vibration
postural dyspnea
postural stimulation of aldosterone
postural stimulation test
postural syncope

posture, squatting
postvalvulotomy syndrome
postvenography phlebitis
postventricular atrial refractory period
    (PVARP)
Potain opening snap in mitral stenosis
Potain sign
potassium
    depressed serum
    ionic
potassium channel blocker
potassium chloride (KCl)
potassium chloride cardioplegia
potassium chloride repletion
potassium chloride solution
potassium concentration, 24-hour urine
potassium deficiency
potassium intoxication
potassium sparing
potassium-sparing diuretics
potassium-sparing effect
potassium wastage
potassium wasting
potassium-43 imaging agent (myocar-
    dial perfusion imaging)
potential
    action
    cardiac action
    membrane
    recruitment
    resting membrane
    tetrodotoxin
    ventricular late (VLP)
potentiation, postextrasystolic
Pottenger sign
Potts anastomosis
Potts anastomosis between descending
    aorta and left pulmonary artery
Potts aortic clamp
Potts aortic-pulmonary artery
    anastomosis

Potts bronchus forceps
Potts bulldog forceps
Potts clamp
Potts coarctation clamp
Potts-Cournand needle
Potts needle
Potts-Niedner clamp
Potts operation
Potts patent ductus clamp
Potts scissors
Potts shunt
Potts right-angled scissors
Potts-Satinsky clamp
Potts 60° angled scissors
Potts-Smith aortic occlusion clamp
Potts-Smith scissors
Potts-Smith side-to-side anastomosis
Potts-Smith tissue forceps
Potts-Smith vascular scissors
Potts technique
Potts thumb forceps
Potts vascular forceps
Potts vascular scissors
pouch
  blind
  pacemaker generator
poudrage
  intrapericardial
  pleural
  talc
pounding, heart
pounding in chest
pounding pain
Poupart ligament
power pack, abdominal
P-P interval
PPA (plexogenic pulmonary
  arteriopathy)
PPAS (peripheral pulmonary artery
  stenosis)
PPD (purified protein derivative)

PPD test
PPH (primary pulmonary hypertension)
PPLO (pleuropneumonia-like
  organisms)
PPM (posterior papillary muscle)
P pulmonale in leads II, III, aVF
P pulmonale syndrome
P-Q interval, short
P:QRS ratio
PRA (plasma renin activity) test
praecox, lymphoedema
PRBCs (packed red blood cells)
preablation
preacinar arterial wall thickness
preangioplasty stenosis
preaortic space, retropancreatic
precapillary pulmonary hypertension
precarious circulation
precarious condition
precatheterization
precautions, universal
precipitant
precipitated
precipitated by exertion, angina
precipitating antibody
precipitating event
precipitating factor
precipitator
precipitously
precipitous rise in blood pressure
preclotted graft
preclotted Meadox woven double
  velour graft
preclotted patch graft
preclot the graft
preclotting of graft
preclude
precluding catheter passage, tortuosity
precordial chest pain
precordial clicking

precordial crunching
precordial discomfort
precordial honk
precordial impulse
precordial impulse amplitude
precordial impulse, bifid
precordial impulse contour
precordial impulse location
precordial knocking
precordial lead
precordial migraine
precordial motion
    heaving
    rocking
    trifid
precordial palpation
precordial thrill
precordial thump
precordial transition zone
precordium
    active
    anterior
    bulging
    lateral
predicated on the assumption
predicted cardiac index
predilection
predispose
predisposed patient
predisposing factors
predominant flow loads
preductal coarctation of aorta
preeclampsia
pre-ejection interval
pre-ejection period (PEP)
pre-excitation (early ventricular
    depolarization)
pre-excitation atrioventricular
    conduction
pre-excitation syndrome
pre-excitation, ventricular

pre-exercise resting supine EKG
preexisting cardiopulmonary disease
preformed clot
preformed curves, catheter with
preformed guide wire
pregnancy-induced hypertension (PIH)
pregnancy-related hypertension
pregnancy, toxemia of
prehypertension
preinfarction angina
preinfarction syndrome
preload
    cardiac
    decreased ventricular
    left ventricular
    ventricular
preload reserve
premature atherosclerosis
premature atrial complex (PAC)
premature atrial contraction (PAC)
premature atrial depolarization
premature atrioventricular junctional
    complexes
premature battery depletion
premature closure of the ductus
    arteriosus
premature complex
    atrial
    junctional
premature contraction
    atrial
    atrioventricular junctional
    ventricular
premature depolarizations, atrial
premature heartbeat (extrasystole)
premature junctional contraction (PJC)
premature mid-diastolic closure of
    mitral valve
premature rewarming, retard
premature valve closure
premature ventricular beats

premature ventricular complex (PVC)
premature ventricular contractions
  (PVC)
  high-amplitude
  monomorphic
premature ventricular depolarizations
premedication
premonitory signs
premonitory symptoms
prenatal corticosteroid treatment
preoperative bronchoscopy
preoperative resting MUGA scan
prep
  Betadine
  Ioban
prepectorally
preperitoneal fat
preponderance, preponderant
prerenal azotemia
prescription (Rx)
presenile gangrene
preservation of native aortic valve
preserve the long thoracic nerve
pressor response, Cushing
pressor therapy
pressure
  airway opening
  alveolar
  ambulant venous (AVP)
  ankle-arm
  AO or Ao (aorta)
  aortic
  aortic root
  arterial (ART or Art.)
  arterial peak systolic
  atmospheres of
  augmentation
  auto positive end-expiratory
  A wave (left or right atrial
    catheterization)
  back

pressure *(cont.)*
  blood (BP)
  brachial artery
  brachial artery cuff
  brachial artery end-diastolic
  brachial artery peak systolic
  C wave (right atrial catheterization)
  capillary
  cardiac filling
  central aortic
  central venous (CVP)
  cerebral perfusion
  chest
  collapse of jugular venous
  continuous positive airway (CPAP)
  coronary artery perfusion (CPP)
  coronary wedge
  critical closing (CCP)
  cuff blood
  diastolic blood (DBP)
  diastolic filling (DFP)
  diastolic perfusion
  diastolic pulmonary artery
  distal coronary perfusion
  Doppler blood
  elevated
  elevated jugular venous
  elevated pulmonary wedge
  end-diastolic
  end-expiratory
  end-inspiratory
  endocardial
  end-systolic (ESP)
  equalized diastolic
  extravascular
  femoral artery (FAP)
  filling
  high blood (HBP)
  high filling
  high interstitial
  high wedge

pressure *(cont.)*
  increased pulmonary arterial
  intracardiac
  intrapericardial
  intrapleural
  intrapulmonary
  intrathoracic
  intraventricular
  intrinsic positive end-expiratory
  in vivo balloon
  jugular venous
  LA (left atrium)
  left atrial (LAP)
  left atrial end-diastolic
  left subclavian central venous
    (LSCVP)
  left ventricular (LV)
  left ventricular cavity
  left ventricular end-diastolic
    (LVEDP)
  left ventricular filling
  left ventricular peak systolic
  left ventricular systolic (LVS)
  left-sided heart
  low wedge
  manual
  maximum inflation
  mean
  mean aortic
  mean arterial (MAP)
  mean atrial
  mean blood
  mean brachial artery
  mean circulatory filling
  mean left atrial
  mean pulmonary artery (MPAP)
  mean pulmonary artery wedge
  mean right atrial
  minimum blood
  PA (pulmonary artery) systolic
  PAD (pulmonary artery diastolic)

pressure *(cont.)*
  PAS (pulmonary artery systolic)
  peak-inflation
  peak regurgitant wave
  peak systolic
  peak systolic aortic (PSAP)
  phasic
  plasma colloid osmotic
  pleural
  positive end-expiratory (PEEP)
  pulmonary arterial wedge (PAWP)
  pulmonary artery (PAP)
  pulmonary artery diastolic (PAD)
  pulmonary artery end-diastolic
    (PAEDP)
  pulmonary artery mean (PAM)
  pulmonary artery peak systolic
  pulmonary artery/pulmonary
    capillary wedge
  pulmonary artery systolic (PAS)
  pulmonary artery wedge (PAWP)
  pulmonary capillary (PCP)
  pulmonary capillary wedge
    (PCWP)
  pulmonary venous capillary (PVC)
  pulmonary venous wedge
  pulmonary wedge
  pulse
  PV (pulmonary vein)
  PVC (pulmonary venous capillary)
  RA (right atrial)
  recoil
  right atrial (RAP)
  right heart
  right-sided heart
  right subclavian central venous
    (RSCVP)
  right ventricular (RVP)
  right ventricular diastolic (RVD)
  right ventricular end-diastolic
  right ventricular peak systolic

pressure *(cont.)*
  right ventricular systolic (RVS)
  right ventricular volume
  RV (right ventricular)
  RVD (right ventricular diastolic)
  RVS (right ventricular systolic)
  segmental lower extremity Doppler
  stump
  subatmospheric
  supersystemic pulmonary artery
  SVC (superior vena cava)
  systemic
  systolic
  systolic blood (SBP)
  torr
  transcutaneous oxygen
  transmyocardial perfusion
  transpulmonary (P_{TP})
  V wave (left or right atrial
    catheterization)
  venous
  wedge
  withdrawal
  X' (prime) wave (right atrial
    catheterization)
  Y wave
  Z point
pressure augmentation
pressure-controlled ventilator
pressure cuff
pressure difference, aortic-left
  ventricular
pressure equalization
pressure flow gradient
pressure gradient
  arteriovenous
  negligible
pressure gradient on pull-back
pressure injector
pressure-flow gradient
pressure-like sensation in chest

pressure loads, pure
pressure measurement
pressure oscillation
pressure overload
pressure pneumothorax
pressure pullback
pressure readings
pressure sensation
pressure support ventilation (PSV)
pressure transducer
pressure waveform
Pressurometer
Presto cardiac device
presumptive diagnosis
presyncopal episode
presyncope
presystolic Austin Flint murmur
presystolic bulge, palpable
presystolic gallop rhythm
presystolic murmur (PSM)
presystolic pulsation
prethrombotic syndrome
pretibial edema
prevention of lung collapse
prevention of thrombus propagation
Price-Thomas bronchial forceps
Prima pacemaker
primary aldosteronism
primary alveolar hypoventilation
primary amyloidosis
primary atypical pneumonia
primary bronchi, right and left
primary chordal dysplasia
primary coccidioidomycosis
primary electrical disease
primary electrical ventricular tachycardia
primary endocardial fibroelastosis
primary hyperparathyroidism
primary hypertension
primary hypertrophic cardiomyopathy

primary hypotension
primary lung neosplasm
primary median sternotomy
primary myocardiopathy
primary pleurisy
primary prosthetic graft infection
primary pulmonary hypertension
primary thrombus
primary tuberculosis
primary varicose veins
primitive ventricle
principal bronchus
principle
   diamond anastomosis
   Doppler
   Fick
   Frank-Starling
   indicator fractionation
P-R interval
   prolongation of
   short
   shortening of
   varying
Prinzmetal angina
Prinzmetal II syndrome
Prinzmetal variant angina
Prism-CL pacemaker
prism method for ventricular volume
proarrhythmia
proarrhythmic effect
proarrhythmic event
probe
   AngeLase combined mapping-laser
   blood flow
   cardiac
   Chandler V-pacing
   cryosurgical
   Doppler flow
   echocardiographic
   electromagnetic flow
   Hagar

probe *(cont.)*
   hand-held exploring electrode
   hand-held mapping
   nasopharyngeal temperature
   nonimaging
   nuclear
   oligonucleotide
   Parsonnet
   pediatric biplane TEE
   sapphire contact
   Siemens-Elema AB pulse
     transducer
   Teflon
   temperature
   transesophageal
probe adhesion to vessel wall
Probe balloon-on-a-wire dilatation
   system, USCI
Probe cardiac device
probe-patent foramen ovale
probing catheter, USCI
procedural risk factors
procedure (see also *method,*
     operation, technique)
   adenosine echocardiography
   arterial switch
   Bentall (for coronary ostial
     revascularization)
   Blalock-Hanlon
   Blalock-Taussig
   Brock
   Cabrol
   Cabrol I anastomosis
   Cabrol I tube graft
   Cabrol II modification of Bentall
   cardiokymography
   Cardiolite scan
   CardioTek (or Cardiotec) scan
   cardiotocography
   CAVH (continuous arteriovenous
     hemofiltration)

procedure *(cont.)*
  Cox maze
  Damus-Norwood
  David
  debanding
  domino
  Edwards-Kerr
  endocardial resection (extended)
  Fick
  flush aortogram
  Fontan repair
  Glenn shunt
  Heineke-Mikulicz
  interventional
  intravenous fluorescein angiography
    (IVFA)
  IVOX artificial lung
  Judkins coronary arteriography
  Ko-Airan bleeding control method
  M-mode echocardiogram
  magnetic resonance angioplasty
    (MRA)
  Mustard
  Nikaidoh
  percutaneous intracoronary
    angioscopy
  pulmonary artery banding
  Quaegebeur modification
  Rashkind balloon atrial septotomy
  Rastan-Konno
  sector scan echocardiography
  Senning
  Sones coronary arteriography
  Todaro tendon resection
  transesophageal echocardiogram
  transfemoral endovascular stented
    graft
  2-D echocardiography
  vectorcardiography
process
  jugular
  left ventricular posterior superior

process *(cont.)*
  prominent xiphoid
  xiphoid
proconvertin blood coagulation factor
prodromal symptoms
prodrome (pl. prodromata)
productive cough
productive phlebitis
products
  fibrin
  fibrin split
profile
  automated physiologic
  biophysical (BPP)
  KDA
  serum lipid
Profile Plus dilatation catheter, USCI
Proflex 5 dilatation catheter
Pro-Flo XT catheter
profound anxiety
profound cardiopulmonary deterioration
profound dyspnea
profound hypertension
profound hypothermia
profound hypothermic circulatory
  arrest (PHCA)
profoundly obtunded infant
profound peripheral eosinophilia
profound shock
profound volume depletion
profound weakness
profunda Dacron patchplasty
profunda femoris artery
profundaplasty
profunda popliteal collateral index
progeria syndrome
prognosis
  equivocal
  excellent
  favorable
  good

prognosis *(cont.)*
  grave
  grim
  guarded
  ominous
  poor
  poor short-term
  unfavorable
Programalith pacemaker
programmability of pacemaker rate
programmable cardioverter-
  defibrillator (PCD)
programmable implantable medication
  system (PIMS)
programmed electrical stimulation
  (PES)
programmed ventricular stimulation
  (PVS)
programmer wand
programming
  bidirectional pacemaker
  over-responsive
  phantom pacemaker
  unidirectional pacemaker
  unresponsive
progression
  inexorable
  poor R wave (PRWP)
progressive angina
progressive anginal syndrome
progressive care unit (PCU)
progressive claudication
progressive coccidioidomycosis
progressive exercise intolerance
progressive hypercapnia
progressive interstitial pulmonary
  fibrosis
progressive intimal thickening
progressively severe fatigue
progressive malignant polyserositis
  with large effusions into pericardium, pleura, and peritoneum

progressive mitral regurgitation
progressive nodular pulmonary fibrosis
progressive parenchymal restriction
progressive pulmonary dystrophy
progressive respiratory distress
progressive shortness of breath
progressive systemic sclerosis
progressive weakness
projection (see also *position, view*)
  anterior
  fingerlike
  LAO (left anterior oblique)
  left lateral
  left posterior oblique
  RAO (right anterior oblique)
  right posterior oblique
  65° LAO
  steep left anterior oblique
  30° LAO
prolapse
  anterior leaflet
  holosystolic
  holosystolic mitral valve
  mitral
  mitral valve (MVP)
  mitral valve leaflet systolic
  posterior leaflet
  systolic
  tricuspid valve
prolapsed mitral valve leaflets
prolapsed tumor through mitral valve
  orifice
prolapsing scallop
prolapsing valve
Prolene suture
proliferating pleurisy
proliferation
  collagen tissue
  connective tissue
  endothelial
  intimal
  myxomatous

proliferative phlebitis
Prolith pacemaker
prolongation
  inspiratory
  QRS interval
  Q-T interval
  Q-T wave
  P-R
prolonged action
prolonged aortic clamping
prolonged bed rest
prolonged clotting time
prolonged ejection time
prolonged expiration
prolonged expiration during quiet
  breathing
prolonged expiratory phase
prolonged in duration
prolonged inspiratory phase
prolonged interval
prolonged left ventricular impulse
prolonged P-R interval
prolonged pulmonary eosinophilia
prolonged Q-T interval, acquired
prolonged Q-T interval syndrome
prolonged rub
prolonged shock
prolonged standing
prominence
  hilar
  mediastinal
prominence of aorta
prominent central pulmonary artery
prominent fourth heart sound
prominent neck pulsations
prominent S_3 (heart sound)
prominent septal lymphatics
prominent systolic venous impulses
prominent fourth heart sound
prominent pulsus paradoxus
prominent third heart sound
prominent U wave

prominent vascular pulsations
prominent ventricular diastolic gallop
prominent xiphoid process
promptly relieved by rest
propagated thrombus
propagation of thrombus
prophylactic antibiotics
prophylactic drug treatment
prophylactic effect
prophylactic implantation of
  pacemaker
prophylactic IVC filter
prophylactic measure
prophylactic pacing
prophylactic penicillin
prophylactic regimen
prophylaxis
  anticoagulant
  endocarditis
  low-dose heparin
  OKT3
  PCP (*Pneumocystis carinii*
    pneumonia)
  routine antimicrobial
  SBE (subacute bacterial
    endocarditis)
  topical antimicrobial
propria, lamina
prostaglandin infusion
prostaglandin synthesis inhibition
prostate carcinoma metastatic to heart
prosthesis (see also *valve*)
  aortic valve
  aortofemoral
  ball-and-cage valve
  ball-cage
  ball valve
  ball-valve type valve
  Baxter mechanical valve
  Beall disk valve
  Beall mitral valve
  bifurcated aortofemoral

prosthesis *(cont.)*
  bileaflet valve
  Bionit vascular
  bioprosthesis
  Björk-Shiley aortic valve
  Björk-Shiley convexo-concave
    60° valve
  Björk-Shiley floating disk
  Björk-Shiley mitral valve
  Björk-Shiley monostrut 72° valve
  Björk-Shiley valve
  bovine pericardial
  Braunwald-Cutter ball valve
  caged ball valve
  Capetown aortic prosthetic valve
  Carpentier annuloplasty ring
  Carpentier-Edwards valve
  collar
  convexo-concave valve
  Cooley Dacron
  Cross-Jones disk valve
  Cutter aortic valve
  Cutter-Smeloff cardiac valve
  DeBakey ball valve
  DeBakey valve
  DeBakey Vasculour
  Delrin frame of valve
  De Vega
  disk valve
  double velour knitted Dacron
  Duromedics aortic valve
  Duromedics heart valve
  femorofemoral crossover
  golf T-shaped polyvinyl
  Hall-Kaster mitral valve
  Hall-Kaster tilting-disk valve
  Hancock aortic valve
  Hancock M.O. II porcine bio-
  Hancock mitral valve
  Hancock porcine heart valve
  intraluminal sutureless
  intravascular

prosthesis *(cont.)*
  Ionescu-Shiley aortic valve
  Ivalon
  Kaster mitral valve
  Kay-Shiley disk valve
  Lillehei-Cruz-Kaster
  Lillehei-Kaster mitral valve
  Lillehei valve
  Lo-Por
  Lo-Por vascular graft
  Magovern ball valve
  Magovern-Cromie
  Meadox woven velour
  Medtronic-Hall heart valve
  Medtronic-Hall tilting-disk valve
  Microknit vascular graft
  Milliknit Dacron
  Milliknit vascular graft
  monostrut cardiac valve
  Neville tracheal and tracheo-
    bronchial
  Omnicarbon heart valve
  Omniscience cardiac prosthesis
  Omniscience heart valve
  Omniscience single leaflet cardiac
    valve
  Omniscience tilting-disk valve
  outflow tract
  polyvinyl
  porcine heterograft
  Rashkind double-disc occluder
  Sauvage filamentous
  Smeloff-Cutter ball valve
  Starr-Edwards
  Starr-Edwards aortic valve
  Starr-Edwards ball valve
  Starr-Edwards disk valve
  Starr-Edwards Silastic ball valve
  stentless porcine aortic valve
  St. Jude Medical aortic valve
  St. Jude Medical bileaflet tilting-
    disk aortic valve

prosthesis *(cont.)*
    Sutter-Smeloff heart valve
    tilting-disk aortic valve
    Toronto SPV bio-
    USCI Sauvage EXS side-limb
    velour collar
    Weavenit (and New Weavenit)
        Dacron prosthesis
    Wesolowski vascular prosthesis
    woven Teflon
prosthesis dehiscence
prosthetic heart valve
prosthetic heart valve poppet
prosthetic valve endocarditis (PVE)
prosthetic valve malfunction
prosthetic valve valvuloplasty
prostigmin and edrophonium chloride
    test (Tensilon)
protamine, heparin reversed with
protamine sulfate, heparin neutralized
    with
protection
    cardiac
    myocardial
protective HDL cholesterol
Protect Point needle
protein
    C-reactive
    guanine-nucleotide-binding
    guanine nucleotide regulatory
    SAA
    streptococcal M
    total
proteinaceous material
protein C deficiency
protein-losing enteropathy
proteinosis
    alveolar
    pulmonary alveolar
protein-rich material
protein S
protein troponin T

proteinuria
Proteus pneumonia
Proteus syndrome
prothrombin consumption test
prothrombin-proconvertin test
prothrombin time (PT)
pro time (PT, prothrombin time)
. protocol
    ACT (activated clotting time)
    advanced cardiac life support
        (ACLS)
    Balke treadmill stress test
    Balke-Ware exercise stress testing
    Balke-Ware treadmill exercise
    Bruce exercise stress testing
    Bruce treadmill exercise stress
    cardiac rehabilitation
    CCU (cardiac care unit)
    chronotropic assessment exercise
        (CAEP)
    Cornell exercise stress testing
    Ellestad treadmill exercise
    exercise
    Kattus treadmill exercise
    LITE (low-intensity treadmill
        exercise)
    Mayo exercise treadmill
    McHenry treadmill exercise
    Mee
    modified Balke treadmill exercise
    modified Bruce treadmill exercise
    modified treadmill
    Naughton-Balke treadmill
    Naughton treadmill exercise
    pacing
    Reeves treadmill exercise
    rule-out MI (myocardial infarction)
        (ROMI)
    Sheffield exercise test
    Sheffield modification of Bruce
        treadmill
    Sheffield treadmill exercise

protocol *(cont.)*
 slow USAFSAM treadmill exercise
 soft rule-out MI
 standard Bruce
 standard Bruce treadmill exercise
 Stanford treadmill exercise
 TIMI II (thrombolysis in myocardial infarction)
 USAFSAM treadmill exercise
 ventilatory muscle training
 Weber exercise stress testing
protodiastolic gallop rhythm
protodiastolic reversal of blood flow
proton density
proton MRI
proton spectroscopy
protopulmonary bilharziasis
prototype drug
prototypical holosystolic murmur
protozoal infestation
protozoal myocarditis
protozoa, tick-borne
protruding atheroma
protrusion, spoonlike (of leaflets)
protuberant abdomen
provocation (see *challenge*)
 aspirin inhalation
 HDM (house dust mites) bronchial
 methacholine bronchial
 oral aspirin
provocative
provocable ischemia
provoked by cold
provoked by dust
provoked by lying down
provoked by smoke
Prower factor X deficiency
proximal anastomosis
proximal and distal portion of vessel
proximal aortic endarterectomy
proximal circumflex artery
proximal clot

proximal coil
proximal coronary sinus (CS)
proximal hypertension
proximal popliteal artery
proximal segment
P-R interval
P-R prolongation
PR segment depression
Pruitt-Inahara balloon-tipped perfusion
 catheter
Pruitt-Inahara carotid shunt
prune juice sputum
pruned appearance of pulmonary
 vasculature
Prussian helmet sign
PRWP (poor R wave progression)
PRx, PRx II ICD
PS (pulmonary sequestration)
PS (pulmonic stenosis)
PSA (pacing system analyzer)
PSAP (peak systolic aortic pressure)
pseudo-Meigs syndrome
pseudoaneurysm, anastomotic
pseudoangina
pseudoclaudication syndrome
pseudocoarctation syndrome
pseudocolor B-mode display
pseudofusion beat
pseudohemophilia, hereditary
pseudohypertrophy of calves
pseudohypoaldosteronism
pseudoincisura
pseudoinfarction
pseudolupus secondary to
 procainamide
pseudomembranous croup
pseudomitral leaflet
Pseudomonas aeruginosa infection
Pseudomonas bronchiectasis
Pseudomonas cepacia
Pseudomonas maltophilia
Pseudomonas pneumonia

pseudoperfusion beats, ventricular
pseudostratified columnar epithelium
pseudotruncus arteriosus
pseudoxanthoma elasticum
pseudoxanthoma elasticum syndrome
P/S (pulmonic/systemic) flow ratio
PSG (peak systolic gradient)
psi, p.s.i. ("sigh") (pounds per square
    inch)
psittacosis
PSM (pansystolic murmur)
PSM (presystolic murmur)
P_2 sound, burying of
PSV (pressure support ventilation)
PSVT (paroxysmal supraventricular
    tachycardia)
PSVT, slow-fast intranodal
psychogenic chest pain syndrome
psychogenic purpura
psychophysiologic hyperventilation
psychosis
    cardiac
    postcardiotomy
psyllium
P synchronous pacing
PT (prothrombin time), prolonged
PTA (percutaneous transluminal
    angioplasty)
PTBD (percutaneous transluminal
    balloon dilatation)
PTC (plasma thromboplastin compo-
    nent)
PTCA (percutaneous transluminal
    coronary angioplasty)
PTCA catheter; catheterization
PTCA coronary angiogram
PTDC (percutaneous transcatheter
    ductal closure)
pterional incision
P terminal force abnormality
pterygoid chest
PTFE (polytetrafluoroethylene)

PTFE arterial graft material
PTFE graft
PTL (posterior tricuspid leaflet)
PTLD (posttransplantation lympho-
    proliferative disorder)
PTMC (percutaneous transvenous
    mitral commissurotomy)
ptosis and miosis (Horner syndrome)
P_{TP} (transpulmonary pressure)
    (mm Hg)
PT/PTT (prothrombin time/partial
    thromboplastin time)
PTT (partial thromboplastin time)
PTT (pulmonary transit time)
puerperium, hemodynamic changes
    during
puerperium myocardiopathy
puff of smoke (moyamoya)
puffer, pink
Puig Massana-Shiley annuloplasty ring
Puig Massana-Shiley annuloplasty
    valve
Pulec and Freedman classification of
    congenital aural atresia
pullback
    left heart
    pressure
pullback across the aortic valve
pullback arterial markings
pullback from ventricle
pullback pressure recording
pullback study
Pulmo-Aide
pulmoaortic canal
pulmogram
pulmolithiasis
pulmonale, cor
pulmonalis
    pleura
    plexus
    vesiculae
pulmonary abscess

pulmonary acid aspiration syndrome
pulmonary acini gigantism
pulmonary alveolar microlithiasis
pulmonary alveolar proteinosis
pulmonary alveolus (pl. alveoli)
pulmonary and cardiac sclerosis
pulmonary angiitis-granulomatosis
   syndrome
pulmonary angiogram, angiography
   digital subtraction
   balloon occlusion
pulmonary arterial circulation
pulmonary arterial hypertension
pulmonary arterial input impedance
pulmonary arterial markings
pulmonary arterial occlusion
pulmonary arterial pressure, increased
pulmonary arterial vent
pulmonary arterial wedge pressure
pulmonary arteries, intraacinar
pulmonary arteriolar vasoconstriction
pulmonary arteriosclerosis
pulmonary arteriovenous aneurysm
pulmonary arteriovenous fistula
pulmonary arteritis
pulmonary artery
   aberrant left
   anomalous
   dilated
pulmonary artery agenesis
pulmonary artery apoplexy
pulmonary artery banding procedure
pulmonary artery catheter-associated
   endocarditis
pulmonary artery catheter, balloon-
   tipped flow-directed
pulmonary artery catheter-related
   bacteremia
pulmonary artery catheter-related
   candidemia
pulmonary artery compression
   ascending aorta aneurysm

pulmonary artery debanding
pulmonary artery end-diastolic
   pressure (PAEDP)
pulmonary artery engorgement
pulmonary artery flotation
pulmonary artery hypertension
pulmonary artery hypoplasia
pulmonary artery incisura
pulmonary artery mycotic aneurysm
pulmonary artery obstruction-Manson
   schistosomiasis
pulmonary artery oxygen saturation
pulmonary artery plication
pulmonary artery pressure (PAP)
pulmonary artery stenosis, peripheral
pulmonary artery wedge pressure
   (PAWP)
pulmonary aspiration of gastric
   contents
pulmonary atresia
pulmonary auscultation
pulmonary autograft procedure
pulmonary AV O_2 difference
pulmonary banding
pulmonary barotrauma
pulmonary bed
pulmonary blood flow
pulmonary blood flow redistribution
pulmonary capillary endothelial cells
pulmonary capillary endothelium
pulmonary capillary hemangiomatosis
pulmonary capillary pressure (PCP)
pulmonary capillary wedge position
pulmonary capillary wedge pressure
   (PCWP)
pulmonary capillary wedge tracing
pulmonary carcinomatosis
pulmonary cartilage
pulmonary cavitation
pulmonary cavity
pulmonary circulation
pulmonary cirrhosis

pulmonary compliance, reduced
pulmonary compression by pleural
fluid or gas
pulmonary congestion
asymmetric
symmetric
pulmonary consolidation
pulmonary contusion
pulmonary cyanosis
pulmonary cystic lymphangiectasis
pulmonary dysfunction, residual
pulmonary dysmaturity
pulmonary edema
acute
cardiogenic
frank
fulminant
high-altitude
interstitial
negative image
neurogenic
noncardiac
noncardiogenic
permeability-type
postoperative
reexpansion
rotating tourniquets for
pulmonary ejection click (PEC)
pulmonary embolectomy
pulmonary embolism (PE)
pulmonary embolus (pl. emboli)
pulmonary emphysema
pulmonary eosinophilia
pulmonary eosinophilia with asthma
pulmonary eosinophilic infiltrates
pulmonary epithelial cells
pulmonary failure
pulmonary fibrosis (see *fibrosis*)
pulmonary fistula, congenital
pulmonary flotation catheter

pulmonary function abbreviations
CC (closing capacity)
C_{dyn} (dynamic lung compliance)
C_{STAT} (static lung compliance)
CV (closing volume)
DL_{CO} (diffusing capacity for
carbon monoxide)
ERV (expiratory reserve volume)
FEV_1 (forced expiratory volume
in 1 second)
FEV_3 (forced expiratory volume
in 3 seconds)
FRC (functional residual capacity)
FVC (forced vital capacity)
FEV_1/FVC ratio
IRV (inspiratory reserve volume)
$MEF_{50\% VC}$ (mid-expiratory flow
at 50% vital capacity)
$MIF_{50\% VC}$ (mid-inspiratory flow
at 50% vital capacity)
MMEF (mean maximal expiratory
flow)
MVV (maximal voluntary
ventilation)
$PaCO_2$ (arterial partial pressure of
CO_2)
PaO_2 (arterial partial pressure of
O_2)
PEF (peak expiratory flow)
P_{TP} (transpulmonary pressure)
Q (perfusion)
R_{AW} (airway resistance)
RV (residual volume)
TLC (total lung capacity)
V (lung volume)
V (ventilation)
V_A (alveolar ventilation)
VC (vital capacity)
VCO_2 (CO_2 production)
VO_2 (O_2 consumption)

pulmonary function tests (PFTs)
  determination of all lung volumes
  diffusing capacity
  flow-volume loop
  maximum inspiratory and
    expiratory pressures
  MVV (maximal voluntary
    ventilation)
  spirometry
pulmonary gangrene
pulmonary gas exchange
pulmonary hemorrhage
pulmonary hilus
pulmonary histiocytosis
pulmonary hypertension
  familial
  hypoxic
  secondary
pulmonary hypoperfusion
pulmonary hypoperfusion unmasked
  by ductus arteriosus closure
pulmonary idiopathic hemosiderosis
pulmonary incompetence
pulmonary infarct (see *infarct*)
pulmonary infarction (see *infarction*)
pulmonary infiltrate (see *infiltrate*)
pulmonary infiltrates, sulfasalazine-
  induced
pulmonary infiltrates with eosinophilia
  (PIE)
pulmonary infiltration eosinophilia
pulmonary insufficiency
pulmonary interstitial emphysema
  (PIE)
pulmonary interstitial idiopathic
  fibrosis
pulmonary Kaposi sarcoma
pulmonary ligament
pulmonary metastasectomy
pulmonary microcirculation
pulmonary microvasculature
pulmonary nodule, solitary

pulmonary obliterative arteriolitis
pulmonary orifice
pulmonary origin of the coronary
  artery, anomalous
pulmonary osteoarthropathy
pulmonary outflow obstruction
pulmonary outflow tract
pulmonary overdistention
pulmonary overexpansion
pulmonary parasites
pulmonary parenchyma
pulmonary parenchymal changes
pulmonary parenchymal disease
pulmonary parenchymal infiltrates
pulmonary parenchymal injury
pulmonary parenchymal window
pulmonary pleura
pulmonary pleurisy
pulmonary plexus
pulmonary rales
pulmonary rhonchi
pulmonary scars
pulmonary schistosomiasis
pulmonary secretions, amber-colored
pulmonary sequestration (PS)
pulmonary sling syndrome
pulmonary sounds in Warthin sign
pulmonary stenosis
pulmonary stenosis-ostium secundum
  defect syndrome
pulmonary stenosis-patent foramen
  ovale syndrome
pulmonary strongyloidiasis
pulmonary suppuration
pulmonary surfactant
pulmonary/systemic flow ratio
pulmonary TB (tuberculosis)
pulmonary thromboembolism (PTE)
pulmonary thrombosis
pulmonary tissue
pulmonary toilet, aggressive
pulmonary toxicity

pulmonary tractotomy
pulmonary trunk
pulmonary trunk idiopathic dilatation
pulmonary trunk murmur
pulmonary tuberculosis (TB)
pulmonary valve
pulmonary valve annulus
pulmonary valve atresia
pulmonary valve atresia-intact
ventricular septum syndrome
pulmonary valve closure
pulmonary valve deformity
pulmonary valve dysplasia
pulmonary valve insufficiency
pulmonary valve stenosis
pulmonary valve stenosis dilation
pulmonary valvular stenosis
pulmonary vascular bed
pulmonary vascular bed impedance
pulmonary vascular disease
pulmonary vascular disease, Heath-
Edwards classification of
pulmonary vascular markings
pulmonary vascular obstruction
pulmonary vascular pattern
pulmonary vascular redistribution
pulmonary vascular reserve
pulmonary vascular resistance (PVR)
increased
Wood units of
pulmonary vascular resistance index
(PVRI)
pulmonary vasculature
pulmonary vasoconstriction, hypoxic
pulmonary vasoreactivity
pulmonary vein apoplexy
pulmonary vein atresia
pulmonary vein, congenital stenosis of
pulmonary vein fibrosis
pulmonary vein stenosis
pulmonary vein wedge angiography
pulmonary veno-occlusive disease

pulmonary venous anomalous
drainage to hepatic vein
pulmonary venous anomalous
drainage mitral stenosis syndrome
pulmonary venous anomalous
drainage to right atrium
pulmonary venous congestion
pulmonary venous connection
partial anomalous
total anomalous
pulmonary venous drainage
pulmonary venous hypertension
pulmonary venous obstruction
pulmonary venous return
pulmonary venous system
pulmonary venous wedge pressure
pulmonary venous-systemic air emboli
pulmonary ventilation
pulmonary vesicles
pulmonary vessels
pulmonary wedge angiography
pulmonary wedge pressure (PWP)
pulmonary wedge elevated
pulmonary wedge resection
pulmonic atresia
pulmonic atresia with intact ventricular
septum
pulmonic component, markedly accentuated
pulmonic component of murmur
pulmonic ejection sound, palpable
pulmonic regurgitation
pulmonic stenosis, peripheral
pulmonic stenosis-ventricular septal
defect
pulmonic stenosis with intact
ventricular septum
pulmonic systolic murmur
pulmonic valve
pulmonic valve dysplasia
pulmonic valve stenosis
pulmonis (also pulmonum), alveoli

Pulmosonic nebulizer
Pulsar NI pacemaker
pulsatile abdominal mass
pulsatile assist device (PAD)
pulsatile cutaneous vascular anomaly
pulsatile flow, dampened
pulsatile mass
pulsatile perfusion
pulsatile tinnitus
pulsatility index (PI)
pulsating empyema
pulsating hepatomegaly
pulsating pain
pulsating pleurisy
pulsating vein
pulsation, pulsations
  capillary
  carotid arterial
  cervical vein
  discrete
  expansile
  hepatic vein
  jugular venous
  large vein
  left ventricular
  lower sternal
  mean venous
  palpable systolic
  precordial
  presystolic
  prominent neck
  prominent vascular
  suprasternal
  transient ectopic
  transmitted carotid artery
  venous (3 cm above the sternal
    angle)
pulsation balloon
pulse, pulses (see also *beat, impulse*)
  abdominal
  abrupt
  absence of

pulse *(cont.)*
  absent
  allorhythmic
  alternating
  anacrotic
  anadicrotic
  anatricotic
  a peak of jugular venous
  apex
  apical
  arterial
  atrial liver
  atrial venous
  atriovenous
  biferious
  bifid arterial
  bigeminal
  bilaterally symmetric
  bisferiens
  bisferious
  bounding arterial
  bounding peripheral
  bounding water-hammer
  brachial
  brisk bifid arterial
  cannon ball
  capillary
  cardiac
  cardiac apex
  carotid
  carotid arterial (CAR)
  catadicrotic
  catatricotic
  centripetal venous
  chaotic
  character of
  collapsing
  Corrigan
  coupled
  C point of cardiac apex
  c wave of jugular venous
  dampened obstructive

pulse *(cont.)*
    delayed femoral
    diastolic collapse of venous
    dicrotic
    dicrotic arterial
    diminished pedal
    diminution of
    distal
    Doppler
    dorsalis pedis
    dorsal pedal
    dropped-beat
    easily palpable
    elastic
    entirely chaotic
    entoptic
    equal
    external carotid
    femoral
    filiform
    formicant
    frequent
    full
    full and equal
    h peak of jugular venous
    hard
    high-tension
    incisura of
    infrequent
    intermittent
    irregular
    irregular but patterned
    irregularly irregular
    jerky
    jugular
    jugular venous
    Kussmaul paradoxical
    labile
    low-tension
    lower extremity
    Monneret
    monocrotic

pulse *(cont.)*
    movable
    nonpalpable
    palpable palmar
    palpable peripheral
    palpable popliteal
    paradoxic
    paradoxical
    parvus
    pedal
    peripheral
    pistol-shot femoral
    pistol-shot radial
    plateau-type
    polycrotic
    popliteal
    posterior tibial
    pressure
    prominent systolic venous
    quadrigeminal
    quick
    Quincke
    Quincke capillary
    radial
    rapid
    reduced
    regular
    regularly irregular
    resting
    retrosternal
    RF
    Riegel
    running
    sharp
    short
    slow
    small water-hammer
    soft
    spike-and-dome
    strong
    symmetric
    synchronous carotid arterial

pulse *(cont.)*
  tardus
  tense
  thready
  tidal wave
  tremulous
  tricrotic
  trigeminal
  trip-hammer
  trough of venous
  ulnar
  undulating
  unequal
  unilateral loss of
  vagus
  venous
  vermicular
  vibrating
  v peak of jugular venous
  water-hammer
  weak peripheral
  wide
  wiry
  x depression of jugular venous
  x descent of jugular venous
  y descent of jugular venous
pulse amplitude
pulse character
pulse count increment
pulse deficit
pulse Doppler interrogation
pulsed Doppler transesophageal
  echocardiography
pulsed Doppler ultrasound
pulsed infrared laser
pulsed laser ablation
pulse duration
pulsed volume recorder (PVR) testing
pulsed-wave Doppler recording
pulse generator of pacemaker (see
  generator)
pulse generator pocket erosion

pulseless bradycardia
pulseless disease
pulseless electrical activity
pulselessness
pulseless syndrome
pulse oximeter
pulse oximetry devices
pulse pressure
pulse rate, baseline standing
pulse reappearance time
pulses altered by changes in position
pulse voltage
pulse volume recording (PVR)
pulse wave
pulse width
pulsus alternans
pulsus bigeminus
pulsus bisferiens (or biferiens)
  (biferious pulse)
pulsus bisferiens
pulsus celer
pulsus paradoxus, prominent
pulsus parvus
pulsus parvus et tardus
pulsus tardus
pulverization
pulverized plaque particulate matter
pump
  angle port
  balloon
  Bard cardiopulmonary support
  BioMedicus
  blood
  BVS (biventricular support) system
  calcium
  cardiac balloon
  Cormed
  Datascope System 90 balloon
  Emerson
  intra-aortic balloon (IABP)
  ion
  Kangaroo

pump *(cont.)*
  muscular venous
  Novacore
  priming of the
  pulmonary artery balloon (PABP)
  push-pull
  sodium
  stroke volume
  sump
  Thoratec
  Travenol
  Travenol infusion
  volumetric infusion
pump failure, Cedars-Sinai classification of
pumping capacity of heart
pumping of the ventricles
pumping, postcardiotomy intra-aortic balloon
pump lung syndrome
pump oxygenator
pump perfusionist
pump reserve
pump standby
pump support
pump technician
punch
  aortic
  circular
  Goosen vascular
  Hancock aortic
  Karp aortic
  Medtronic aortic
  Sweet sternal
puncture
  arterial
  blind percutaneous (of subclavian vein)
  groin
  iatrogenic
  percutaneous
  transseptal

puncture *(cont.)*
  venous
  ventricular
pupillary constriction
pupils, Argyll Robertson
pure pressure loads
Puritan-Bennett ventilator
Purkinje arborization
Purkinje cells
Purkinje cell tumor
Purkinje fibers
Purkinje network
Purmann method
purple toes syndrome
purpura
  Henoch-Schönlein
  posttransfusion
  Schönlein-Henoch
  thrombotic thrombocytopenic
pursed-lip breathing
purse-stringing effect
purse-string suture
purulent bronchitis
purulent endocarditis
purulent exudate in pleural cavity
purulent pericardial exudate
purulent pericarditis
purulent pleurisy
purulent sputum
push-pull pump syndrome
pus in pleural cavity
putrid empyema
putrid odor
putrid sputum
PV (pulmonic valve)
PVARP (postventricular atrial refractory period)
PVB (premature ventricular beat)
PVC (premature ventricular contraction)
  bigeminal
  early-cycle

PVC *(cont.)*
  monomorphic
  multifocal
  multiform
  paired
  unifocal
  PVCs in a bigeminal pattern
PVD (peripheral vascular disease)
PVE (prosthetic valve endocarditis)
P vector
PVER (paced ventricular evoked
  response)
PvO_2 (venous oxygen tension)
PVOD (pulmonary veno-occlusive
  disease)
PVR (peripheral vascular resistance)
PVR (pulmonary vascular resistance)
PVR (pulse volume recorder)
PVRI (pulmonary vascular resistance
  index)
PVS (programmed ventricular
  stimulation
PW (posterior wall)
PW (pulse width)
P wave
  bifid
  biphasic
  broadened
  depressed
  diphasic
  flattened
  inverted

P wave *(cont.)*
  low-amplitude
  nonconducted
  notched
  peaked
  pointed
  retrograde
  tall
  terminal negativity of
  upright
  widened
P wave amplitude
PWT (posterior wall thickness)
pyelography, excretory intravenous
pyknic
pyogenic bacteria
pyopericardium pericarditis
pyopneumothorax
pyothorax
PYP (pyrophosphate) myocardial scan
pyramidal hemorrhagic zone
pyramid method for ventricular
  volume
pyridine sulfonylurea class of drugs
pyridoxilated stroma-free hemoglobin
  (SFHb)
pyriform (piriform) sinus
pyrogen reaction
pyroglycolic acid sutures
pyrophosphate (PYP) myocardial scan
pyrosis (heartburn)

Q, q

Q (cardiac ouput)
Q (perfusion)
QCA (quantitative coronary arteriography)
Q-cath catheterization recording system
QEEG (quantitative electro-encephalography)
Q fever endocarditis
Q-H interval of jugular venous pulse
QO_2 (oxygen consumption)
QOL (quality of life) index
Q Port
QR pattern
QRS complex (see also *complex*)
  fusion
  narrow
  normal
  normal voltage
  preexcited
  slurring of
  wide
QRS complex duration
QRS duration
QRS interval
QRS loop, counterclockwise superiorly oriented frontal

QRS score
QRS synchronized shock
QRS-T angle, wide
QRS-T complex
QRS-T interval
QRS vector
QRS vertical axis
QS complex
QS deflection
Q-Stress treadmill
QS wave
QS_2 (total electromechanical systole on phonocardiogram)
QS_1, QS_2 interval
Q-T_c interval (corrected QT interval)
Q-T interval prolongation
Q-T interval sensing pacemaker
Q-T prolongation
Q-T syndrome, long
Q-U interval
quadrangulation of Frouin
quadrigeminy
quadripolar catheter
quadripolar electrode catheter
quadripolar steerable electrode catheter
quadruple rhythm

Quaegebeur modification of Carpentier
  repair
Quain fatty degeneration of the heart
Quain fatty heart
quality of A_2, tambour
quality of breath sounds
quality of life (QOL) index
Quanticor catheter
quantification
quantify
quantitation of ischemic muscle
quantitative analysis
quantitative coronary arteriography
quantitative electroencephalography)
  QEEG
Quantum pacemaker
quasitransmural endocardial incision
Quénu-Muret sign
Quick method
Quick one-stage prothrombin time test
Quick test
quiescent heart, electromechanically
Quik-Prep, Quinton
Quincke angioedema disease

Quincke capillary pulsations
Quincke disease
Quincke edema
Quincke pulse
Quincke sign
quinolone antibiotics
quinolones
quinsy
Quinton catheter
Quinton computerized exercise EKG
  system
Quinton electrode
Quinton PermCath
Quinton Quik-Prep
Quinton-Scribner shunt
Quinton vascular access port
Q wave
  large
  left precordial
  nondiagnostic
  pathologic
  septal
Q wave infarctions
Q wave in the right precordial leads

R, r

Raaf Cath (vascular catheter)
RAAPI (resting ankle-arm pressure
index)
RACAT (rapid acquisition computed
axial tomography)
racemaker (runaway artificial
pacemaker)
rachitic rosary
racing of heart
RAD (reactive airways disease)
RAD (reversible airways disease)
RAD (right axis deviation)
radial artery catheter
radial artery graft
radial artery to cephalic vein
anastomosis
radial artery to cephalic vein fistula
radial pulse
radial vascular thermal injury
radiate ligament
radiating chest pain
radiating to axilla
radiating to the clavicle
radiation fibrosis
radiation-induced pericarditis
radiation nephritis
radiation pericardial disease

radiation pneumonitis
radiation toxicity syndrome
radical, hydroxyl
radicular arteries
radicularis anterior magna, arteria
radicularis magna
radiculitis, cervical
radio frequency (rf) field
radioactive aerosol
radioactive fibrinogen scan
radioactive labeling
radioactive string markers
radioactive xenon gas inhalation
radioactivity in lungs
radioenzymatic technique
Radiofocus Glidewire
radiofrequency ablation (RFA)
transaortic
transseptal
radiofrequency ablation therapy
radiofrequency catheter ablation
(RFCA, RCA)
radiofrequency energy
radiofrequency modification,
transcatheter
radiographic control
radiographic pincushion distortion

radioimmunoassay (RIA)
radioisotope (see *contrast medium*)
radioisotope lung scan
radiolabeled fibrinogen
radiolucent foci
radionuclear venography
radionuclide angiocardiography,
  equilibrium
radionuclide angiogram (RNA)
radionuclide cineangiography
radionuclide gated blood pool scanning
radionuclide ventriculography, bicycle
  exercise
radiopaque wire of counteroccluder
  buttonhole
radiotracer
RAE (right atrial enlargement)
Raeder-Arbitz syndrome
ragpicker's disease
railroad track sign
rake retractor
rale, rales
  amphoric
  atelectatic
  basilar
  bibasilar
  border
  bronchial
  bubbling
  cavernous
  cellophane
  clicking
  coarse
  collapse
  consonating
  crackling
  crepitant
  diffuse
  diffuse inspiratory crepitant
  dry
  expiratory

rale *(cont.)*
  extrathoracic
  fine
  fine crepitant
  guttural
  gurgling
  hollow
  inspiratory
  laryngeal
  marginal
  metallic
  mucous
  musical
  moist
  pleural
  post-tussive
  pulmonary
  sibilant
  sonorous
  sticky
  subcrepitant
  tinkling
  tracheal
  Velcro
  vesicular
  wet
  whistling
rale de retour (rattle of return)
rale indux (crepitant rale)
rale muqueux (subcrepitant sound)
rale redux (subcrepitant sound)
rales clear with coughing
rales clear with deep breathing
rales, rhonchi, or wheezes
rales, wheezes, rhonchi, or rubs
Raman spectroscopy
ramp atrial pacing
ramp decrement
ramping
ramp overdrive pacing
ramp pacing

ramp technique of atrial pacing
ramus branch
ramus intermedius artery branch
ramus medialis branch
ramus medianus
Randall stone forceps for thrombo-
    endarterectomy
Rand microballoon
R and S wave pattern over precordium,
    reversal of
Raney clamp
range, therapeutic (of drug)
RAO (right anterior oblique)
RAO position for cardiac catheteriza-
    tion
RAO view on cardiac catheterization
RA (right atrium) oxygen saturation
RAP (right atrial pressure)
raphe
rapid atrial pacing
rapid breathing
rapid deceleration injury
rapid early repolarization phase
rapid filling phase
rapid filling wave
rapid fluid expansion
rapid heartbeat
rapid inspiratory flow rates
rapid oscillatory motion
rapid pulse
rapid repolarization phase
rapid respirations
rapid respiratory rate
rapid sequence intravenous pyelogram
    (IVP)
rapid shallow breathing
rapid thoracic compression technique
rapid ventricular rate
rapid ventricular response
RA (right atrial) pressure
RAS (rotational atherectomy system)

Rashkind atrial septostomy
Rashkind balloon atrial septostomy
Rashkind balloon atrial septotomy
Rashkind blade septostomy
Rashkind cardiac device
Rashkind double-disc occluder
Rashkind double umbrella device
Rashkind-Miller atrial septostomy
Rashkind occluder
Rashkind septostomy balloon catheter
Rasmussen mycotic aneurysm
rasp (raspatory)
    Alexander-Faraheuf rib
    Doyen rib
    Haight
rasping bruit
rasping cough
rasping sound
raspy
RAST (radioallergosorbent) test
Rastan-Konno procedure
Rastelli atrioventricular canal defect
    (type A, B, or C)
Rastelli operation for correction of
    large ventricular septal defects
rate
    aldosterone secretion
    atrial (AR)
    auricular
    basic
    circulation
    echo intensity disappearance
    erythrocyte sedimentation (ESR)
    exercise-induced heart
    glomerular filtration
    heart (HR)
    intrinsic heart
    KVO (keep vein open)
    left ventricular filling
    magnet
    maximal heart

rate *(cont.)*
    maximum predicted heart (MPHR)
    peak exercise heart
    peak expiratory flow (PEFR)
    peak filling (PFR)
    percent of predicted
    predetermined heart
    predicted maximum heart
    pulse
    rapid respiratory
    rapid ventricular
    reduced glomerular filtration
    respiratory
    resting heart
    sed (sedimentation)
    sinus
    slew (SR)
    standby
    stroke ejection
    systolic ejection (SER)
    target heart
    time-to-peak filling (TPFR)
    variable response
    ventricular
    washout
    Westergren sedimentation
rate-adaptive pacemaker
rate and incline of treadmill
rate and rhythm of heartbeat
rate and rhythm, regular (RRR)
rated capacity of cardiac pump
rate hysteresis
rate limit
rate-modulated pacemaker
rate-responsive pacemaker, permanent
rate-sensing lead
RATG (rabbit antithymocyte globulin)
rating of perceived exertion (RPE)
ratio
    a/A
    AH:HA

ratio *(cont.)*
    AO:AC (aortic valve opening to
        aortic valve closing)
    aortic root
    cardiothoracic (CTR)
    CK:AST
    conduction (number of P waves to
        number of QRS)
    E:A (on echocardiography)
    ESP-ESV
    ESWI-ESVI (end-systolic wall
        stress index to end-systolic
        volume)
    FEV_1–FVC; FEV_1 to FVC
    I–E (inspiration to expiration)
    I–E (inspiratory to expiratory)
    inverse inspiratory–expiratory time
    LA–AR (left atrium/aortic root)
    left ventricular systolic time
        interval
    maximum diameter to minimum
        diameter
    mean total cholesterol to HDL
    orifice-to-annulus
    P–S flow (pulmonic–systemic)
    P:QRS
    PASP–SASP (pulmonary to sys-
        temic arterial systolic pressure)
    pulmonary–systemic blood flow
    pulmonary to systemic flow
    R/S amplitude
    R/S wave
    risk–benefit
    RV6:RV5 voltage
    RVP–LVP (right ventricular to left
        ventricular systolic pressure)
    septal to free wall
    T–D (thickness to diameter of
        ventricle)
    VLDL-TG to HDL-C
rattle, death

rattling bruit
rattling cough
rattling sound
Rauchfuss triangle
rauwolfia derivative
R$_{AW}$ (airway resistance)
raw irritated throat
rawness in chest
Raynaud disease
Raynaud gangrene
Raynaud phenomenon
Raynaud syndrome
Ray-Tec x-ray detectable sponge
RBBB (right bundle branch block)
RBC (red blood cell) count
RBC indices
   MCH (mean corpuscular
     hemoglobin)
   MCHC (mean corpuscular
     hemoglobin concentration)
   MCV (mean corpuscular volume)
RBC, technetium-99m-labeled
RCA (right coronary artery)
RCA (rotational coronary
   atherectomy)
RCM (restricted cardiomyopathy)
RDS (respiratory distress syndrome)
RDW (red cell diameter width)
reabsorbable suture
reaccumulation
reaction (see also *effect, phenomenon,*
   test)
   allergen-induced bronchial
   allergic
   allograft
   anaphylactic
   anaphylactoid
   atopic
   cell-mediated
   cytotoxic
   delayed

reaction *(cont.)*
   Eisenmenger
   foreign body
   granulomatous
   homograft
   hypersensitivity
   immune-complex-mediated
   inflammatory
   inflammatory granulomatous
   Jaffé rate
   Koch
   Liebermann-Burchard
   pneumococcus capsule swelling
   pyrogen
   tuberculin
   vagal
reaction recovery time
reactive airways disease (RAD)
reactive airways dysfunction syndrome
reactive arterioles
reactive disease of smooth muscle
reactive hyperemia
reactivity, bronchial
Reader paratrigeminal syndrome
Real coronary artery scissors
real-time chirp Z transformer
real-time Color Flow Doppler imaging of blood flow
real-time images
real-time 2-D Doppler flow-imaging
real-time ultrasonography
ream out (verb)
rebound, heparin
rebreather, partial
rebreathing mask
recalcitrant
recanalization
   argon laser
   laser
   percutaneous transluminal coronary
   peripheral laser (PLR)

recanalization technique
recanalized artery
recanalized ductus
recanalizing
receptor
  adrenergic
  airway epithelial irritant
  alpha
  alpha-adrenergic
  $alpha_1$-adrenergic
  beta
  beta-adrenergic
  $beta_1$-adrenergic
  $beta_2$-adrenergic
  decreased beta-adrenergic
  juxtacapillary
  LDL
  small airways stretch
recessed balloon septostomy catheter
recession of eyeball
recession, rib
recipient (noun)
recipient heart
reciprocal changes
reciprocal depression of ST segments
reciprocating atrioventricular
  tachycardia
reciprocating conduction
reciprocating permanent atrioventricular junctional tachycardia
reciprocating rhythm
reciprocating tachycardia
recirculation
recoarctation of the aorta
recognizable trigger
recoil
  arterial
  catheter
  elastic
recoil pressure
recombinant hemoglobin (rHbl.l)

reconstitution of blood flow in artery
reconstitution via a profunda
reconstitution via collaterals
reconstruction
  aortic
  Dor
  gated 3-D
  patch graft
  respiration gated 3-D
  three-dimensional
  transannular patch
reconstruction of aorta
recording
  color Doppler
  continuous-wave Doppler
  pullback pressure
  pulsed-wave Doppler
  simultaneous
recording electrode
recovery of donor organs for transplantation
recovery period of myocardium
recovery time
  corrected sinus node
  sinus node
recovery, uneventful
recrudescence
recrudescent toxoplasmosis
recruitment
recruitment potential
rectus muscle split longitudinally
rectus sheath incised
rectus sheath pocket
recumbency
recumbent
recurrent bronchiectasis
recurrent cardiac arrest
recurrent ductus
recurrent episodes
recurrent intractable ventricular tachycardia

recurrent laryngeal nerve
recurrent, not-so-sudden cardiac death
recurrent pulmonary embolism
recurrent respiratory infections (RRI)
recurring ectopic beats
red-cedar asthma
red cell aplasia
red cell diameter width (RDW)
reddish brown sputum
red hepatization of lung
Redifocus guide wire
RediFurl TaperSeal IAB catheter
redirection of inferior vena cava
redistributed thallium scan
redistribution
    flow
    pulmonary blood flow
    pulmonary vascular
redistribution myocardial image
redistribution of pulmonary vascular
    blood flow
red-streaked sputum
red tissues
reduced alveolar ventilation
reduced breath sounds
reduced cardiac output
reduced circulation
reduced compliance of chamber
reduced diffusing capacity
reduced exercise tolerance
reduced glomerular filtration rate
reduced peripheral pulses
reduced plasma volume
reduced pulmonary compliance
reduced stroke volume
reduced systemic cardiac output
reduction, afterload
reduction in thoracic volume
reduction of blood viscosity
redundant aortic leaflets
redundant carotid artery

redundant chordae tendineae
redundant mitral valve leaflets
redundant scallop of posterior annulus
Reed annuloplasty technique
Reed ventriculorrhaphy
re-endothelialization
reentrant circuit
reentrant loop
reentrant rhythm
reentrant supraventricular tachycardia
reentrant tachycardia
reentry
    anisotropic
    atrial
    atrioventricular (AV) nodal
    Bachmann bundle
    bundle branch (BBR)
    functional
    intra-atrial
    SA nodal
    sinus nodal
reentry circuit
Reeves treadmill exercise protocol
reexpansion of lung
reexpansion pulmonary edema
referred pain
REFI (regional ejection fraction
    image)
refill, capillary
reflectant
reflection
    epicardial
    pericardial (on x-ray)
reflectivity, high
reflex (see also *phenomenon*, *sign*)
    abdominocardiac
    Abrams heart
    Aschner
    atriopressor
    Bainbridge
    baroreceptor

reflex *(cont.)*
  Bezold-Jarisch
  bregmocardiac
  carotid sinus
  Churchill-Cope
  conditioned
  coronary
  Cushing
  deep tendon (DTR)
  diving
  Erben
  heart
  hepatojugular
  Hering-Breuer
  hyperactive carotid sinus
  inverted oculocardiac
  Livierato
  Lovén
  McDowall oculovagal
  oculocardiac
  psychocardiac
  pulmonocoronary
  vagal
  vascular
  vasopressor
  viscerocardiac
reflex cough
reflex syncope
Reflotron bedside theophylline test
reflux
  abdominojugular
  acid
  hepatojugular
reflux esophagitis
refractoriness, ventricular
refractory angina
refractory asthma
refractory congestive heart failure
refractory heart failure
refractory hypertension
refractory hypoxemia

refractory period of myocardium
  (see also *period*)
  effective
  functional
  relative
refractory to medical therapy
refractory to treatment
refractory ventricular fibrillation
refractory ventricular tachycardia
Reg. (regurgitation)
regimen
  antirejection
  desensitizing
  exercise
  prophylactic
  stepped-care antihypertensive
region
  aortic annular
  dark
  perihilar
regional compliance
regional ejection fraction image
  (REFI)
regional left ventricular function
regional myocardial uptake of thallium
regional perfusion by mixed venous
  blood
regional venous hypertension
regional ventricular function
regional wall motion abnormality,
  left ventricular
regional wall motion assessment
Regional Organ Procurement Agency
  (ROPA)
regression
  multiple logistic
  plaque
  spontaneous
  univariate logistic
regular irregularity
regular rate and rhythm

regular rate and rhythm without gallop
  or rub
regular sinus rhythm (RSR)
regulation
  defective volume
  volume
regurgitant CV waves
regurgitant flow
regurgitant jet
regurgitant lesion
regurgitant mitral valve murmur
regurgitant murmur
regurgitant orifice
regurgitant orifice area (ROA)
regurgitant pandiastolic flow
regurgitant pocket
regurgitant stream
regurgitant velocity
regurgitant volume
regurgitation (Reg.)
  aortic (AR)
  aortic valve
  congenital
  congenital aortic
  congenital mitral (CMR)
  Dexter-Grossman classification of
  mitral
  Grossman scale for
  ischemically mediated mitral
  massive aortic
  mitral valve
  pansystolic mitral
  paravalvular
  physiologic
  pulmonary
  pulmonic (PR)
  pulmonic valve
  silent
  transient tricuspid (of infancy)
  tricuspid (TR)
  tricuspid orifice

regurgitation *(cont.)*
  tricuspid valve
  trivial mitral
  valvular (VR)
regurgitation of sour fluid
rehabilitation, cardiac
rehabilitation exercises
Rehbein rib spreader
Rehfuss tube
rehydrated
Reichek method of calculating end-
  systolic wall stress
Reilly bodies
reimplantation, coronary ostial
reimplantation technique
reinfarction
reinforced second sound
Reinhoff clamp
Reinhoff-Finochietto rib spreader
reintimalization
Reiter disease
rejection
  borderline severe
  chronic
  chronic humoral
  focal moderate
  hyperacute
  low moderate
  resolved
  resolving
  severe acute
rejection crisis
relapse
relapsing polychondritis
relation
  end-diastolic pressure-volume
  end-systolic pressure-volume
  force-frequency
  force-length
  force-velocity
  Frank-Starling (of the heart)

relationship
  anecdotal
  Frank-Starling
relative hypoxia
relative refractory period (RRP)
relative shunt flow
relaxation
  isovolumic (IVR)
  period of isovolumic
relaxation time (in MRI scan)
  T1
  T2
relaxing factor, endothelium-derived
Relay pacemaker
release, Valsalva
relieved by antacids
relieved by rest, angina
remission
  clinical
  spontaneous
remnant
  ductal
  heart
remodeling of thrombus
remote history
removable Herbst appliance
renal arteriography
renal artery aneurysm
renal artery occlusion
renal atrophy
renal cholesterol embolization
  syndrome
renal cocktail
renal cortex, patchy atrophy of
renal duplex scan
renal dyspnea
renal failure
  chronic
  postoperative
renal function impairment
renal hemangiopericytoma
renal hypertension

renal parenchymal disease
renal sclerosis
renal shutdown
renal thromboendarterectomy,
  transaortic
renal vasculitis
renal vein renin, differential
renal vein thrombosis
Rendu-Osler-Weber disease or syndrome (also *Weber-Osler-Rendu*)
renin
  circulating
  differential renal vein
  plasma
renin activity, suppressed plasma
renin-angiotensin system
renin-dependent hypertension
renin levels, serum
renin-secreting tumor
renin suppression
renovascular disease
renovascular hypertension
Rentrop infusion catheter
reocclusion, postthrombolytic coronary
repair (see also *operation*)
  aortic valve (AV)
  Barbero-Marcial
  Brom
  Fontan
  hemitruncus
  infrarenal aortic
  intraventricular tunnel
  Takeuchi
  Trusler
  tunnel
repeated bouts of coughing
repeated sneezing
reperfuse
reperfusion
  controlled aortic root
  coronary
  normokalemic

reperfusion in acute myocardial
   infarction
reperfusion injury of postischemic
   lungs
reperfusion therapy
repetition time (TR)
repetitive maximal inspiratory maneuvers against closed shutter
repetitive monomorphic ventricular
   tachycardia
repetitive sneezing
replacement
   aortic root
   aortic valve (AVR)
   ascending aneurysm
   mitral valve (MVR)
   orthotopic total heart
repletion
repolarization
   atrial
   early
   early rapid
   final rapid
   transient
   ventricular
repolarization phase, rapid early
reproducible pain
rescue defibrillation
rescue shock
resectability
resection (see also *operation*)
   aneurysm
   endocardial
   endocardial-to-epicardial
   infundibular
   lung
   selective subendocardial
   subaortic
   Todaro tendon
   transmural
   video-assisted thoracoscopic

resection *(cont.)*
   wedge (of lung)
   wedge-shaped sleeve aneurysm
reserve
   cardiac
   contractile
   coronary flow (CFR)
   diastolic
   left ventricular systolic functional
   myocardial perfusion (MPR)
   preload
   pulmonary vascular
   pump
   regional contractile
   stenotic flow (SFR)
   systolic
   ventricular
reserve force
reserve mechanism, heart rate
reservoir
   cardiotomy
   peripheral venous
residua
residual deficit, significant
residual gradient
residual plaque
residual pulmonary dysfunction
residual volume (RV)
residual volume/total lung capacity
   (RV/TLC)
resilient artery
reinfection tuberculosis
resistance
   airway (R_{AW})
   arteriolar
   calculated
   coronary vascular
   decreased peripheral vascular
   decreased systemic
   expiratory
   fixed pulmonary valvular

resistance *(cont.)*
  increased airways
  increased cerebral vascular
  increased outflow
  increased peripheral
  increased pulmonary vascular
  index of runoff
  lead
  multidrug
  multiple drug
  nasal airway
  peripheral
  peripheral vascular (PVR)
  pulmonary
  pulmonary arteriolar
  pulmonary vascular (PVR)
  systemic
  systemic vascular (SVR)
  total peripheral (TPR)
  total pulmonary (TPR)
  vascular
  vascular systemic
  Wood units index of
resistive breathing through fixed
  orifice
resistivity
resolution stage
resolved (or resolving) rejection
resonance
  bandbox
  cough
  cracked-pot
  skodaic
  tympanic
  vesicular
  vesiculotympanic
  vocal
  whispering
  wooden
resonant frequency
resonant percussion note

resorption, fluid
resorption of dependent edema fluid
respiration
  abdominal
  absent
  accelerated
  accessory muscles of
  amphoric
  artificial
  asthmoid
  Austin Flint
  Biot
  Bouchut
  bronchial
  bronchocavernous
  bronchovesicular
  cavernous
  cerebral
  Cheyne-Stokes
  cogwheel
  collateral
  controlled diaphragmatic
  Corrigan
  costal
  deep
  diaphragmatic
  divided
  electrophrenic (EPR)
  forced
  gasping
  granular
  grunting
  harsh
  Holger Nielsen artificial
  indefinite
  inhibited
  interrupted
  jerky
  Kussmaul
  Kussmaul-Kien
  labored

respiration *(cont.)*
  meningitic
  metamorphosing
  mouth-to-mouth
  nervous
  paradoxical
  periodic
  puerile
  rapid
  rude
  Schafer artificial
  Seitz metamorphosing
  shallow
  Silvester artificial
  slow
  splinting
  stertorous
  supplementary
  suppressed
  thoracic
  transitional
  tubular
  unlabored
  vesiculocavernous
  vicarious
  wavy
  wheezing
  whistling
respiration gated three-dimensional
  reconstruction
respirations per minute
respirator (see *ventilator*)
  BABYbird
  Better Breathing HEPA-tech half-
    mask
  Bird
  cabinet
  cuirass
  Engström
  tank
  volume

respiratory acidosis
respiratory alkalosis
respiratory arrest
respiratory assist, mechanical
respiratory bronchiole
respiratory complications
respiratory compromise
respiratory decompensation
respiratory-dependent pacemaker
respiratory depression and apnea from
  drug overdose
respiratory distress at rest
respiratory distress syndrome (RDS)
  of newborn
respiratory distress with grunting
respiratory droplets
respiratory effort
respiratory embarrassment
respiratory excursions full and equal
respiratory failure, hypoxemic
respiratory flora, moderate growth of
  normal
respiratory frequency
respiratory infection, self-limiting
respiratory insufficiency
respiratory irritants
respiratory isolation
respiratory modulation of vascular
  impedance
respiratory muscle weakness
respiratory noise
respiratory physical therapy
respiratory rate (RR)
respiratory spasm
respiratory status, compromised
respiratory stertor
respiratory stridor
respiratory syncytial virus (RSV)
respiratory therapy
respiratory tract obstruction,
  mechanical

Respirgard II nebulizer
respirologist
Respironics CPAP machine
response
  abnormal ejection fraction
  baroreceptor-mediated
  blunted chronotropic
  cardioinhibitory
  controlled ventricular
  Cushing pressor
  early asthmatic
  humoral
  hypotensive
  late asthmatic
  rapid ventricular
  slow ventricular
  torque
  tyramine
  vagal
  vasoactive
  vasoconstrictor
  vasodepressor
  vasodilatory
  ventricular
  visuomotor
  Wenckebach upper rate
  whole body inflammatory
response rate, variable
responsiveness, airway
Res-Q AICD (automatic implantable
  cardioverter-defibrillator)
rest
  angina at
  breathlessness at
  ectopic (of thyroid tissue)
  embryonic cell (in the septum)
rest angina
rest dyspnea
rest force
rest images
rest LV function
rest pain

rest-related angina
rest RV function
rest thallium-201 myocardial imaging
Restcue CC Dynamic Air Therapy
re-stenosis after angioplasty
resting electrocardiogram
resting end-systolic wall stress
resting heart
resting heart rate
resting imaging
resting MUGA scan, preoperative
resting phase of cardiac action
  potentials
resting pulse
resting-redistribution thallium-201
  scintigraphy
resting regional myocardial hypoperfusion
restoration of sinus rhythm
restricted fluid intake
restriction
  dietary sodium
  exercise
  fluid
restrictive bulbo-ventricular foramen
restrictive cardiac syndrome
restrictive cardiomyopathy
restrictive defect
restrictive hemodynamic syndrome
restrictive hemodynamics
restrictive lung disease
restrictive myocardial disease
restrictive-obstructive lung disease,
  mixed
restrictive pattern
restrictive pericarditis
restrictive ventilatory defect
restrictive ventilatory pattern
results
  hemodynamic
  suboptimal
resuscitate, resuscitated

resuscitation
  cardiac
  cardiopulmonary (CPR)
  closed chest cardiopulmonary
  fluid
  mouth-to-mouth
resuscitative devices
resuscitative thoracotomy
resuscitator, cardiopulmonary
resuture
retained secretions
retard premature rewarming
retention
  carbon dioxide (CO_2)
  fluid
  salt
  sodium
  water
reticularis, livedo
reticulation
reticulocyte count
reticuloendothelial system
reticulogranular appearance
reticulogranular pattern
reticulonodular infiltrates
reticulum, sarcoplasmic
retinal angioid streaks
retinal exudate
retinopathy, hypertensive
retracted leaflets
retraction
  chest-wall
  clot
  costal
  inspiratory
  intercostal
  late systolic
  midsystolic
  mild subcostal
  postrheumatic cusp
  sternocleidomastoid
  sternum

retraction *(cont.)*
  substernal
  suprasternal
  systolic
retraction on inspiration, chest
retraction wave
retractor
  Allison lung
  Ankeney sternal
  Army-Navy
  atrial
  Beckman
  Bookwalter
  Burford
  Cooley atrial
  Crawford aortic
  Cushing vein
  Davidson scapular
  Deaver
  DeBakey-Cooley
  Favaloro sternal
  Finochietto
  Garrett
  Gelpi
  Green
  Haight-Finochietto rib
  hand-held
  Harrington
  Hartzler rib
  Himmelstein sternal
  IMA (inferior mesenteric artery)
  Kelly
  Kirklin atrial
  leaflet
  lung
  malleable
  malleable ribbon
  Miller-Senn
  Ochsner
  ophthalmic
  rake
  Richardson

retractor *(cont.)*
  Sachs vein
  Sauerbruch
  self-retaining
  Semb lung
  Senn
  small rake
  sternal
  U.S. Army
  vein
  Volkmann
  Weitlaner
retractor system
  Omni tract
  self-retaining table-mounted
retraction wave
Retract-o-tape
retrocardiac infiltrate
retrocardiac space
retroesophageal right subclavian artery
retroesophageal subclavian artery
retrofascial
retrograde aortogram
retrograde arterial catheterization
retrograde atherectomy
retrograde atrial activation mapping
retrograde blood flow across valve
retrograde blood velocity
retrograde conduction
retrograde coronary sinus infusion
retrograde fashion
  advanced in a
  catheter advanced in a
retrograde femoral arterial approach
retrograde filling of vessels
retrograde infusion of cardioplegic
  solution
retrograde injection
retrogradely (backward)
retrograde percutaneous femoral artery
  approach for cardiac catheterization

retrograde perfusion
retrograde refractory period
retrograde ventriculoatrial conduction
retropancreatic preaortic space
retroperfusion
  coronary sinus
  synchronized
retroperitoneal approach
retroperitoneal fibrosis, perianeurysmal
retroperitoneal hematoma
retroperitoneal space
retroperitoneal tunnel
retroperitoneal tunneling
retropharyngeal abscess
retrosternal chest pain
retrosternal pain
return
  anomalous
  anomalous pulmonary venous
  central arterial
  infracardiac type total anomalous
    venous
  paracardiac type total anomalous
    venous
  pulmonary venous
  supracardiac type total anomalous
    venous
  systemic venous
  total anomalous pulmonary venous
  total anomalous venous
    venous
return of sinus rhythm
return to baseline
REV procedure (intraventricular
  repair of anomalies of ventriculoarterial connection)
revascularization
  coronary
  coronary ostial
  heart
  infrainguinal

revascularization *(cont.)*
  myocardial
  percutaneous
  surgical
revascularized
reversal of ventricular tachycardia
reversal, shunt
reversed arm leads
reversed coarctation
reversed differential cyanosis
reverse distribution
reversed greater saphenous vein
reversed splitting
reversed 3 sign
reversed with protamine, heparin was
reverse immunoassay
reversible airways disease (RAD)
reversible atrial pacing
reversible defect
reversible ischemia
reversible obstructive airway disease
  (ROAD)
reversible ventriclar fibrillation
reversible ventriclar tachycardia (VT)
rewarm
rewarming, retard premature
Reynolds number
Reynolds vascular clamp
RF (radiofrequency)
RFA (radiofrequency ablation)
RFCA (radiofrequency catheter
  ablation)
RF-generated thermal balloon catheter
RFP (rapid filling period)
RF (rapid filling) pulses
RFW (rapid filling wave)
RF wave of cardiac apex pulse
RF (rheumatic fever)
rhabdomyoblast
rhabdomyoma of heart
rhabdomyosarcoma, cardiac
rhabdomyosarcoma of the heart

rHb1.1 (recombinant hemoglobin)
RHD (rheumatic heart disease)
rhEPO or rHuEPO (recombinant
  human erythropoietin)
rheumatic adherent pericardium
rheumatic aortic insufficiency
rheumatic aortic stenosis
rheumatic aortitis
rheumatic carditis
rheumatic chorea
rheumatic endocarditis
rheumatic fever (RF)
rheumatic heart disease (RHD)
rheumatic lesion
rheumatic myocarditis
rheumatic nodule
rheumatic pericarditis
rheumatic pneumonia
rheumatic valvular deformity
rheumatic valvulitis
rheumatism, articular
  acute
  subacute
  desert
rheumatoid-arthritis-associated
  interstitial lung disease
rheumatoid arthritis (RA) factor
rheumatoid arthritis-pneumoconiosis
rheumatoid lung disease
rheumatoid lung silicosis
rheumatoid nodule
rheumatoid pericarditis
rheumatoid pneumoconiosis
Rh-null syndrome
rhomboideus muscle
rhomboid major muscle
rhonchi (pl. of rhonchus)
  coarse
  coarse sibilant expiratory
  high-pitched
  humming
  low-pitched

rhonchi *(cont.)*
 musical
 post-tussive
 post-tussive inspiratory
 pulmonary
 scattered
 sibilant
 sonorous
 whistling
rhonchi on forced exhalation
rhonchus (pl. rhonchi)
rHuEPO or rhEPO (recombinant
 human erythropoietin)
rhythm
 accelerated atrioventricular (AV)
  junctional
 accelerated idioventricular (AIVR)
 atrial escape
 atrial gallop
 atrioventricular junctional escape
 atrioventricular nodal
 AV (atrioventricular)
 AV junctional
 AV nodal (idionodal)
 AVNR (atrioventricular nodal)
 baseline
 bigeminal
 cardiac
 coronary nodal
 coronary sinus (CSR)
 coupled
 dual
 ectopic
 embryocardia
 escape
 fibrillation
 gallop
 idioventricular (IVR)
 irregularly irregular heart
 junctional
 junctional escape
 mu

rhythm *(cont.)*
 nodal
 nodal escape
 normal sinus (NSR)
 paced
 pacemaker
 parasystolic
 pendulum
 predominant
 presystolic gallop
 protodiastolic gallop
 pulseless idioventricular
 quadruple
 reciprocal
 reciprocating
 reentrant
 regular
 regular sinus (RSR)
 regularly irregular heart
 sinoatrial
 sinus
 sinusoidal irregular
 slow escape
 supraventricular
 systolic
 tic-tac
 transitional
 triple
 ventricular
 wide complex
rhythm disturbance
rhythmical
rhythmic auscultatory cadence
rhythmicity
rhythm runs, benign idioventricular
rhythm strip
RIA (radioimmunoassay)
rib, ribs
 hypoplastic horizontal
 retracted
rib approximator, Bailey
rib guillotine

rib notching
rib recession
rib-resecting incision
rib spaces, narrowed
rib spreader
Richardson retractor
richly cellular exudate
Rickettsia burnetii infection
rickettsial myocarditis
rickettsial pneumonia
ridge
  broad maxillary
  fibromuscular
  septal
  supra-aortic
  supracoronary
riding embolus
Ridley syndrome
Riegel pulse
Riesman myocardosis
right and retrograde left heart
  catheterization
right-angle chest tube
right-angle clamp
right-angled telescopic lens
right ankle indices
right anterior oblique (RAO) position
right anterior oblique projection
right aortic arch with mirror image
  branching
right atrial appendage
right atrial chamber
right atrial enlargement
right atrial extension of uterine
  leiomyosarcoma
right atrial patch positioned over the
  right atrioventricular sulcus
right atrial pressure (RAP)
right atrial sarcoma
right atrioventricular valve
right atrium
right axis deviation

right border of heart
right bundle branch block with left
  anterior (or posterior) hemiblock
right bundle branch heart block
  (RBBB)
right coronary artery, dominant
right coronary cusp
right coronary plexus (of heart)
right femoral artery
right fibrous trigone
right first intercostal space
right free-wall pathway
right-handedness, ventricular
right heart catheter
right heart failure
right heart pressure
right internal jugular artery
right internal mammary anastomosis
right Judkins catheter
right-left disorientation
right main stem bronchus
right middle lobe lingula
right middle lobe subsegments
right middle lobectomy
right minithoracotomy
right second intercostal space
right semilunar valve
right-sided empyema
right-sided heart failure
right-sided pneumonia
right subclavian artery, retroesophageal
right to left shunt of blood
right-to-left shunt with pulmonic
  stenosis
right upper lobe
right upper sternal border
right ventricle
  augmented filling of
  double-outlet
  parchment
  Taussig-Bing double-outlet

right ventricle adherent to posterior
table of sternum
right ventricle outflow tract
right ventricle-pulmonary artery
conduit
right ventricle-to-ear time
right ventricular assist device (RVAD)
right ventricular bypass tract
right ventricular cardiomyopathy,
arrhythmogenic
right ventricular chamber
right ventricular coil
right ventricular conduction defect
right ventricular dysplasia, arrhythmogenic
right ventricular ejection fraction
(RVEF)
right ventricular end-diastolic volume
(RVEDV)
right ventricular endocardial sensing
lead
right ventricular endomyocardial
biopsy
right ventricular end-systolic volume
(RVESV)
right ventricular failure
right ventricular hypertrophy (RVH)
right ventricular hypoplasia
right ventricular impulse, hyperdynamic
right ventricular inflow view
right ventricular infundibulectomy
right ventricular infundibulum
right ventricular lift
right ventricular myocardial aplasia
right ventricular obstruction, intraventricular
right ventricular outflow obstruction
right ventricular outflow tract
right ventricular overload
right ventricular patch positioned over
the atrioventricular sulcus

right ventricular pressure (RVP)
right ventricular preponderance
right ventricular stroke work (RVSW)
right ventricular stroke work index
(RVSWI)
right ventricular systolic time interval
right vocal cord
rigor, frank
Riley-Day syndrome
rimlike calcium distribution
RIND (reversible intermittent or
ischemic neurologic deficit)
Rindfleisch, fold of
ring
aortic subvalvular
atrioventricular
Carpentier
congenital (of aortic arch)
Crawford suture
double-flanged valve sewing
Duran annuloplasty
mitral
mitral valve
prosthetic valve sewing
prosthetic valve suture
Puig Massana-Shiley annuloplasty
Sculptor flexible annuloplasty
sewing
supra-annular suture
supravalvar
tricuspid valve
universal valve prosthesis sewing
valve
vascular
ring dissector
ring of Vieussens
ring shadows with air-fluid levels
ripple, triple
risk
formidable
surgical
risk/benefit ratio

risk factors
  cardiac risk
  incremental
  patient
  procedural
risk index, Detsky modified cardiac
Riva-Rocci manometer
Rivero-Carvallo maneuver or sign
Riviere sign
R-lactate enzymatic monotest
RMVT (repetitive monomorphic
  ventricular tachycardia)
RNA (radionuclide angiogram), gated
RNS terminal
RNV (radionuclide ventriculogram)
ROA (regurgitant orifice area)
ROAD (reversible obstructive airway
  disease)
roaring in ears
Robertson sign
Robicsek Vascular Probe (RVP)
Robinson catheter
robust
Rochester-Mixter artery forceps
rocking precordial motion
Rocky Mountain spotted fever
Rodriguez-Alvarez catheter
Rodriguez catheter
roentgenkymography
roentgenogram, chest
roentgenographic control
roentgenographic silhouette
Roger bruit
Roger disease
Roger murmur
Roger syndrome
Roger ventricular septal defect
Rokitansky disease
R/O (rule out)
Rolleston rule for systolic blood
  pressure
Romano-Ward syndrome

Romberg-Wood syndrome
Romhilt-Estes score for left ventricu-
  lar hypertrophy
ROMI (rule out myocardial infarc-
  tion); also ROMIed
rongeur
  Bethune
  Cushing
  Giertz
  Kerrison
  Sauerbruch
  Semb
R on T (R wave on T wave)
R on T phenomenon on EKG
R on T ventricular premature
  contraction
roof, Dacron
roof of coronary sinus
room air
room air arterial blood gases
root
  aortic
  dilated aortic
root of lung
ROPA (Regional Organ Procurement
  Agency)
rope-like cord (in thrombophlebitis)
ropy sputum
Roques syndrome
rose fever
Rosenbach syndrome
Rosen-Castleman-Liebow syndrome
Rosen guide wire
Rosenthal syndrome
Ross operation
Rostan asthma
Rostan syndrome
Rotablator atherectomy device
ROTACS guide wire
rotating burr
rotating tourniquets for pulmonary
  edema

rotation
  counterclockwise
  neck
rotation therapy, continuous lateral
rotational atherectomy system (RAS)
rotational coronary atherectory (RCA)
Rotch sign in pericardial effusion
Rotex II biopsy needle
Rothschild sign in tuberculosis
Roth spots
Roticulator, suture
Roubin-Gianturco flexible coil stent
rougeur, simple (erythema)
roughened pleurae
roughened state of pericardium
roughening of lining of artery
rough murmur
rough zone
Rougnon de Magny syndrome
Rougnon-Heberden angina pectoris
rounded border of lung
roundworm infestation
routine antimicrobial prophylaxis
roving hand-held bipolar electrode
Royal Flush angiographic flush
  catheter
Royer-Wilson syndrome
Rozanski precordial lead placement
  system
RPA (right pulmonary artery)
RPE (rating of perceived exertion)
R-P interval
rpm (rotations per minute)
RPV (right pulmonary vein)
RR (respiratory rate)
RR cycle
RR interval
RR' (RR prime) pattern
RRI (recurrent respiratory infections)
RRP (rate-responsive pacing)
RRP (relative refractory period)
RRR (regular rate and rhythm)

rS deflection
RS complex (also rS complex)
RSCVP (right subclavian central
  venous pressure)
RS4 pacemaker
RSR (regular sinus rhythm)
R/S ratio; wave ratio
RSR' triphasic pattern (on EKG)
RS-T segments
RSV (regurgitant stroke volume)
RSV (respiratory syncytial virus)
R-to-R scanning
rt-PA (recombinant tissue plasminogen activator) thrombolysis
RT segment, elevated
RTV total artificial heart
R-2 defibrillator pads
rub
  coarse friction
  creaking friction
  faint friction
  friction
  grating friction
  harsh friction
  loud friction
  pericardial
  pericardial friction
  pleural
  pleural friction
  pleuritic
  prolonged
  scratchy friction
  shuffling friction
  soft friction
rubber band, Vesseloops
rubber, vulcanizing silicone
rubbery mass
rubbery sputum
rubbing sound
rubedo
rubella, maternal
rubeola

Rubinstein-Taybi syndrome
rubor, dependent
rubrous
ruddy cyanosis
rudimentary outlet chamber
rudimentary ventricular chamber
Ruel forceps
rufous
rule
    Simpson
    Trusler
rule of bigeminy
rule out (R/O)
rule out myocardial infarction (ROMI)
rumble
    Austin Flint
    booming
    crescendo
    diastolic
    mid-diastolic (or middiastolic)
    protodiastolic
rumbling murmur
Rumel catheter
Rumel myocardial clamp
Rumel thoracic forceps
Rumel tourniquet
Rummo syndrome
Rundles-Falls syndrome
runaway pacemaker
runoff
    absent
    aortic
    arterial
    digital
    distal
    inadequate
    single-vessel
    suboptimal
    three-vessel
    two-vessel
    vessel
runoff arteriogram

runoff resistance, index of
runoff vessel
runoff views, aortofemoral arteri-
    ography with
runs of arrhythmia
runs of atrial fibrillation
runs of PVCs (premature ventricular
    contractions)
runs of tachycardia
runs of ventricular tachycardia,
    spontaneously occurring
runs of VPCs (ventricular premature
    contractions)
runting syndrome
rupture
    abdominal aortic aneurysm
    arterial
    cardiac
    chordae tendineae
    chordal
    contained aneurysmal
    interventricular septal
    myocardial
ruptured aneurysm
ruptured aortic cusp
ruptured capillaries
ruptured chordae
ruptured chordae tendineae
ruptured emphysematous bleb
ruptured thoracic duct
rupture of arch
    papillary muscle
    plaque
    ventricular free wall
    ventricular septal
    vessel
rupture of blebs on surface of lungs
rupture of bullae on surface of lungs
rupture of emphysematous bleb
rupture of emphysematous bulla in
    apex of lung
rupture of heart muscle

rupture of lung
rupture of membranes (ROM)
rupture of myocardium
rupture with bleeding
Russell-Silver syndrome
Russian tissue forceps
rusty sputum
RV (residual volume)
RVA (right ventricular apical) electro-
gram
RVAD (right ventricular assist
device), Thoratec
RVBF (reversed vertebral blood flow)
RVCD (right ventricular conduction
defect)
RVD (right ventricular diastolic)
pressure
RVD (right ventricular dimension)
RVE (right ventricular enlargement)
RVEDP (right ventricular end-
diastolic pressure)
RVEDV (right ventricular end-
diastolic volume)
RVEF (right ventricular ejection
fraction)
RVESV (right ventricular end-systolic
volume)
RVFW (right ventricular free wall)
RVH (right ventricular hypertrophy)

RVID (right ventricular internal
diameter)
RVM (right ventricular mass)
R voltage
RVOT (right ventricular outflow tract)
RVP (right ventricular pressure)
RVP (Robicsek vascular probe)
RVP–LVP (right ventricular to left
ventricular systolic pressure) ratio
RV (right ventricle) pressure
RVS (right ventricular systolic)
pressure
RV strain
RVSTI (right ventricular systolic time
interval)
RVSW (right ventricular stroke work)
RVSWI (right ventricular stroke work
index)
RV/TLC (residual volume/total lung
capacity)
R' (R prime) wave
R wave (on EKG)
low-amplitude
tall right precordial
upright
r wave of jugular venous pulse
R wave progression, poor (on EKG)
R wave upstroke, slurred (on EKG)
Rx (prescription) therapy

S, s

S$_1$ (first heart sound)
S$_1$ amplitude
S$_1$Q3 pattern
S$_1$Q3T3 pattern
S$_1$-S$_2$ interval (heart sounds)
S$_1$-S$_3$ interval (heart sounds)
S$_1$-S$_2$-S$_3$ pattern (heart sounds)
S$_2$ (second heart sound)
  audible expiratory splitting of
  fixed splitting of
  paradoxical splitting of
  physiologically split
S$_3$ (third heart sound)
  audible
  palpable
  prominent
S$_3$ gallop
S$_4$ (fourth heart sound)
S$_4$ abolished by breath holding
S$_4$ abolished by sitting up
S$_4$ abolished by standing up
S$_4$, exaggerated
S$_4$ palpable
SA (sinoatrial)
SAA protein
SAB (sinoatrial block)
Sabathie sign

sac
  air
  alveolar
  aneurysmal
  false
  heart
  pericardial
  pleural
  terminal air
  wrapped aneurysmal
saccular appearance, lobulated
saccular bronchiectasis
saccular mass
sacculated pleurisy
Sachs vein retractor
Sack-Barabas syndrome
saclike spaces
sacrospinalis muscle
SACT (sinoatrial conduction time)
saddle embolism or embolus
Sade modification of Norwood
  procedure
SaECG (signal-averaged electrocardiogram)
sagging ST segment
sagittal image
sagittal plane loop

443

sagittal tomogram
Sahli method of measuring hemoglobin calorimetrically
saint (see *St. Jude, St. Thomas*)
Salibi carotid artery clamp
salicylate ingestion
salient history
salient physical findings
saline
  cold
  half normal (0.45% NaCl)
  heparinized
  iced
  normal (0.9% NaCl)
  topical cold
saline flush
saline irrigation
saline lavage
saline loading
saline solution
Salkowski test
sallow
salmonellosis
salt edema
salt intake, excessive
salt-restricted diet
salt restriction
salt retention
salvage of limb
salvage of myocardium
salvage therapy
salvo of echoes
salvo of premature ventricular
  complexes
salvo of ventricular tachycardia
Salzman test
SAM (systolic anterior motion) on
  2-D echocardiogram
sampling, adrenal vein
Samuels forceps
Samuels hemoclip
SAN (sinoatrial node)

Sanchez-Cascos cardioauditory
  syndrome
sandbag
Sanders sign in constrictive pericarditis
Sandrock test for thrombosis
sandwich patch closure, anterior
sandwich technique
Sanfilippo syndrome
sanguineous exudate
sanguineous pleural exudate
San Joaquin Valley coccidioidomycosis
San Joaquin Valley disease
San Joaquin Valley fever
SA (sinoatrial)
SA nodal reentry tachycardia
SA node (also called *sinus*)
Sansom murmur
Sansom rhythmical murmur
Sansom sign in pericardial effusion
SaO_2 (arterial oxygen saturation)
saphenofemoral junction
saphenous varices
saphenous vein
  greater
  reversed greater
saphenous vein bypass graft
saphenous vein bypass graft disease
saphenous vein graft (SVG)
saphenous vein incompetence
sapphire contact probe
saralasin infusion
sarcoid, Boeck
sarcoidosis
sarcoma
  cardiac
  endobronchial Kaposi
  intrathoracic Kaposi
  Kaposi epicardial
  myocardial infiltration by Kaposi
  pulmonary Kaposi
  right atrial
sarcomere, A bands of

sarcoplasmic reticulum
Sarns aortic arch cannula
Sarns electric saw
Sarns two-stage cannula
Sarns ventricular assist device
Sarns wire-reinforced catheter
Sarot artery forceps
Sarot bronchus clamp
SAS (supravalvular aortic stenosis)
Satinsky aortic clamp
Satinsky scissors
Satinsky vascular clamp
Satinsky vena cava clamp
satisfactory threshold
saturated fats
saturation
  aortic oxygen
  arterial oxygen (SaO_2)
  decreased arterial hemoglobin
  low oxygen
  mixed venous
  oxygen (O_2)
  oxyhemoglobin
  PA (pulmonary artery) oxygen
  RA (right atrium) oxygen
Sauerbruch retractor
Sauerbruch rib shears
Sauerbruch rongeur
sausaging of a vein
Sauvage arterial graft
Sauvage filamentous prosthesis
Sauvage filamentous velour Dacron
  arterial graft material
saw
  Gigli
  Hall sternal
  oscillating sternotomy
  Sarns electric
  sternotomy
  Stryker
sawtooth configuration

Sawyer-Jones syndrome
SB (sinus bradycardia)
SBE (subacute bacterial endocarditis)
SBE prophylaxis
SBF (systemic blood flow)
SBP (systolic blood pressure)
SBSP (simultaneous bilateral spontaneous pneumothorax)
SC (systolic click)
SCAD (spontaneous coronary artery
  dissection)
SCA-EX catheter with rotating blades
SCA-EX ShortCutter catheter with
  rotating blades
scalar EKG
scale (see *index*, *score*)
  Borg (perceived exertion)
  Abbreviated Injury
scalene node biopsy
scalenus anterior muscle
scalenus anticus muscle hypertrophy
scalenus anticus syndrome
scalenus minimus
scalloped commissure
scalloped luminal configuration
scalloping
scallop of posterior annulus, redundant
scallop, prolapsing
scalp edema
scalp electrode
scalpel, ultrasonic
scalp pH
scan
  attenuation
  Captopril-stimulated renal
  Cardiolite ([99mTc] sestamibi)
  Cardiotec or CardioTec ([99mTc]
    teboroxime)
  cine CT (computed tomography)
  cine view in MUGA (cinemato-
    graph in multiple gated
    acquisition)

scan *(cont.)*
  computerized tomography (CT)
  dipyridamole thallium-201
  duplex
  gated equilibrium blood pool
  high-resolution computed
    tomography
  hot spot
  125I (I 125) fibrinogen
  131I-iodocholesterol
  131I meta-iodobenzylguanide
    (131I-MIBG)
  isotope-labeled fibrinogen leg
  MUGA (multiple gated acquisition)
  blood pool radionuclide
  myocardial perfusion
  perfusion and ventilation lung
  perfusion lung
  PET
  31P nuclear magnetic resonance
  PYP (pyrophosphate technetium)
    myocardial
  radioactive fibrinogen
  radionuclide gated blood pool
  redistributed thallium
  renal duplex
  rest thallium-201
  resting MUGA
  R to R
  scintillation
  serial duplex
  SPECT thallium
  stress thallium
  99mTc glucoheptonate
  99mTc pyrophosphate myocardial
  thallium
  ultrafast CT
  ventilation lung
  ventilation-perfusion lung
scan decrement
scan pacing

scanty findings
scanty mucoid sputum
scapula, inferior tip of
scar
  arrhythmogenic
  dense
  infarcted
  myocardial
  nonviable
  pulmonary
  scarred
  well-demarcated
  zipper
scar formation on myocardium
scarification of pleura
Scarpa method
Scarpa triangle
scarred fibrotic media
scarring
  apical
  interstitial
  selective
scarring of valve
scar tissue
scattered rhonchi
scattering of sound waves
SCD (sudden cardiac death)
Schafer artificial respirations
Schatz-Palmaz tubular mesh stent
Schede operation for leg varicose
  veins
Schede resection of thorax for chronic
  empyema
Schede thoracoplasty
Scheie syndrome
Schellong-Strisower phenomenon
Schepelmann sign in dry pleurisy
Schick sign of tuberculosis
Schick stridor heard on expiration
Schiff test
Schistosoma haematobium

schistosoma infection
Schistosoma japonicum
Schistosoma mansoni
schistosomiasis
  cardiopulmonary
  Manson
  pulmonary
schistosomiasis japonica syndrome
Schlichter test
Schmincke-Bernheim syndrome
Schneider catheter
Schneider PTCA instruments
Schneider-Shiley catheter
Schneider Wallstent
Schneider wire
Schnidt clamp
Schnidt passer
Scholten endomyocardial biopsy
  forceps
Scholten endomyocardial bioptome
Schonander film changer
Schonander technique
Schönenberg syndrome
Schönlein disease
Schönlein purpura
Schoonmaker femoral catheter
Schoonmaker multipurpose catheter
Schroeder syndrome
Schrötter syndrome
Schuco nebulizer
Schultz modification of the
  Liebermann-Burchardt reaction for
  cholesterol
Schultze test
Schultze acroparesthesia
Schumaker aortic clamp
Schwarten balloon dilatation catheter
Schwarten LP guide wire
Schwartz clamp
Schwartz test for patency of deep
  saphenous veins
sciatic artery, persistent

Sci-Med Express balloon
Sci-Med SSC "Skinny" catheter
SciMed Express Monorail balloon
SciMed membrane oxygenator
scimitar deformity
scimitar-shaped flap
scimitar-shaped shadow
scimitar sign on chest radiograph
scimitar syndrome
scimitar vein
Scinticore multicrystal scintillation
  camera
scintigram, scintigraphy
  AMA-Fab (antimyosin monoclonal
    antibody with Fab fragment)
  dipyridamole thallium-201
  dual intracoronary
  exercise stress-redistribution
  exercise thallium
  gated blood pool
  indium-111 (^{111}In)
  infarct-avid hot-spot
  ^{131}I-19-iodocholesterol
  labeled FFA (free fatty acid)
  metaiodobenzylguanidine (MIBG)
  microsphere perfusion
  myocardial
  myocardial cold-spot perfusion
  myocardial perfusion
  NEFA (non-esterified fatty acid)
  planar thallium
  pulmonary
  pyrophosphate
  resting-redistribution thallium-201
  SPECT thallium
  ^{99m}Tc-PYP (pyrophosphate)
  thallium perfusion
  thallium-201 myocardial
scintillation camera
scintillation, migrainous-like
scintillation scan
scintirenography

scintiscan (scintigraphy)
scintiscanning of lungs
scissors
  bandage
  Beall circumflex artery
  Church
  coronary artery
  Crafoord thoracic
  curved
  DeBakey endarterectomy
  DeBakey valve
  DeMartel vascular
  Diethrich coronary
  Diethrich valve
  dissecting
  Duffield
  Finochietto thoracic
  Haimovici arteriotomy
  Harrington-Mayo thoracic
  hook
  Howell coronary
  iris
  Kantrowitz vascular
  Karmody venous
  Lincoln
  Lincoln-Metzenbaum
  Litwak mitral valve
  Mayo
  Metzenbaum
  microvascular
  Mills arteriotomy
  Nelson
  Potts right-angled
  Potts 60° angled
  Potts-Smith vascular
  Real coronary artery
  right-angle
  Satinsky
  Smith
  Snowden-Pencer
  Spencer
  Stille-Mayo

scissors *(cont.)*
  straight
  Strully
  valve
  Westscott
  Willauer thoracic
  Wilmer
SCL (sinus cycle length)
SCLC (small-cell lung cancer)
sclerae
  blue
  bluish coloration of
scleroderma
sclerosing breast periphlebitis
sclerosing breast phlebitis
sclerosing mediastinitis
sclerosis
  arterial
  arteriocapillary
  arteriolar
  calcified
  coronary
  endocardial
  medial calcific
  Mönckeberg
  progressive systemic
  pulmonary and cardiac
  renal
  segmental vein
  subendocardial
  tuberous
  valvular
  vascular
  venous
sclerosis of aorta
sclerotherapy
sclerotic coronary arteries
sclerotic degeneration
SCOOP 1 transtracheal oxygen
  catheter
SCOOP 2 catheter with distal and
  side openings

scooping, nonspecific (on EKG)
scope, Jako anterior commissure
score
   CASS
   Detsky modified cardiac risk index
   Dripps-American Surgical
     Association
   Estes EKG
   Gensini coronary artery disease
   Goldman
   Goldman cardiac risk index
   mean wall motion
   QRS
   Romhilt-Estes left ventricular
     hypertrophy
   Selvester QRS
   TAPSE (tricuspid annular plane
     systolic excursion)
   wall motion
scoring, CASS
scotoma
scout films
scratch
   Means-Lerman
   systolic
scratchy friction rub
scratchy murmur
scratchy throat
screen, collagen vascular
screw-in lead
screw-in lead pacemaker
screw-on epimyocardial lead
screw-on lead
scrub typhus
Sculptor flexible annuloplasty ring
SCV-CPR (simultaneous compression-
   ventilation CPR)
SD (standard deviation)
SDBP (systemic diastolic blood
   pressure)
SDPS (protamine solution)
SE (standard error)

seagull bruit
seagull murmur
seal and suction
sealant, fibrin
seated, valve is
Sebastiani syndrome
secondary atrioventricular heart block
secondary bacterial infection
secondary cartilaginous joint
secondary chordal dysplasia
secondary coccidioidomycosis
secondary endocardial fibroelastosis
secondary erythrocytosis
secondary extravasation of intravascular contents
secondary hypertension
secondary lymphedema
secondary median sternotomy
secondary myocardiopathy
secondary pacemaker
secondary pleurisy
secondary venous insufficiency
second branch of artery
second component
second-degree atrioventricular block
second diagonal branch
second-hand smoke
second heart sound, loud pulmonic
   component
second heart sound, single
second intercostal space
second left interspace
second order chordae
second pulmonic sound, accentuated
second sound followed by opening
   snap
second sound, reinforced
secretion
   ACTH
   ADH (antidiuretic hormone)
   amber-colored pulmonary
   bronchial

secretion *(cont.)*
  liquification of
  mucopurulent
  nonpurulent pulmonary
  retained
  thickened
secretion-filled medium-sized bronchi
sector echocardiography
secundum and sinus venosus defects
secundum atrial septal defect (ASD)
sed (sedimentation) rate
sedentary lifestyle
sedimentation rate, Wintrobe
Seecor pacemaker
seesaw (to-and-fro) murmur
segment
  akinetic
  amplitude and slope of ST
  angulated
  anterior
  anterior basal
  anterobasal
  anterolateral
  apex
  apical
  arterial
  bronchopulmonary
  coarcted
  contiguous
  depressed PR
  depressed ST
  diaphragmatic
  distal
  elevated RT
  elevated ST
  endarterectomized
  expansile aortic
  hypokinetic
  infarcted lung
  inferior
  inferior basal
  inferoapical

segment *(cont.)*
  inferoposterior
  nonfilling venous
  noninfarcted
  posterior
  posterobasal
  posterolateral
  P-R
  proximal
  RS-T
  septal wall
  septum
  ST
  ST-T
  superior
  Ta
  TQ
  upsloping ST
  venous
segmental atelectasis
segmental bowel infarction
segmental bronchi
  cardiac
  lateral
  lateral basal
  medial
  medial basal
  posterior
  posterior basal
  superior
segmental bronchus
segmental ischemia
segmental lesion
segmental limb pressure
segmental lower extremity Doppler
  pressures
segmental orifice
segmental perfusion abnormality
segmental plethysmography
segmental pneumonia
segmental resection
segmental vein sclerosis

segmental wall motion
    akinetic
    dyskinetic
    hyperkinetic
    hypokinetic
segmental wall motion abnormality
segmentectomy of lung
segs (segmented neutrophils)
Sehrt clamp
Sehrt compressor
SEI (subendocardial infarction)
Seitz bronchial inspiration
Seitz sign
seizure
Seldinger needle
Seldinger percutaneous technique
Seldinger technique, modified
selective arteriogram
selective cannulization
selective coronary arteriography
selective coronary cineangiography
selective scarring of posterobasal
    portion of left ventricle
selective vascular ligation
selective visualization
self-expanding stent
self-inhibition, pacemaker
self-limited
self-limiting respiratory
    infection
self-positioning balloon
self-retaining retractor
self-retaining table-mounted retractor
    system
Selman clamp
Selman vessel forceps
Selverstone cardiotomy hook
Selverstone carotid clamp
Selvester QRS score
SEM (systolic ejection murmur)
Semb forceps
Semb lung retractor

Semb rongeur
semicircularis, linea
semiclosed endarterectomy
semi-Fowler position
semilateral position
semilunar (aortic and pulmonary)
    valves
semilunar aortic valve regurgitation
semilunar pulmonic valve regurgitation
semilunar valve cusp
senescent aortic stenosis
Sengstaken-Blakemore tube
senile arteriosclerosis
senile emphysema
senile myocarditis
senile nevus
Senning atrial baffle repair
Senning intra-atrial baffle
Senning operation for transposition
Senn retractor
sensation
    flip-flop
    fluttering
    globus
    pressurelike
    squeezing
    suffocating
sensing
    afterpotential
    integrated bipolar
    intrinsic
    pacemaker
    R wave
sensing error
sensing sensitivity
sensing specificity
sensing spike
sensing threshold
sensing wire
sensitivity
    airway
    baroreflex

sensitivity *(cont.)*
  pacemaker
  sensing
Sensolog pacemaker
sensor, sensors
  Hall-effect position
  minute ventilation
  muscle activity
  respiration
  temperature
  vibration
Sensor Kelvin pacemaker
Sensor-Medics metabolic cart
sensorium
sensory impairment
sentinel nodes
SEP (systolic ejection period)
separation
  aortic cusp
  leaflet
sepsis
  catheter-related (CRS)
  gram-negative
  overwhelming
septa
  alveolar
  thickened alveolar
septal accessory pathway
septal amplitude
septal arcade
septal band
septal cardiac defect
septal collateral
septal cusp of right atrioventricular
  valve
septal defect
  atrial
  atrioventricular
  interventricular
septal dip
septal hypertrophy, asymmetric

septal hypokinesis
septal hypoperfusion on thallium scan
septal infarction
septal leaflet
septal necrosis
septal papillary muscle
septal pathway
septal perforation
septal perforator branch
septal perforators
septal ridge
septal separation
septal thickness
septal wall thickness
septation
septectomy
  atrial
  Blalock-Hanlon atrial
  Blalock-Hanlon partial atrial
septic bronchitis
septic emboli
septic embolization
septic embolus
septic endocarditis
septic lung syndrome
septic myocarditis
septic pelvic thrombophlebitis with
  emboli
septic phlebitis
septic pleurisy
septic pulmonary emboli
septic pulmonary infarction
septic shock
septic thrombosis
septic tonsillitis
septicemia
septomarginal trabecula
septostomy
  balloon
  balloon and blade
  balloon atrial

septostomy *(cont.)*
  blade
  blade and balloon atrial
  blade atrial
  Mullins transseptal blade and
    balloon atrial
  Park blade and balloon atrial
  Rashkind balloon
  Rashkind balloon atrial
  Rashkind blade
  Rashkind-Miller atrial
  transcatheter knife blade atrial
septotomy, balloon atrial
septum (pl. septa)
  anteroapical trabecular
  asymmetric hypertrophy of
  atrial
  atrioventricular
  bronchial
  bulbar
  canal
  conal
  conus
  dyskinetic
  infundibular
  intact ventricular
  interatrial (IAS)
  interventricular (IVS)
  membranous
  muscular atrioventricular
  sinus
  thickened
  ventricular
septum primum
septum secundum
sequela (pl. sequelae)
  clinical
  significant
sequence
  A-B-C (airway, breathing, circula-
    tion) (in cardiopulmonary
    resuscitation)

sequence *(cont.)*
  C-A-B (circulation, airway,
    breathing) (in cardiopulmonary
    resuscitation)
  conventional pulse
  echo-planar
  gradient-echo imaging
  gradient-echo pulse
  Klippel-Feil
  spin-echo imaging
sequential balloon inflation
sequential bypass graft
Sequential Compression Device,
  Kendall
sequential dilatations
sequential graft
sequential in situ bypass
sequential monophasic shocks
sequential obstruction
sequential pacing
sequestered lobe of lung
sequestration, third space
Sequicor pacemaker
sequoiosis asthma
SER (systolic ejection rate)
serial cardiac isoenzymes
serial changes
serial CPK and LDH isoenzymes
serial cut film technique
serial duplex scan
serial EKG tracings
serial electrophysiologic testing (SET)
serial lesions
serial samples of blood
serial tracings
seriography
Seroche syndrome
serofibrinous pleurisy
seroma, graft
seropurulent pleurisy
serosanguineous fluid
serosum, pericardium

serotonin
serous exudate
serous exudation
serous pericarditis
serous pericardium
serous pleurisy
serrated catheter
Serratia marcescens
serratus anterior muscle
serum aspergillus precipitins
serum cardiac enzymes
serum cryptococcal antigen
serum electrophoresis
serum iron
serum lactate level, elevated
serum lipid level
serum lipid profile
serum magnesium
serum myoglobin (Mb) concentration
serum phosphorus level
serum potassium concentration
serum prothrombin conversion
   accelerator (SPCA)
serum renin levels
Servelle-Martorell syndrome
servomotor
sessile plaque
sestamibi technetium-99m stress test
SET (serial electrophysiologic testing)
7E3 monoclonal antiplatelet antibody
17-hydroxylase deficiency
seventh intercostal space
7-3 rule
severe acute rejection
severe cardiopulmonary failure
severe exertion
severe infarction
severe oxygen debt
severe respiratory distress
sewing ring
sew-on lead
SF wave of cardiac apex pulse

SFA (subclavian flap aortoplasty)
SFA (superficial femoral artery)
SFHb (stroma-free hemoglobin,
   pyridoxilated)
SFR (stenotic flow reserve)
SGOT (serum glutamic-oxaloacetic
   transaminase)
SGPT (serum glutamic-pyruvic
   transaminase)
shadow
   bat's wing (on x-ray)
   butterfly (on x-ray)
   cardiac
   discoid
   fusiform
   hilar
   large thymus (obscuring cardiac
     silhouette)
   linear
   Ponfick
   toothpaste
   tramlines
   tumorlike
   widened heart
shadowing, acoustic
Shadow over-the-wire balloon catheter
shag, aortic
shagging of cardiac borders
shaggy aorta syndrome
shake test
shaking chills
shaking sound
shallow breathing
shallow respirations
shapeable guide wire
Shapiro sign
sharp border of lung
sharp carina
sharp dissection
sharp pain
sharp pulse
sharp, stabbing pain

sharp waves
shaver catheter
Shaver-Ridell syndrome
Shaver syndrome
shears
   Bethune rib
   Gluck rib
   Sauerbruch rib
   Shoemaker rib
   Stille-Giertz rib
sheath
   angioplasty
   arterial
   catheter
   check-valve
   Cook transseptal
   Cordis
   femoral artery
   French
   guiding
   Hemaquet
   introducer
   Mullins
   Mullins transseptal
   peel-away
   rectus
   Silastic
   tearaway
   transseptal
   USCI angioplasty guiding
   vascular
   venous
sheath and side-arm
sheath with side-arm adapter
sheath-dilator, Mullins transseptal
sheathless insertion technique
sheepskin boot
Sheffield exercise test protocol
Sheffield modification of Bruce
   treadmill protocol
Sheffield treadmill exercise protocol
Sheldon catheter

shell, ejection
shepherd's hook or crook deformity
Shibley sign
shift
   mediastinal
   ST segment
   superior frontal axis
shift to the left (white blood cells)
shift to the right (white blood cells)
shifting pacemaker syndrome
Shiley guiding catheter
Shiley-Ionescu catheter
Shiley tracheotomy tube
Shimazaki area-length method
shivering
SHJR4s (side-hole Judkins right,
   curve 4 French, short)
shock
   advanced cardiogenic
   bacteremic
   biphasic
   biphasic electrical
   cardiogenic
   circulatory
   committed defibrillation
   DC electrical
   diastolic
   defibrillation
   distributive
   40 joule rescue
   hemorrhagic
   hypovolemic
   initial
   joule
   noncardiogenic
   obstructive
   pleural
   pneumonia-induced septic
   postcardiotomy
   postoperative
   profound
   prolonged

shock *(cont.)*
  QRS synchronized
  rescue
  septic
  sequential monophasic
  simultaneous
  spurious
  toxic
  vasogenic
  viremic
shock blocks
shocking electrode
shocking lead
shock lung
shock lung syndrome
shocky appearance
Shoemaker rib shears
Shone anomaly
Shone syndrome
short P-Q interval
short P-R interval
short rib-polydactyly syndrome
Short syndrome
short-acting bronchodilators
short-axis parasternal view
short-axis plane
short-axis plane on echocardiography
short-axis slice
short-axis view
shortening
  fractional myocardial
  mean rate of circumferential
shortness of breath (SOB)
shortness of breath at rest
shortness of breath with low-level
  exercise
short pulse
shortwindedness
shots, guiding
shoulder-hand syndrome
shoulder of the heart
shower of echoes

Shprintzen velocardiofacial syndrome
shrinkage, graft
shudder, carotid
shudder of carotid arterial pulse
shuffling friction rub
shunt
  aorta to pulmonary artery
  aorticopulmonary
  aortopulmonary
  apicoaortic
  arteriovenous (A-V)
  ascending aorta to pulmonary
    artery
  bidirectional
  Blalock
  Blalock-Taussig
  Buselmeier
  cardiac
  cardiovascular
  Davidson
  descending aorta-pulmonary artery
  descending thoracic aorta to
    pulmonary artery
  dialysis
  extracardiac
  extracardiac right-to-left
  Glenn
  Gore-Tex
  Gott
  Holter
  intracardiac
  intracardiac right-to-left
  intracardial
  intrapericardial aorticopulmonary
  intrapulmonary
  ISCI
  Javid
  Javid endarterectomy
  left-to-right
  modified Blalock-Taussig
  net
  peritoneovenous

shunt *(cont.)*
  portacaval
  portasystemic vascular
  Potts
  Pruitt-Inahara carotid
  Quinton-Scribner
  reversed (right-to-left)
  right-to-left (reversed)
  subclavian artery to pulmonary
    artery
  subclavian-pulmonary
  Sundt
  supracardiac
  systemic-pulmonary artery
  vena cava to pulmonary artery
  venoarterial
  ventriculoatrial
  ventriculopleural
  Wakabaushi
  Waterston
  Waterston-Cooley
shunted blood
shunt flow
  anatomic
  physiologic
  relative
shunting
  aortopulmonary
  atrial right-to-left
  central aortopulmonary
  intracardiac
  intrapulmonary
  venoarterial
shunting of blood
  left-to-right
  marked
  right-to-left
shunt reversal
shutdown, renal
shuttle technique, bronchoscopic
Shy-McGee-Drager syndrome
SI (sinus irregularity)

SI (stroke index)
sibilant rales
sibilant rhonchi
sicca
  laryngitis
  pericarditis
sickle cell anemia
sickle cell–thalassemia disease
sickle cell trait
sickle chest syndrome
sicklemia
sickling test
sickness
  acute mountain
  altitude
  decompression
  hypobarism-acute mountain
  mountain
sick sinus node
sick sinus syndrome (SSS)
  extrinsic
  intrinsic
SICOR (computer-assisted cardiac
  catheter recording system)
side-arm adapter, sheath with
side-arm pressure port
side-biting clamp
side branch occlusion
side-by-side transposition of great
  arteries
side-hole catheter
siderosis, welder's
siderotica, pneumoconiosis
sidewinder catheter
side-to-side anastomosis
SIDS (sudden infant death syndrome)
Siemens-Albis bicycle ergometer
Siemens electrode
Siemens-Elema AB pulse transducer
  probe
Siemens-Elema pacemaker
Siemens-Pacesetter pacemaker

Siemens PTCA/open heart table
Siemens Servo 900C ventilator
sieve, vena caval
Siewert syndrome
sighing
sighing breathing
sighing dyspnea
sigmoid omentum
sign
    Abrahams
    ace of spades (on angiogram)
    amputation
    angel wing
    antler (on x-ray)
    aortic arch aneurysm
    aortic nipple
    apical cap
    applesauce
    Auenbrugger
    Baccelli (of pleural effusion)
    bagpipe
    Bamberger
    Becker
    Bethea
    Biermer
    Biot
    Bird
    Bouillaud
    Bozzolo
    Branham
    Branham arteriovenous fistula
    Braunwald
    Broadbent
    Broadbent inverted
    Brockenbrough
    Brockenbrough-Braunwald
    Cardarelli
    cardinal
    cardiorespiratory
    carotid string
    Carvallo
    Castellino

sign *(cont.)*
    Cegka
    Claybrook
    clenched fist
    Corrigan
    cortical
    coughing
    crescent
    Cruveilhier
    cuff
    D'Amato
    de la Camp
    Delbet
    Delmege
    de Musset (aortic aneurysm)
    de Mussey (pleurisy)
    d'Espine
    Dorendorf
    Drummond
    Duroziez
    E (on x-ray)
    Ebstein
    Ellis
    Ewart
    Federici
    figure 3
    finger tip
    Fischer
    Fleischner
    focal neurologic
    Frank
    Franz
    Friedreich
    Fürbringer
    Gerhardt
    Glasgow
    gloved finger
    gooseneck (on x-ray)
    Grancher
    Greene
    Grocco
    Grossman

sign *(cont.)*
Gunn crossing
Hall
Hamman
Hamman pneumopericardium
Heim-Kreysig
Hill
Homans
Hoover
Hope
Huchard
Jaccoud
Jackson
jugular
Jürgensen
Karplus
Katz-Wachtel
Kellock
knuckle
Korányi
Korányi-Grocco
Kussmaul
Kussmaul venous
Laënnec
Lancisi
Landolfi
Levine
liver-jugular
Livierato
Livierato abdomino-cardiac
Mahler
Mannkopf
McGinn-White
Meltzer
Moschcowitz (of arterial occlusive
    disease)
Müller (Mueller) aortic
    regurgitation
Musset (de Musset)
Nicaladoni-Branham
Oliver-Cardarelli
ominous

sign *(cont.)*
Osler
pad
patent bronchus
Paul
Perez
Pfuhl
Pfuhl-Jaffé
Pins
plumb-line
Potain
Pott
Pottenger
premonitory
Prevel
Prussian helmet
Quénu-Muret
Quincke
rabbit ear
railroad track
reversed 3 (on x-ray)
Rivero-Carvallo
Riviere
Robertson
Rotch
Rothschild
Sabathie
Sanders
Sansom
Schepelmann
Schick
scimitar
Seitz
Shapiro
Shibley
Skoda
Smith
spinal
square-root
Sterles
Sternberg
3

sign *(cont.)*
  trapezius ridge
  Traube aortic regurgitation
  vein
  vital
  Weill
  Westermark
  Williams
  Williamson
  wind sock (echocardiogram)
  Wintrich
signal
  Doppler
  magnetic resonance
  mosaic-jet
signal-averaged electrocardiogram
  (SaECG)
signal blooming
signal dephasing
signal intensity
signal magnification
signal void
signature, echo
signif (significant)(ly)
significant axis deviation
significant, clinically
significant residual deficit
significant sequelae
Sigvaris compression stockings
Silastic bead embolization
Silastic catheter
Silastic electrode casing
Silastic H.P. tissue expander
Silastic loop
Silastic sheath
Silastic tape
Silastic tubing
Silastic vessel loop
"sil-ee-um" (psyllium)
silent ischemia
silent mitral stenosis
silent myocardial infarction

silent ischemia
silent patent ductus arteriosus
silent regurgitation
silhouette
  cardiac (large thymus shadow
    obscuring)
  enlarged cardiac
  luminal
  roentgenographic
  widened cardiac
silhouette image
silhouette technique
silicoarthritis
silicone dioxide inhalation
silicone rubber, vulcanizing
Silicore catheter
silicosis
  complicated
  conglomerate
  infective
  non-nodular
  rheumatoid lung
  simple
  simple nodular
silicotic fibrosis of lung
silicotic lung
silicotic mediastinitis
silicotic nodule with central necrosis
silicotic visceral pleura
silicotuberculosis
silk sutures
Silk guide wire
silo-filler's disease
silo-filler's lung
silver finisher's lung
silver polisher's lung
Silver-Russell syndrome
Silver syndrome
Silverman II syndrome
silver wire effect
silver wiring
Silvester artificial respirations

SIMA (single internal mammary
  artery) reconstruction
Simmons-type sidewinder catheter
Simon foci
Simon nitinol percutaneous IVC filter
simple acroparesthesia
simple arteriovenous anastomosis
simple arteriovenular anastomosis
simple rougeur (erythema)
simple silicosis
simplex, xanthoma tuberosum
Simplus catheter
Simplus PE/t dilatation catheter
Simpson atherectomy
Simpson atherectomy catheter
Simpson atherectomy device, PET
  balloon
Simpson Coronary AtheroCath (SCA)
  system
Simpson method to calculate LV
  volume and LVEF
Simpson peripheral AtheroCath
Simpson-Robert catheter
Simpson rule method for ventricular
  volume
Simpson rule volume method
Simpson Ultra-Low Profile II balloon
  catheter
simultaneous balloon inflation
simultaneous bilateral spontaneous
  pneumothorax (SBSP)
simultaneous individual stapling (SIS)
simultaneous pacing and coronary
  blood flow measurement
simultaneous pacing and coronary
  sinus lactate sampling
simultaneous recording
simultaneous shocks
simultaneous waveforms, truncated
  exponential
SIMV (synchronized intermittent
  mandatory ventilation)

sine-wave pattern on electrocardiogram
Singh-Vaughn-Williams classification
  of arrhythmias
single atrium
single atrium syndrome
single-bore cannula
single-cannula atrial cannulation
single-chamber pacing
single-channel ECG
single extrastimuli
single-lung transplantation
single-outlet heart
single pleurisy
single second heart sound
single-slice long-axis tomograms
Singleton-Merten syndrome
single ventricle
single ventricle syndrome
single ventricle with pulmonic stenosis
single-vessel disease
single-vessel runoff
Singley forceps
singultus
sinistrocardia
sinoatrial (SA)
sinoatrial block
sinoatrial branch
sinoatrial bundle in heart
sinoatrial conduction time (SACT)
sinoatrial exit block
sinoatrial heart block
sinoatrial node (SA or S-A node)
    Flack
    Koch
sinoatrial node artery
sinoatrial node dysfunction
sinoatrial node infarction
sinoatrial rhythm
sinoauricular heart block
sinoauricular node
sinobronchitis

sinotubular junction
sinus
  accessory
  aortic
  aortic valve
  carotid
  coronary (CS)
  coronary (of Valsalva)
  distal coronary (DCS)
  left coronary
  middle coronary (MCS)
  noncoronary
  oblique
  pericardial
  Petit
  proximal coronary (PCS)
  pulmonary
  subeustachian
  transverse
  Valsalva
  venous
sinus arrest
sinus aneurysm, aortic
sinus arrhythmia
sinus beat, post-PVC
sinus bradycardia
sinus cycle length (SCL)
sinus exit block
sinus impulse
sinus-initiated QRS complex
sinus irregularity (SI)
sinusitis-bronchiectasis syndrome
sinus mechanism
sinus nodal reentry
sinus node automaticity
sinus node depression
sinus node dysfunction
sinus node recovery time, corrected
sinus node reentry
sinus of Morgagni
sinus of pulmonary trunk

sinus of Valsalva
sinus of venae cavae
sinusoidal irregular rhythm
sinusoids
sinus pause
sinus retroperfusion, coronary
sinus rhythm, normal
sinus rhythm return
sinus segment
sinus septum
sinus slowing
sinus tachycardia
sinus venarum cavarum
sinus venosus defect
sinus venosus syndrome
sinus venous defect
sirolimus
SIS (simultaneous individual stapling)
  lobectomy
site
  arrhythmogenic
  de-airing
site of maximal intensity
sitting-up view
situs
  atrial
  D-loop ventricular
  L-loop ventricular situs
situs ambiguus of atria
situs atrialis solitus
situs concordance
situs inversus totalis
situs solitus
  atrial
  visceral
situs viscerum inversus
sixth intercostal space
60° left anterior oblique projection
sizer, prosthetic valve
sizing, balloon
Sjögren syndrome

skeletal emphysema
skin blanching with pressure
skin prick test, DPT-positive
skin, taut
skin testing
skin wheal (*not* weal)
skin wheal diameter
Skinny dilatation catheter
Skinny over-the-wire balloon catheter
skipped beat
skipping a heartbeat
skodaic bruit
skodaic resonance
skodaic tympany
Skoda sign
sl (slight)(ly)
slate-gray cyanosis
slave balloon
slaved programmed electrical
    stimulation
slaved PS
SLE (systemic lupus erythematosus)
sleep apnea, obstructive
sleep dysfunction
slew rate (SR)
slice
    apical short-axis
    basal short-axis
    horizontal long-axis
    mid-ventricular short-axis
    short-axis
    tomographic
    vertical long-axis
slice format
sliding plasty
sling
    pericardial
    pulmonary artery
    vascular
sling ring complex
Slinky catheter

slip-in connection
slipping rib syndrome
slitlike costomediastinal recess
slitlike lumen
slitlike opening
slitlike orifice
slit-shaped vessel lumen
sliver of aneurysmal wall
SLMD (symptomatic left main
    disease)
slope
    closing (on echo)
    D to E (of mitral valve)
    decreased E to F (E-F)
    disappearance
    E to F (of mitral valve)
    flat diastolic
    flattened E to F
    opening (on echo)
    ST/HR (ST segment/heart rate)
slope of valve opening
slot blot analysis
sloughing of skin from necrosis
slow-channel blocking drugs
slow-fast atrioventricular node reentry
    tachycardia
slow-fast tachycardia
slow filling wave
slow-flow lesions
slow-flow malformation
slow-flow vascular anomaly
slowing of electrical conduction
slowing of heart rate
slow inspiration, inhalation by
slow-pathway conduction
slow-pathway modification
slow-reacting substance of anaphylaxis
    (SRS-A)
SLP (systolic pressure determination)
sludging of blood
sluggishly flowing blood

slush
ice
topical cooling with ice
SM (systolic murmur)
SMA (Sequential Multiple Analyzer)
chemistry panel (SMA-6,
SMA-12, SMA-17, SMA-20)
albumin
alkaline phosphatase
ALT (alanine aminotransferase)
(formerly SGPT)
AST (aspartate aminotransferase)
(formerly SGOT)
BUN (blood urea nitrogen)
calcium
cholesterol
creatinine
glucose
LDH (lactic dehydrogenase)
phosphorus
SGOT (now AST)
SGPT (now ALT)
sodium
total protein
triglyceride
uric acid
SMA (superior mesenteric artery)
small airway dysfunction
small airways stretch receptors
small airways study, peripheral
small aorta syndrome
small cardiac vein
small-cell carcinoma of the lung
small-cell lung cancer (SCLC)
small cuff syndrome
small defibrillating patch
small feminine aorta
small-lunged emphysema
Small Particle Aerosol Generator
nebulizer
small patch lead
small rake retractor

small saphenous vein
small water-hammer pulse
SMAP (systemic mean arterial
pressure)
smart defibrillator
SmartNeedle
smear, fungal
Smec balloon catheter
Smeloff-Cutter ball-cage prosthetic
valve
Smeloff prosthetic valve
Smith-Lemli-Opitz syndrome
Smith-Magenis syndrome
Smith murmur
Smith scissors
Smith sign
smoke inhalation
smokelike echoes
smoker respiratory syndrome
smoker's cough
smoking, pack-years of cigarette
smooth glistening membrane
smooth muscle, reactive disease
SMT (septomarginal trabeculum)
Sn-mesoporphyrin (SnMP)
Sn-protoporphyrin
snake graft
snap
high-pitched opening
mitral opening
opening (OS)
palpable opening
valvular
snare, caval
sneezing
frequent
paroxysmal
repeated
repetitive
staccato
Snider match test for pulmonary
ventilation

sniffles
snorer, nonapneic
snowman deformity
Snowden-Pencer forceps
Snowden-Pencer scissors
snowman appearance of heart
   (on x-ray)
snowplow effect
snowplow occlusion
SNRT (sinus node recovery time)
snuff taker's pituitary disease
snugged down, suture
SO$_2$ (oxygen saturation)
soaked in thrombin, coil
soap bubble appearance of exudate
SOB (shortness of breath)
sodium
   decreased exchangeable
   erythrocyte
sodium channel blocker
sodium concentration, 24-hour urine
sodium content of foods
sodium-induced asthma
sodium nitroprusside
sodium pertechnetate Tc 99m
sodium retention
sodium-restricted diet
soft friction rub
SOF-T guide wire
soft heart sounds
Softip diagnostic catheter
soft murmur (low grade)
Softouch guiding catheter
soft pulse
Softrac
soldier's heart syndrome
soldier's patches of pericardium
soldier's spot
soleal vein
soleus muscle
solid edema of lung
solitary lung nodule

solitary mass
solitary pulmonary nodule
solitus
   atrial situs
   situs
   visceral situs
Solo catheter with Pro/Pel coating
Solomon syndrome
solution (see *medications*)
   albumin
   antibiotic
   balanced salt
   bibiotic
   cardioplegic
   cold blood hyperkalemic
      cardioplegic
   cold cardioplegic
   cold lactated Ringer's
   cold topical saline
   cooling
   colloid
   crystalloid cardioplegic
   dextran and saline
   dextran, saline, papaverine, and
      heparin
   fixative
   hand-agitated
   hemostatic
   heparinized saline
   hyperkalemic crystalloid
      cardioplegic
   hyperosmotic
   ice slush
   ice-cold physiologic
   intracellular-like, calcium-bearing
      crystalloid (ICS)
   leukocyte-depleted terminal blood
      cardioplegic
   normal saline (NS)
   papaverine
   physiologic
   potassium chloride

solution *(cont.)*
    priming
    saline
    uncrystallized cardioplegic
somatic symptoms
somatic tremor
somatomedin C
somatostatin
somatotropin-releasing hormone
somnolence
Sondergaard cleft (interatrial groove)
Sones arteriography technique
Sones brachial cutdown technique
Sones cardiac catheter
Sones cardiac catheterization
Sones Cardio-Marker catheter
Sones cineangiography technique
Sones coronary arteriography
Sones coronary cineangiography
Sones guide wire
Sones Hi-Flow catheter
Sones selective coronary arteriography
sonicated albumin microbubbles
sonicated contrast medium
Sonifer sonicating system
sonogram, -graphy
sonography, Acuson computed
sonolucent area or zone
sonorous rales
sonorous rhonchi
Sonos 500 2.5 MHz ultrasonographic
    transducer
Sorin pacemaker
Sorin prosthetic valve
soroche
SOS guide wire
Soto USCI balloon
souffle
    cardiac
    continuous mammary
    funic
    funicular

souffle *(cont.)*
    mammary (sound on auscultation)
    systolic mammary
sound (see also *bruit, fremitus,*
    murmur, rale)
    abnormal heart
    absent breath
    adventitious breath
    adventitious heart
    adventitious lung
    A₂ (aortic closure) heart
    amphoric breath
    aortic ejection
    aortic second
    atrial
    atrial gallop
    auscultatory
    bandbox
    Beatty-Bright friction
    bell
    bellows
    booming diastolic rumble
    bottle
    brass
    breath
    bronchial breath
    bronchovesicular breath
    cannon
    cat mewing
    cavernous breath
    clapping
    clear ringing musical note
    cogwheel breath
    coin
    cracked-pot sound
    crackling
    diastolic
    discrete
    distant breath
    distant heart
    dull wooden nonmusical note
    eddy

sound *(cont.)*
  ejection (E)
  faint breath
  filing
  first heart (S_1)
  fixed splitting of second heart
  flapping
  flapping rustle
  fourth heart (S_4)
  friction
  gallop
  heart
  hippocratic
  humming top
  inspiratory-expiratory breath
  Korotkoff heart
  light crackling
  M_1 (mitral valve closure) heart
  mammary souffle
  metallic
  muffled breath
  muffled heart
  new leather
  P_2 (pulmonic closure) heart
  pacemaker heart
  paradoxical splitting of second heart
  paradoxically split S_2
  parchment
  parchment rubbing
  peacock
  percussion
  pericardial friction
  physiologic heart
  physiologic splitting of second heart
  physiologic third heart
  pistol-shot
  pistol-shot femoral
  pleuritic
  popping
  prominent third
  prosthetic valve

sound *(cont.)*
  pulmonary component of second heart
  pulmonic ejection
  rasping
  rattling
  reduced
  reduced breath
  ringing
  rippling
  rubbing
  rustle of silk
  rustling
  S_1 (first heart sound)
  S_2 (second heart sound)
  S_3 (third heart sound)
  S_4 (fourth heart sound)
  sail
  sawing
  second heart (S_2)
  second pulmonic
  shaking
  single second heart
  snapping
  souffle (heart puffing sound)
  splashing
  split
  split apical first
  succussion
  summation (SS)
  suppressed
  systolic ejection
  systolic grating
  T_1 (tricuspid valve closure) heart
  tambour (drum)
  third heart (S_3)
  tick-tack
  to-and-fro
  transitory
  tubular breath
  tumor plop heart
  tympanitic

sound *(cont.)*
  ubiquitous
  valvular ejection
  ventricular filling (third heart
    sound)
  ventricular gallop
  vesicular breath
  water-wheel
  weak heart
  white
  widely split second heart
  wood
sound reflector
source, defibrillator power
Southern blot analysis or test
Southern blot hybridization
Southwestern blot test
S/P (status post)
space
  anatomical dead
  antecubital
  apical air (on x-ray)
  Burns
  dead
  echo-free
  epicardial
  fifth intercostal
  first intercostal
  fourth intercostal
  free pericardial
  His perivascular
  Holzknecht
  intercellular
  intercostal
  interpleural
  interstitial
  intravascular
  left fifth intercostal space
  left intercostal (LICS)
  peribronchial alveolar
  pericardial
  pleural

space *(cont.)*
  Poiseuille
  popliteal
  posterior septal
  retrocardiac
  retropancreatic preaortic
  right first intercostal
  right second intercostal
  second intercostal
  seventh intercostal
  sixth intercostal
  third intercostal
space-occupying lesions
spade-shaped valvotome
sparkling appearance of myocardium
spasm
  bronchial
  catheter-induced
  catheter-induced coronary artery
  coronary
  coronary artery (CAS)
  diffuse arteriolar
  inspiratory
  postbypass
  respiratory
  vascular
  venous
spasm of bronchial smooth muscles
spasmodic croup
spasmodic rhinorrhea
spastic contractions
spastic heart
spatula, spatulated, spatulating
SPCA (serum prothrombin conversion
  accelerator)
specificity, sensing
specimen collecting device
speckle, blood
speckled pattern
SPECT (single photon emission
  computed tomography)
SPECT thallium scan

SPECT thallium scintigram
SPECT thallium test
SPECT tomography
Spectraflex pacemaker
spectral Doppler
spectral analysis
spectral pattern
Spectranetics excimer laser for
    coronary angioplasty
Spectraprobe-Max probe
Spectrax programmable Medtronic
    pacemaker
Spectrax SXT pacemaker
spectroscopy
    fluorescence
    magnetic resonance
    NMR (nuclear magnetic resonance)
    proton
specular echo
Speedy balloon catheter
spell
    anginal
    cyanotic hypoxic
    fainting
    hypercyanotic
    hypoxemic
    hypoxic
    pallid breath-holding
    sneezing
    syncopal
    tetrad
    violent sneezing
Spencer stitch curved scissors
Spens syndrome
sphenoidal sinusitis
spherical lesion
spherical mass
spherocytosis, hereditary
sphincter incontinence
sphingolipidosis
sphygmography
sphygmomanometer, cuff

spider angiomata
spider cells
spider nevus (pl. nevi)
spider x-ray view
spike
    atrial
    H and H' (H prime)
    sensing
    wave
spike-and-dome configuration
spike-dome configuration
spike-Q interval
spiking fever
spin density
spin-echo imaging sequence
spin-echo sequence
spinal needle
spinal sign in pleurisy
spindle, aortic
spindle-shaped arterial
spindly limbs
Spinhaler turbo-inhaler
spinocerebellar ataxia
spiral dissection
spiral position
spiraling dissection
spirals, Curschmann
spirochetal infection
spirochetal myocarditis
spirometer
    incentive
    Tissot
spirometry
    FEV$_1$ (forced expiratory volume
        in 1 second)
    full-volume loop
    FVC (forced vital capacity)
    MMEF (mean maximal expiratory
        flow)
spirometry after bronchodilator
spirometry before bronchodilator
spitting up blood

splanchnic vasculature
splanchnic vessels
splashing bruit
splash, succussion
splenic flexure syndrome
splenic follicular arteriolitis
splenic hilar vasculitis
splenomegaly
  Opitz thrombophlebitic
  persistent
  postcardiotomy lymphocytic
splenorenal anastomosis
splenorenal arterial bypass graft
splint, pneumatic
splinter hemorrhage
splinting
splinting of the chest
splinting on deep breathing
splinting respirations
splint-type tear
split apical first sound
splitting
  audible
  fixed
  narrow expiratory
  narrow inspiratory
  paradoxic
  paradoxic respiratory
  physiologic
  plaque
  reversed
  widened respiratory
splitting of S_1 or S_2 heart sounds
splitting of first heart sound, wide
splitting of second heart sound, wide
sponge
  Collostat hemostatic
  4 x 4
  laparotomy
  papaverine-soaked
  Ray-Tec
  stick

sponge and needle counts
sponge dissector
spongiosa of mitral valve
spontaneous breathing
spontaneous cardioversion
spontaneous closure of defect
spontaneous coronary artery dissection
  (SCAD)
spontaneous echo contrast
spontaneous infantile ductal aneurysm
spontaneous pneumothorax
spontaneous regression
spontaneous remission
spontaneous subsidence
spontaneous tension pneumothorax
spontaneous transient vasoconstriction
spoon forceps
spoonlike protrusion of leaflets
sporadic hypertriglyceridemia
spores, fungal hyphae and
spot
  Brushfield
  cold
  hot
  milk
  Roth
  soldier's
  Tardieu
spot-film fluorography
spray-as-you-go anesthesia technique
spray, lidocaine
spreader
  Bailey rib
  Burford rib
  Burford-Finochietto rib
  Davis rib
  DeBakey rib
  Favaloro-Morse rib
  Finochietto rib
  Haight rib
  Harken rib
  Lemmon sternal

spreader *(cont.)*
  Lilienthal rib
  Medicon
  Miltex rib
  Morse sternal
  Nelson rib
  Rehbein rib
  Reinhoff-Finochietto rib
  Tuffier rib
  Weinberg rib
  Wilson rib
Spring catheter with Pro/Pel coating
spring-loaded vascular stent
S-QRS interval
spur, calcific
spurious findings
spurious polycythemia
spurious shocks
sputum (pl. sputa)
  abundant
  albuminoid
  blood-flecked
  blood-tinged
  bloody
  brick-red in color
  brown
  chunky
  clear
  clear viscous
  copious
  dark
  fetid
  foul-tasting
  frothy at the top (of layered)
  gelatinous
  gelatinous mottled
  globular
  grayish
  green
  green-yellow
  greenish and turbid in the middle
    (of layered)

sputum *(cont.)*
  greenish-yellow
  icteric
  moss-agate
  mucoid
  mucopurulent
  nonfetid
  nummular
  opalescent
  pink
  pinkish
  prune juice
  purulent
  putrid
  red-streaked
  reddish brown
  ropy
  rubbery
  rusty
  scant, scanty
  tenacious
  thick
  thick with pus at the bottom (of
    layered)
  viscid
  viscous
  watery
  white
  whitish
  yellow
  yellowish-green
sputum aeroginosum
sputum cruentum
sputum culture and sensitivity
sputum eosinophilia
sputum induction
sputum of bronchial asthma
sputum-producing cough
squamous cell carcinoma of lung
squamous endothelium
squamous epithelium, stratified
squamous metaplasia

squared-off thorax
square-root sign in chronic constrictive
   pericarditis
squatting and prompt standing
squatting posture
squatting to relieve dyspnea
squeaking murmur
squeezing pain
squeezing sensation
SR (slew rate)
Srb syndrome (no vowel)
SRS-A (slow-reacting substance of
   anaphylaxis)
SRT (segmented ring tripolar) lead
SS (summation sound)
SS-A (Ro) antibody
SS-B (La) antibody
SSS (sick sinus syndrome)
SSS (subclavian steal syndrome)
ST (sinus tachycardia))
stab wound incision
stab wound, separate
stabilized human umbilical vein,
   Biograft
stabilized human umbilical vein graft
stable angina
stable, hemodynamically
stable vital signs
staccato sneezing
Stack autoperfusion balloon
Stack perfusion coronary dilatation
   catheter
stacked tomograms
stage
   congestion
   resolution
staged closure
Stage I–VII of Bruce protocol
stagnant hypoxia
stain
   acid-fast bacilli (AFB)
   Gram

stain (cont.)
   Pneumocystis carinii pneumonia
      (PCP)
stainless steel mesh stent
stainless steel staples
stainless steel wire suture
staircase phenomenon
Stairmaster mobile stairs
stamina
STA-MCA (superficial temporal
   artery-middle cerebral artery)
   bypass procedure
standard Bruce protocol
standard calorimetric assays
standard deviation (SD)
standard error (SE)
standardization wave
standard Lehman catheter
standard limb leads
standard modality
standard patch lead
standby pacemaker
standby, pump
standby rate
standstill
   atrial
   cardiac
   ventricular
Stanford classification of aortic
   dissection
Stanford left ventricular bioptome
Stanford treadmill exercise protocol
Stanicor pacemaker
stannosis
stannous pyrophosphate
staphcidal drug
staphylococcal bacteremia
staphylococcal myocardiits
staphylococcal pericarditis
staphylococcal pharyngitis
staphylococcal pleurisy
staphylococcal pneumonia

staphylococcal pneumonitis
staphylococci (pl. of staphylococcus)
staphylococcus
  coagulase-negative
  coagulase-positive
  Staphylococcus aureus infection
stapler
  Auto-Suture surgical
  Auto-Suture Premium TA-55
    surgical
  endoscopic articulating (EAS)
  endoscopic multifeed (EMS)
  TA-90
staples
  stainless steel
  TA-30 4.5 mm
Starcam camera
Starling curve
Starling law of the heart
Starling mechanism
Starnes operation
Starr-Edwards aortic valve prosthesis
Starr-Edwards ball valve prosthesis
Starr-Edwards cardiac valve prosthesis
Starr-Edwards disk valve prosthesis
Starr-Edwards mitral prosthesis
Starr-Edwards pacemaker
Starr-Edwards Silastic valve
Starr-Edwards valve prosthesis
star-shaped vessel lumen
stasis dermatitis
stasis edema
stasis of blood flow
stasis of blood in veins
stasis skin changes
stasis ulcers
stasis, venous
state
  hypercoagulable
  hyperdynamic
  inotropic
Statham electromagnetic flowmeter

Statham strain-gauge transducer
static exercise
static gangrene
static lung
static lung compliance (C_{STAT})
stationary arterial waves
stationary bicycle
STAT shock delivery
status
  acid-base
  ambulatory
  DNAR (Do Not Attempt
    Resuscitation)
  DNR (Do Not Resuscitate)
  functional
  no CRP
  ventricular
status anginosus
status asthmaticus
status dysraphicus
status post (S/P)
stay sutures
ST depression
  downsloping
  horizontal
  reciprocal
steal
  arterial
  coronary artery
  subclavian
steal in angio-osteohypertrophic
  syndrome
steal phenomenon
steam autoclaved
Steell murmur
steep left anterior oblique view
steep Trendelenburg position
steerable catheter
steerable electrode catheter
steering, electronic independent beam
Steerocath catheter
Steidele complex

Steidele syndrome
Steinert disease
stellar nevus
stellate ganglion block
stellectomy
Stellite ring material of prosthetic
    valve
stem bronchus
Stemphylium lanuginosum
stenocardia
stenoses (pl. of stenosis)
stenosing ring of left atrium
stenosis
    acquired mitral
    American Heart Association
        classification of
    aortic (AS)
    aortic valvular
    aortoiliac
    atypical aortic valve
    bicuspid valvular aortic
    branch pulmonary
    bronchial
    buttonhole mitral
    calcific aortic
    calcific bicuspid valvular
    calcific mitral
    calcific senile aortic valvular
    calcific valvular
    carotid artery
    common pulmonary vein
    congenital aortic
    congenital aortic valvular
    congenital mitral
    congenital pulmonary
    congenital subaortic
    congenital subvalvular aortic
    congenital supravalvular aortic
    congenital tricuspid
    congenital valvular aortic
    coronary artery
    coronary luminal

stenosis *(cont.)*
    coronary ostial
    critical
    critical coronary
    critical valvular
    cross-sectional area
    culprit
    diffuse
    discrete
    discrete subaortic
    discrete subvalvular aortic (DSAS)
    dynamic subaortic
    eccentric
    external iliac
    femoropopliteal atheromatous
    fibromuscular subaortic
    fishmouth mitral
    fixed-orifice aortic
    flow-limiting
    focal
    focal eccentric
    granulation
    hemodynamically significant
    high-grade
    hypercalcemia supravalvular aortic
    hypertrophic infundibular
        subpulmonic
    hypertrophic subaortic
    idiopathic hypertrophic subaortic
        (IHSS)
    infrainguinal bypass
    infrarenal
    infundibular
    infundibular pulmonary
    infundibular pulmonic
    infundibular subpulmonic
    innominate artery
    interrenal
    linear
    luminal
    membranous
    membranous subvalvular aortic

stenosis *(cont.)*
  mitral (MS)
  mitral valve
  multifocal short
  muscular subaortic
  napkin-ring
  noncalcified
  noncalcified coronary
  noncritical
  nonrheumatic aortic
  nonrheumatic valvular aortic
  ostial
  peripheral arterial
  peripheral pulmonary artery
    (PPAS)
  peripheral pulmonic
  post-PTCA
  postangioplasty
  preangioplasty
  pulmonary
  pulmonary artery
  pulmonary artery branch
  pulmonary valve
  pulmonary valvular
  pulmonary vein
  pulmonic (PS)
  pulmonic (with intact ventricular
    septum)
  relative mitral
  renal artery
  rheumatic aortic
  rheumatic aortic valvular
  rheumatic mitral
  rheumatic tricuspid
  segmental
  senescent aortic
  severe
  silent mitral
  subaortic
  subclavian artery
  subinfundibular pulmonary
  subpulmonary

stenosis *(cont.)*
  subpulmonic
  subpulmonic infundibular
  subtle mitral
  subvalvar aortic
  subvalvular aortic
  subvalvular congenital aortic
  supra-aortic
  supraclavicular aortic stenosis
  suprarenal
  supravalvar aortic
  supravalvular
  supravalvular aortic (SAS, SVAS)
  supravalvular pulmonic
  tapering
  tight
  tricuspid (TS)
  tricuspid valve
  true mitral
  tubular
  tunnel subaortic
  tunnel subvalvular aortic
  unicusp aortic
  valvar aortic
  valvular aortic
  valvular pulmonic
stenosis area
stenosis diameter
stenosis length
stenosis of coronary orifices
stenosis of saphenous vein
stenosis of unicuspid aortic valve
stenosis with a spastic component
stenotic but patent tricuspid valve
stenotic coronary artery
stenotic isthmus
stenotic lesion
stenotic valve
stent
  activated balloon expandable
    intravascular
  balloon-expandable

stent *(cont.)*
  balloon-expandable flexible coil
  balloon-expandable intravascular
  biodegradable
  coil vascular
  Cordis tantalum
  Dacron
  endoluminal
  Gianturco
  Gianturco-Roubin flexible coil
  heat-expandable
  helical coil
  interdigitating coil
  intravascular
  Medivent vascular
  nitinol thermal memory
  Palmaz balloon-expandable
  Palmaz balloon-expandable iliac
  Palmaz vascular
  Palmaz-Schatz
  Palmaz-Schatz coronary
  polymeric endoluminal paving
  Roubin-Gianturco flexible coil
  Schatz-Palmaz tubular mesh
  self-expanding
  spring-loaded
  spring-loaded vascular
  stainless steel mesh
  Strecker balloon-expandable
  Strecker tantalum
  thermal memory
  Ultraflex self-expanding
  Wallstent spring-loaded
  Wiktor
  wire-mesh self-expandable
  zig-zag
stent deployment
stent embolization
stent expansion
stenting, intracoronary
stent migration
stent-mounted allograft valves

stent-mounted heterograft valve
stentless porcine aortic valve
stentless valve
stent placement, intracoronary
stent recanalization
stent thrombosis
stent-vessel wall contact
stepdown unit
stepped-care antihypertensive regimen
stepup (or step-up)
Steri-Drape
sterilely prepped and draped
Steri-Strips
Sterles sign
sternal angle
sternal angle of Louis
sternal articulations, pain in
sternal border
  left
  lower left
  mid-left
sternal cartilage
sternal edge
sternal joint
sternal lift
sternal marrow
sternal pleural reflection
sternal reflection
sternal splitting
sternal wire suture
Sternberg myocardial insufficiency
Sternberg pericarditis
Sternberg sign in pleurisy
Sterneedle tuberculin test
sternoclavicular angle
sternoclavicular joint
sternoclavicular junction
sternocleidomastoid muscle
sternocleidomastoid retraction
sternocostal joint
sternocostal surface of heart
sternohyoid muscle

sternopericardial ligament
sternothyroid muscle
sternotomy
  median
  midline
  primary median
  secondary median
sternotomy incision
sternum
  anterior bowing of
  burning sensation over
  nonunion of operated
sternum retraction
sternutation
steroid dependent
steroid-eluting active fixation lead
steroidogenesis, adrenal
steroids
  adrenal
  parenteral
stertorous breathing
stertor, respiratory
Stertzer brachial guiding catheter
Stertzer-Myler extension wire
stethoscope
  bell of
  diaphragm of
  nuclear
Stevens-Johnson syndrome
Stewart-Hamilton technique for cardiac
  output
ST/HR slope (ST segment/heart rate)
STI (systolic time interval)
stick (venipuncture or arterial
  puncture)
stick tie
sticky exudate
sticky rales
stiff heart syndrome
stiffness
  lung
  ventricular

stiff noncompliant lungs
stigmata of stroke
Still early systolic murmur
Stille-Crawford clamp
Stille-Giertz rib shears
Stille-Mayo scissors
Still murmur
stimulant, alpha-adrenoceptor
stimulation
  atrial single and double extra-
    inotropic
  programmed electrical (PES)
  programmed ventricular (PVS)
  slaved programmed electrical
  transvenous electrode (of atrium)
  ventricular single and double extrastimulation threshold of pacemaker
stimulator
  Bloom DTU 201 external
  Bloom programmable
stimuli (pl. of stimulus)
  afterpotential
  noxious
  paired
  premature
S-T interval
stippling of lung fields
stitch (see *suture*)
St. Jude bileaflet prosthetic valve
St. Jude composite valved conduit
St. Jude Medical bileaflet valve
St. Jude Medical composite graft
St. Jude valve prosthesis
stockings
  antiembolism
  compression
  elastic
  Jobst
  Jobst-Stride support
  Jobst-Stridette support
  Sigvaris compression
  Stride support

stockings *(cont.)*
  TED (thromboembolic disease)
  thigh-high compression
  Vairox high compression vascular
  VenES II Medical
  Zimmer antiembolism support
Stokes-Adams attack
Stokes-Adams disease
Stokes-Adams syndrome
stoma
  coronary artery
  tracheostomy
stone heart phenomenon
stone heart syndrome
Stoney method
Stoney technique
stony mass
stooped posture
stopcock
stoppage of heart
stored energy
stored ventricular electrogram
Storz needle cannula
straddling atrio-ventricular valves
straddling embolus
straddling of tricuspid valve
straight AP pelvic injection
straight-back syndrome
straight biopsy cup forceps
straight chest tube
straight flush percutaneous catheter
straight Hasson grasper
strain
  left ventricular (LV)
  right ventricular (RV)
  Valsalva
strain gauge, mercury-in-Silastic
straining heart muscle
strain pattern on EKG
strandy pulmonic infiltrate
strap cells
strap muscle

straw, fungus-laden
strategy
  alpha-stat
  pH-stat
stratified clot
stratified squamous epithelium
Strauss method
straw-colored fluid
streaking, coarse
streaks
  atherosclerotic fatty
  retinal angioid
stream, regurgitant
Strecker balloon-expandable stent
Strecker tantalum stent
strep throat
streptococcal carditis
streptococcal empyema
streptococcal M proteins
streptococcal pericarditis
streptococcal pleurisy
streptococcal sore throat
streptococcus (pl. streptococci)
  alpha
  anhemolytic
  beta
  gamma
  group A, B, C (etc.)
  hemolytic
  indifferent
  nonhemolytic
  viridans
Streptococcus (S.)
Streptococcus hemolyticus
Streptococcus mitis
Streptococcus pneumoniae
Streptococcus pyogenes
Streptococcus sanguis
Streptococcus scarlatinae
Streptococcus viridans
streptokinase resistance test
streptokinase thrombolysis

stress
   mechanical
   occupational
   pharmacologic
stress erythrocytosis
stress images
stress imaging
stress management
stress perfusion and rest function by
   sestamibi-gated SPECT
stress test
   dipyridamole thallium
   isometric exercise
   Persantine thallium
   submaximal
stress testing of cardiac response
stress thallium scan
stress thallium-201 myocardial
   imaging
stress ulcer
stress-induced
stress-injected sestamibi-gated SPECT
   with echocardiography
stretch, abnormal airways
STRETCH cardiac device
stretched lung
stricture, anastomotic
Stride support stockings
stridor
   mild to moderate
   postextubation
   respiratory
stridulous breathing
stringlike bands of fibrous tissue
string-of-beads appearance
string sign
strip
   cardiac monitor
   EKG monitor
   felt
   rhythm
   transtelephonic rhythm

stripe, paraspinal pleural
stripper
   Alexander rib
   Babcock vein
   Dunlop thrombus
   Emerson vein
   endarterectomy
   external vein
   internal vein
   Matson rib
   Mayo vein
   Meyer vein
   Nabatoff vein
   olive-tipped
   Trace vein
   vein
   Webb vein
stripper with bullet end
stripping of multiple communicators
stripping of perforators and communicators
stripping, varicose vein
stroke
   cardiogenic embolic
   embolic
   thromboembolic (TE)
stroke distance, Doppler-derived
stroke ejection rate
stroke force
stroke index (SI)
stroke power
stroke syndrome
stroke volume (SV)
   adequate
   augmented
   back
   cardiac
   decreased
   reduced
stroke volume index (SVI)
stroke volume pump
stroke work

stroma
stroma-free hemoglobin solution
Strongyloides stercoralis infection
strongyloidiasis, pulmonary
structural weakness of bronchial wall
 supports
structures
 central hilar
 superior mediastinal
Strully scissors
strut
 tricuspid valve
 valve
 valve outflow
strut chordae
Stryker saw
ST segment abnormality
ST segment alteration
ST (segment) and T wave abnormalities (same as ST-T wave)
ST segment coved
ST segment depressed
ST segment depression
 downsloping
 exercise-induced
 horizontal
 reciprocal
 slight
 upsloping
ST segment displacement
ST segment distortion
ST segment elevated
ST segment elevation
 marked
 slight
ST segment isoelectric
ST segment monitoring
ST segment sagging
ST segment shift
ST segment upsloping
ST segment vector forces

ST-T abnormalities
ST-T wave changes
ST vector
ST wave
Stuart blood coagulation factor
Stuart-Prower blood coagulation factor
Stuart-Prower factor X deficiency
study (see also *procedure, test, trial*)
 APRICOT (aspirin versus coumadin
  in prevention of reocclusion and
  recurrent ischemia after success-
  ful thrombolysis)
 Bogalusa Heart
 cardiac wall motion
 cardiovascular radioisotope scan
  and function
 carotid duplex
 Coronary Artery Surgery (CASS)
 Doppler flow
 electromagnetic blood flow
 electrophysiologic (EP)
 enzyme
 Familial Atherosclerosis Treatment
  (FATS)
 first-pass
 Framingham
 gated blood pool
 GISSI (Italian Group for the Study
  of Survival in Myocardial
  Infarction)
 International (of Infarct Survival)
  (ISIS)
 MILIS (Multicenter Investigation
  for the Limitation of Infarct
  Size)
 Oslo
 parameter
 periorbital Doppler
 PIOPED (Prospective Investigation
  of Pulmonary Embolism
  Diagnosis)

study *(cont.)*
  pull-back
  STILE (Surgery versus Thrombo-
    lysis for Ischemia of the Lower
    Extremity)
  TIMI-IIA (Thrombolysis in
    Myocardial Infarction)
  TIMI-IIB (Thrombolysis in
    Myocardial Infarction)
  TOPS (Treatment of Post-
    Thrombolytic Stenoses)
  virology
  wall motion
stump of a resected bronchus
stump pressure
stunning, myocardial
stuporous
Sturge-Weber syndrome
stylet
  straight
  transseptal
Stylus cardiovascular suture
Stypven time test for deficiency of
  factor X
sub (subendocardial)
subacute allergic pneumonia
subacute bacterial endocarditis (SBE)
subacute bronchopneumonia
subacute cardiac tamponade
subacute constrictive pericarditis
subacute interstitial myocarditis
subacute mountain sickness
subadventitial plane
subadventitial tissue
subannular mattress sutures
subannular placement of sutures
subannular region
subaortic curtain
subaortic glands
subaortic muscle
subaortic resection
subaortic stenosis, discrete

subarachnoid hemorrhage, diffuse
subatmospheric pressure
subcapsular hematoma
subcarina (pl. subcarinae)
subclavia, ansa
subclavian approach for cardiac
  catheterization
subclavian artery
subclavian artery stenosis
subclavian flap aortoplasty (SFA)
subclavian loop
subclavian peel-away sheath
subclavian-pulmonary shunt
subclavian steal syndrome (SSS)
subclavian turndown technique
subclavian vein, blind percutaneous
  puncture of
subclavian vein catheterization
subclavicular approach
subcommissural suture annuloplasty of
  neo-aortic valve
subcortical intracerebral hemorrhage
subcostal approach
subcostal artery
subcostal branch
subcostal nerve
subcostal retractions, mild
subcostal window
subcrepitant rales
subcutaneous array electrode
subcutaneous emphysema
subcutaneous hemangioma
subcutaneous patch
subcutaneous patch electrode
subcutaneous pocket
subcutaneous sutures
subcutaneous tissue
subcutaneous tunnel
subcutaneous veins
subcuticular closure
subcuticular layer
subcuticular skin closure

subendocardial fibroelastosis
subendocardial infarct
subendocardial infarction (SEI)
subendocardial injury
subendocardial ischemia
subendocardial myocardial infarction
subendocardial necrosis
subendocardial resection
subendocardial sclerosis
subendocardium
subendothelial hyalinization
suberosis
   cork worker's
   maple-bark worker's
subeustachian sinus
subfascially
subglottic area
subglottic edema
subinfundibular pulmonary stenosis
subintimal cleavage plane
subintimal dissection
subisthmic coarctation, atypical
subjective symptoms
sublingual nitroglycerin
sublingual varices
submassive pulmonary embolism
submaximal exercise
submaximal exercise test
submaximal stress test
submersion syndrome
submucous resection
submuscular patch lead
suboptimal results
suboptimal runoff
suboptimal visualization
suboptimally visualized
subpectoral implantation of pulse
   generator
subpectoral pocket
subperiosteal resection
subphrenic abscess
subpleural bleb

subpleural curvilinear lines
subpulmonary conus underdevelop-
   ment
subpulmonic fluid
subpulmonic infundibular stenosis
subpulmonic obstruction
subpulmonic outflow
Subramanian clamp
subrectus placement
subsegment of lung
subsegmental bronchus
subsegmental perfusion abnormality
subsegments, right middle lobe
subsidence, spontaneous
substances, paramagnetic
substernal angle
substernal burning discomfort
substernal chest pain
substernal discomfort
substernal pain
substernal retractions
substitute, oxygenated perfluorocarbon
   blood
subtherapeutic theophylline level
subtle mitral stenosis
subtotal graft excision
subtotal lesion
subtraction films, manual
subvalvular aneurysm
subvalvular aortic obstruction
subvalvular aortic stenosis
subvalvular congenital aortic stenosis
subvalvular obstruction
subxiphoid approach
subxiphoid echocardiography view
subxiphoid implantation
subxiphoid incision
subxiphoid view
successful conversion
succussion sound
succussion splash
sucking pneumothorax

Sucquet-Hoyer anastomosis
Sucquet-Hoyer canal
suction
  Frazier
  nasotracheal
suction bottle
suction line, aortic vent
suction tip
  Andrews
  Yankauer
suction-type electrode
sudden blockage of coronary artery
sudden cardiac death (SCD)
sudden death, adult
sudden infant death syndrome (SIDS)
suffocating chest pain
suffocating sensation
suffocating thoracic dystrophy
Sugita right angle aneurysm clamp
Sugiura vascular surgery procedure
  for esophageal varices
suitable candidate
sulcus (pl. sulci)
  atrioventricular
  posterior interventricular
  pulmonary
sulcus terminalis
sulfasalazine-induced pulmonary
  infiltrates
sulfonamides
sulfonylureas
sulfur colloid, technetium bound to
SULP II catheter
Sumida cardioangioscope
summation beat
summation gallop (S_3 and S_4)
summation sound (SS)
summit, ventricular septal
sump catheter
sump drain
sump pump
Sundt-Kees clip for aneurysms

Sundt shunt
Super-9 guiding cardiac device
superdominant left anterior descending
  artery
superfcal femoral artery
superficial breast phlebitis
superficial cardiac dullness
superficial cardiac plexus
superficial crepitation
superficial femoral artery
superficial femoral artery occlusion
superficial femoral vein
superficial posterior compartment
superficial vein
superimposed bronchial infection
superimposed mycoplasma pneumonia
superimposed pulmonary infection
superior border of heart
superior border of rib
superior bronchus
superior caval defect
superior caval obstruction
superior costotransverse ligament
superior epigastric artery
superior genicular artery
superior intercostal artery
superior intercostal vein
superior lobe of lung
superior margin of inferior rib
superior marginal defect
superior mediastinal structures
superior mediastinum
superior mesenteric artery (SMA)
superior mesenteric artery syndrome
superior phrenic branch
superior pulmonary vein
superior segment
superior thoracic aperture
superior thyroid artery
superior vena cava lead
superior vena cava obstruction
superior vena cava, penetrating injury to

superior vena cava syndrome
supernormal conduction
supernormal excitation
superoinferior heart
superolaterally
superoxide dismutase
superselective embolization
SuperStat hemostatic agent
supersystemic pulmonary artery
  pressure
supervene
supine bicycle exercise treadmill
supine hypotensive syndrome
supine hypotensive syndrome of
  pregnancy
supplemental oxygen
supply
  accessory blood
  collateral
support
  hemodynamic
  inotropic
  mechanical circulatory
  mechanical ventilatory
  pump
  temporary percutaneous cardio-
    pulmonary
  ventilatory
supportive therapy
suppressed breath sounds
suppressed cough reflex
suppressed plasma renin activity
suppression
  overdrive
  renin
suppression of arrhythmia
suppression of breath sounds
suppurative pericarditis
suppurative phlebitis
suppurative pleurisy
suppurative pulmonary infection
supra-annular constriction

supra-annular suture ring
supra-aortic ridge
supra-aortic Takayasu arteritis
supra-aortic stenosis
supra-aortic trunk
supracardiac shunt
supracardiac type total anomalous
  venous return
supraceliac aorta
supraceliac aorta-femoral artery
  bypass graft
supraceliac aorta-visceral artery
  bypass graft
supraceliac aortic bypass graft
supraceliac aortofemoral bypass graft
supraclavicular aortic stenosis,
  uncomplicated
supraclavicular lymph nodes
supraclavicular murmur
supraclavicular nerve
supraclavicular node
supraclavicular systolic murmur
supraclavicular triangle
supraclinoid internal carotid artery
supracoronary ridge
supracristal defect
supracristal septal defect
supracristal ventricular defect
supracristal ventricular septal defect
supradiaphragmatic aorta
supraglottic edema
supra-Hisian (or suprahisian) block
supramesocolic
suprapleural membrane
suprarenal aneurysm, mycotic
suprarenal stenosis
suprasternal bulging
suprasternal notch
suprasternal notch incision
suprasternal notch thrill
suprasternal notch view on echocardiogram

suprasternal retraction on inspiration
suprasternal window
supravalvar aortic stenosis syndrome
supravalvar ring
supravalvular aortic stenosis (SAS,
    SVAS)
    Brom repair of
    congenital
supravalvular aortic stenosis syndrome
supravalvular aortogram
supravalvular mitral stenosis
supravalvular pulmonic stenosis
supraventricular arrhythmia
supraventricular crest (SVC)
supraventricular ectopic levels
supraventricular ectopic pacemaker
supraventricular rhythm
supraventricular tachyarrhythmia (SVT)
supraventricular tachycardia (SVT),
    inducible sustained orthodromic
supraventricular tachydysrhythmias
supraventricularis, crista
surface coils
surface cooling initiated by circulating
    water
surface, endothelial
surface-induced deep hypothermia
surface phagocytosis
surface tension of lungs
surfactant
    bovine lavage extract
    heterologous
    homologous
    natural
    pulmonary
    synthetic
surfactant activity
surfactant deficiency
surfactant depletion
surgery (see *operation*)
    invasive
    minimally invasive (MIS)

surgery *(cont.)*
    palliative
    video-assisted thoracic (VATS)
surgical cardiac tamponade
surgical emphysema
surgical extirpation
surgical field
surgical intervention
surgically curable hypertension
surgically induced complete heart
    block
Surgical Nu-Knit
surgical revascularization
surgical venous interruption
Surgicel gauze
Surgidine
Surgilase 150 laser
Surgilase CO$_2$ laser
Surgilene suture
Surgilon suture
Surgitool 200 prosthetic valve
surveillance
susceptible, susceptibility
suspended heart syndrome
sustained anterior parasternal motion
sustained apical impulse
sustained hypertension
sustained left ventricular heave
sustained or nonsustained reciprocating
    tachycardia
Sutter-Smeloff heart valve prosthesis
suture (also *stitch*)
    absorbable
    alternating blue and white mattress
    anchoring
    angle
    atraumatic
    Auto Suture
    basting
    black
    blue and white mattress
    blue and white Tycron

suture *(cont.)*
  braided
  braided silk
  bridle
  buried
  cardiovascular silk
  catgut
  chromic
  chromic catgut
  circular
  circumferential
  coated
  collagen
  continuous
  cotton
  Dacron
  Dacron-bolstered
  deep
  Deklene
  Dermalene
  Dermalon
  Dexon
  Dexon Plus
  double-armed
  doubly ligated
  dural tenting
  end-to-side
  EPTFE (expanded polytetrafluoro-
    ethylene) vascular
  Ethibond
  Ethicon
  Ethiflex
  Ethilon
  everting
  everting mattress
  figure-of-8
  Flexon steel
  Frater
  Gregory stay
  gut
  guy
  heavy silk

suture *(cont.)*
  heavy wire
  horizontal
  horizontal mattress
  imbricating
  intermittent
  interrupted
  interrupted pledgeted
  intracuticular
  inverted
  inverting
  Lembert
  locked
  locking
  loop
  mattress
  mattress-type
  Maxon
  Mersilene
  Mersilene braided nonabsorbable
  monofilament absorbable
  monofilament nylon
  monofilament polypropylene
  nonabsorbable
  noneverting
  Novofil
  Nurolon
  nylon
  over-and-over
  over-and-over whip
  patch-reinforced mattress
  PDS Vicryl
  pericostal
  Perma-Hand
  plain
  plastic
  pledgeted
  pledgeted Ethibond
  pledgeted mattress
  Polydek
  polypropylene
  pop-off

suture *(cont.)*
Potts tie
preplaced
Prolene
pursestring or purse-string
pyroglycolic acid
reabsorbable
retention
running
seromuscular-to-edge
silk
simple
single-armed
skin staples
stainless steel wire
staples
stay
Steri-Strips
sternal wire
stitch
subannular mattress
subcutaneous
subcuticular
Surgilene
Surgilon
synthetic
Teflon
Teflon-pledgeted
Teflon-pledgeted mattress
tenting
Tevdek
Tevdek pledgeted
through-and-through
through-and-through continuous
through-the-wall mattress
Ti-Cron
traction
transfixion
Trumbull
Tycron
U double-barrel

suture *(cont.)*
umbilical tape
undyed
vertical
Vicryl
whipstitch
white
white silk
wire
suture bites
sutureless electrode lead
sutureless myocardial electrode
suture ligature
suture Roticulator
Suture Strip Plus
SV (stroke volume)
SVAS (supravalvular aortic stenosis)
SVC (superior vena cava)
SVC (supraventricular crest)
SVG (saphenous vein graft)
SVI (stroke volume index)
SvO_2 (venous oxygen saturation)
SVPC (supraventricular premature
    contraction)
SVR (systemic vascular resistance)
SVRI (systemic vascular resistance
    index)
SVT (supraventricular tachyarrhythmia)
SVT (supraventricular tachycardia)
swallowed electrode
swallow syncope
swallowing, difficulty
Swan aortic clamp
Swan-Ganz balloon-flotation catheter
Swan-Ganz flow-directed catheter
Swan-Ganz guide wire TD catheter
Swan-Ganz pacing TD catheter
Swan-Ganz pulmonary artery catheter
Swan-Ganz technique for cardiac
    catheterization
Swan-Ganz thermodilution catheter

S wave
  deep
  slurred
  systolic
  wide
sweats, drenching
Sweet sternal punch
swelling, ankle
swelling resolves overnight
SWI (stroke work index)
Swing DR1 DDDR pacemaker
swirling smokelike echoes
swiss roll technique
Swiss cheese appearance
Swiss cheese ventricular septal defect
swollen throat
swollen tissues
Swyer-James syndrome
Swyer-James unilateral hyperlucency
  of lung
Sydenham chorea
Sydenham cough
Symbion cardiac device
Symbion/CardioWest 100-mL total
  artificial heart (TAH)
Symbion J-7 70-mL ventricle total
  artificial heart (TAH)
Symbion Jarvik-7 artificial heart
Symbion pneumatic assist device
Symbios pacemaker
symbolic convention, Van Praagh
symmetric pulmonary congestion
symmetrical chest or thorax
symmetrical mediastinal adenopathy
symmetrical phased array
sympathetic chain
sympathectomy
  cardiac
  high thoracic left
  lumbar
  periarterial
  regional cardiac

sympathetic trunk
sympathicotonic orthostatic
  hypotension
sympathomimetic activity
sympathomimetic amines, cardiac
sympathomimetic drug
symphysis pubis
symptomatic digitalis-induced
  bradyarrhythmia
symptomatology
symptom complex
symptom-free period
symptom-limited exercise test
symptom reproduced with exertion
symptoms
  brachiocrural
  Buerger
  Burghart
  cardinal
  characteristic
  cognitive
  concomitant
  constitutional
  equivocal
  faciobrachial
  factitious
  nostril
  objective
  Oehler
  pathognomonic
  premonitory
  prodromal
  somatic
  subjective
  Tar
  transitory
  vegetative
symptom triad, classical
synchronicity
synchronized DC cardioversion
synchronized intermittent mandatory
  ventilation (SIMV)

synchronous carotid arterial pulse
synchronous mode of pacemaker
synchrony
    atrioventricular (AV)
    loss of AV (atrioventricular)
    out of
    ventricular
syncopal attack
syncopal spell
syncope
    Adams-Stokes
    afferent nerve stimulation
    arrhythmia-induced
    cardiac
    cardiogenic
    cardioinhibitory carotid sinus
    carotid sinus
    cerebral carotid sinus
    cerebrovascular
    cough
    defecation
    deglutition
    diver's
    drug-induced
    effort
    exertional
    glossopharyngeal
    glossopharyngeal-vagal
    malignant vasovagal
    micturition
    near
    neurally mediated
    neurocardiogenic
    neuroregulatory
    ocular cardiac reflex
    orthostatic
    positional
    postprandial
    post-tussive
    postural
    pressor-postpressor

syncope *(cont.)*
    reflex
    swallow
    temporal lobe
    tussive
    vagal
    vagal carotid sinus
    vago-vagal
    vasodepressor
    vasodepressor carotid sinus
    vasovagal
    vertiginous
    X
syncope anginosa
syncytial virus, respiratory
syncytium
    circular
    horseshoe-shaped
syndactyly
syndrome
    AAIR pacemaker
    Aase
    Abramo-Fiedler
    absent pulmonary valve
    acid-pulmonary-aspiration
    Acosta (or D'Acosta)
    acute aortic regurgitation
    acute coronary
    acute febrile mucocutaneous lymph
        node
    Adams-Stokes
    adult respiratory distress (ARDS)
    Afelius
    Alagille
    ALCAPA (anomalous origin of left
        coronary artery from the
        pulmonary artery)
    Aldrich
    Alexander
    allergic alveolitis
    Alport

syndrome *(cont.)*
   alveolar capillary block
   Angelman
   angina
   angina decubitus
   angina intermedia
   angina with normal coronaries
   anginal
   anomalous first thoracic rib
   anterior chest wall
   antiphospholipid (APS)
   aorta coarctation
   aortic arch
   aortic arch calcification-osteo-
      porosis-tooth-buds hypoplasia
   aortic arch hypoplasia
   aortic bifurcation
   Apert
   apical systolic click-murmur
   Archer
   Arneth
   arrythmogenic right ventricular
      dysplasia
   arteriohepatic dysplasia
   arthropathy-camptodactyly
   atherosclerotic occlusive
   athletic heart
   atypical chest pain
   autoerythrocyte sensitization
   Ayerza
   Baader
   bagassse worker
   Barlow
   Bartter
   basilar artery
   Becker
   beer and cobalt
   beer drinker
   Behçet
   Bernard-Soulier
   Bernheim
   Bernheim-Schmincke

syndrome *(cont.)*
   Beuren
   bird fancier's
   Blackfan-Diamond
   Bland-Garland-White
   blue finger
   blue toe ("trash foot")
   blue velvet
   Bouillaud
   Bouveret-Hoffmann
   Bradbury-Eggleston
   bradycardia-tachycardia
   brady-tachy (slang for
      bradytachycardia)
   bradytachycardia
   bradytachydysrhythmia
   Brett
   Brock
   Brock middle lobe
   bronchial cartilage absence-
      bronchiectasis-bronchomalacia
   bronchial carcinoma myasthenia
   bronchiectasis-megaesophagus-
      osteopathy
   bubbly lung
   buckled innominate artery
   Budd-Chiari
   Burke
   caisson
   capillary leak
   capillary leakage
   Caplan
   carcinoid
   cardiac neurosis
   cardiac radiation
   cardiac-limb
   cardioauditory
   cardiocutaneous
   cardiofacial
   cardioinhibitory carotid sinus
   cardiopathia nigra
   cardiovascular-arm

syndrome *(cont.)*
  cardiovocal
  carnitine deficiency
  carotid sinus (CSS)
  Carpenter
  cat eye
  Cayler
  Ceelen-Gellerstedt
  celiac artery compression
  celiac axis
  cervical aorta
  Chandra-Khetarpal
  Charcot-Weiss-Baker
  CHARGE (colobomas, choanal
    atresia, mental and growth
    deficiency, genital and ear
    anomalies)
  Chiari-Budd
  cholesterol pericarditis
  chronic hyperventilation
  Churg-Strauss
  circulatory hyperkinetic
  Clarke-Hadfield
  Clerc-Levy-Cristeco (CLC)
  click
  click-murmur
  CLC (Clerc-Levy-Cristeco)
  cobbler chest
  Cockayne
  Colinet-Caplan
  concealed Wolff-Parkinson-White
  congenital central hypoventilation
  Conn
  Conradi-Hünermann
  Corvisart
  cork worker
  Cornelia de Lange
  coronary artery steal
  coronary steal
  Corrigan
  Cossio-Berconsky
  costal margin

syndrome *(cont.)*
  costochondral junction
  costoclavicular
  costosternal
  cotton-mill fever
  CREST (calcinosis cutis,
    Raynaud's phenomenon,
    esophageal dysmotility,
    sclerodactyly, telangiectasia)
  cri du chat (short-arm deletion-5)
  croup
  Cruveilhier-Baumgarten
  Curracin-Silverman
  Cushing
  cutis laxa
  Cyriax
  Da Costa
  Davies
  Davies-Colley
  declamping shock
  defibrinating
  DeGimard
  de Lange
  De Martini-Balestra
  Demons-Meigs
  Determann
  Diamond-Blackfan
  DiGeorge
  dilantin
  diphasic postcardiotomy
  disseminated intravascular
    coagulation
  Doehle-Heller
  double outlet–left ventricle (DOLV)
  double outlet–right ventricle (DORV)
  Down
  Dressler
  Dusard
  dysbarism
  Dysshwannian
  Eaton-Lambert
  Edwards

syndrome *(cont.)*
effort
Ehlers-Danlos
Eisenmenger
elfin facies
Elliotson
Ellis-van Creveld
Elsner
eosinophil lung
eosinophilia-myalgia
eosinophilia-pulmonary tuberculosis
Erdheim I
erythrocyte autosensitization
external carotid steal
factor III platelet deficiency
Fahr-Volhard
Fallot
Fanconi-Hegglin
fat embolism (FES)
Feldaker
fibrinogen-fibrin conversion
Fiedler
Fissinger-Rendu
flapping valve
floppy valve
florid Marfan
Fluckiger
Foix-Alajouanine
Forney
Forrester
Friedel Pick
Frimodt-Moller
fulminant acute eosinophilic
    pneumonia-like
extrinsic sick sinus
funnel chest
Gaisböck
Gallavardin
gastrocardiac
giving up-given up
GLH (Green Lane Hospital)
Goldenhar

syndrome *(cont.)*
Goodpasture
Gorlin
Gouley
Gowers
Graham-Burford-Mayer
Gregoire blue
Gsell-Erdheim
Guillain-Barré
Hale
Hamman
Hamman-Rich
hand-heart
Hantavirus pulmonary
Harbitz
Harbitz-Mueller
Harkavy
Hayem-Widal
heart and hand
heart-hand II
Heberden
Hegglin
hemangioma-thrombocytopenia
hemopleuropneumonia
heterotaxy
Hippel-Lindau
Hislop-Reid
holiday heart
hollow chest
Holmes
Holt-Oram
homocystinuria
Horner
Hughes-Stovin
Hunter
Hurler
Hutchinson-Gilford progeria
Hutinel-Pick
hyperdynamic heart
hypereosinophilic
hyperkinetic heart
hypersensitive carotid sinus

syndrome *(cont.)*
   hypersensitive xiphoid
   hyperviscosity
   hypogenetic lung
   hypoplastic aorta
   hypoplastic left-heart (HLHS)
   hypoplastic left ventricle
   hypoplastic right-heart
   idiopathic hypereosinophilic
   idiopathic long QT interval
   iliocaval compression
   immotile cilia
   incomplete Kartagener
   incontinentia pigmenti
   infantile
   inferior vena cava
   inframammary
   intercoronary steal
   intermediate coronary
   intrinsic sick sinus
   ischemic heart
   ischemic heart disease
   Ivemark
   Janus
   Jervell and Lange-Nielsen
   Jervell-Lange-Nielson
   Jeune
   Jeune-Tommasi
   Kabuki make-up
   Kaposi-Besnier-Libman-Sacks
   Kartagener
   Kasabach-Merritt
   Kast
   Katayama
   Kawasaki
   Kearns-Sayre
   Kearns-Shy
   Kemp-Elliot-Gorlin
   King
   Klauder
   Klein-Waardenburg
   Klippel-Feil

syndrome *(cont.)*
   Klippel-Trénaunay
   Klippel-Trénaunay-Weber
   Kugelberg-Welander
   Kurtz-Sprague-White
   Kussmaul
   Labbé
   LAMB (lentigines, atrial myxoma,
      blue nevi)
   Lambert-Eaton
   Laslett-Short
   Laubry-Pezzi
   Laurence-Moon-Biedl
   Laurence-Moon-Biedl-Bardet
   lazy leukocyte
   Leitner
   Lenegre
   LEOPARD
   Leriche
   Lev
   Lewis
   LGL (Lown-Ganong-Levine) variant
   Lian-Siguier-Welti venous
      thrombosis
   Libman-Sacks endocarditis
   Liddle
   locked lung
   Löffler (Loeffler) endomyocardial
   Loehr-Kindberg
   long QT (LQTS)
   long QTc interval
   low cardiac output
   low-flow
   Lown-Ganong-Levine (LGL)
   low-output
   low-renin essential hypertension
   low salt
   lupus-like
   Lutembacher
   Macleod
   Maffucci
   mal de Meleda

syndrome *(cont.)*
  Malin
  Manson schistosomiasis-pulmonary
    artery obstruction
  manubriosternal
  maple-bark worker
  Marable
  Marchiafava-Micheli
  Marfan
  marfanoid hypermobility
  Marie-Bamberger
  Maroteaux-Lamy
  Martorell
  Martorell-Fabre
  MAS (Morgagni-Adams-Stokes)
  Master
  maternal hypotension
  maternal rubella
  Maugeri
  McArdle
  MCLS
  Meadows
  Meigs
  Meigs-Cass
  Mendelson
  Ménière
  midaortic
  middle aortic
  middle lobe
  midsystolic click–late systolic
    murmur
  milk leg
  Miller-Dieker
  Millikan-Siekert
  Minot–von Willebrand
  mitral click
  mitral click-murmur
  mitral regurgitation–chordal
    elongation
  mitral valve prolapse
  Mönckeberg
  Mohr

syndrome *(cont.)*
  Monday fever
  Mondor
  Monge
  Morgagni-Adams-Stokes (MAS)
  Morquio
  Morquio I
  mort d'amour
  Moschowitz
  Mounier-Kuhn
  Moynahan
  MSA (multiple system atrophy)
  mucocutaneous lymph node
  mulibrey nanism
  multiple system atrophy (MSA)
  myxoma with facial freckling
  nail-patella
  NAME (nevi, atrial myxoma,
    myxoid neurofibroma,
    ephelides)
  nervous heart
  nonhypertension
  Noonan
  nutrition heart
  organic dust
  organic dust toxic
  Ormond
  Ortner
  Osler-Libman-Sacks
  osteogenesis imperfecta
  pacemaker
  pacemaker twiddler's
  Page
  Paget-Schrötter (Schroetter)
  Paget-von Schrötter
  Pallister-Hall
  paraneoplastic
  parchment heart
  Parkes Weber
  Patau (trisomy 13)
  pectoralis major
  Penderluft

syndrome *(cont.)*
pericardiotomy
pericarditis-liver pseudocirrhosis
perinatal respiratory distress
peripheral cholesterol embolization
PF-III (platelet factor III)
Pick
pickwickian
PIE (pulmonary infiltrate-
eosinophilia)
pigeon breeder's
placental transfusion
P mitrale
Poland sequence
Polhemus-Schafer-Ivemark
polyangiitis overlap
popliteal artery entrapment
Porter
post-cardiac injury
postcardiotomy
postcardiotomy psychosis
postcoarctation
postcommissurotomy
posterior fossa compression
post-MI
postmyocardial infarction
postperfusion
postperfusion lung
postpericardiotomy
postphlebitic
postthrombotic
postvalvulotomy
P pulmonale
preexcitation
preinfarction
prethrombotic
primary mitral valve prolapse
Prinzmetal II
progeria
progressive anginal
prolonged QT interval
Proteus

syndrome *(cont.)*
pseudoclaudication
pseudocoarctation
pseudo-Meigs
pseudoxanthoma elasticum
psychogenic chest pain
pulmonary acid aspiration
pulmonary sling
pulmonary stenosis-ostium
secundum defect
pulmonary stenosis-patent foramen
ovale
pulmonary valve atresia-intact
ventricular septum
pulmonary venous anomalous
drainage-mitral stenosis
pulseless
pump lung
purple toes
push-pull pump
QT
radiation toxicity
Raeder-Arbitz
Raynaud
reactive airways dysfunction
renal cholesterol embolization
Rendu-Osler-Weber
respiratory distress (of newborn)
restrictive cardiac
restrictive hemodynamic
Rh-null
Ridley
Riley-Day
Roger
Romano-Ward
Romberg-Wood
Roques
Rosen-Castleman-Liebow
Rosenbach
Rosenthal
Rostan
Rougnon de Magny

syndrome *(cont.)*
Royer-Wilson
Rubinstein-Taybi
Rummo
Rundles-Falls
runting
Russell-Silver
Sack-Barabas
Sanchez-Cascos cardioauditory
Sanfilippo
Sawyer-Jones
scalenus anticus
Scheie
schistosomiasis japonica
Schmincke-Bernheim
Schönenberg
Schroeder
Schrötter (Schroetter)
scimitar
septic lung
Seroche
Servelle-Martorell
shaggy aorta
Shaver
Shaver-Ridell
shifting pacemaker
shock lung
Shone
short rib-polydactyly
Short
shoulder-hand
Shprintzen
Shy-Drager
Shy-McGee-Drager
sick sinus (SSS)
Siewert
Silver
Silverman II
Silver-Russell
single atrium
single ventricle
Singleton-Merten

syndrome *(cont.)*
sinus venosus
sinusitis-bronchiectasis
Sjögren
slipping rib
small aorta
small cuff
Smith-Lemli-Opitz
smoker respiratory
soldier's heart
Solomon
Spens
splenic flexure
Srb (no vowel)
Steidele
Stevens-Johnson
stiff heart
Stokes-Adams
stone heart
straight-back
stroke
subclavian steal (SSS)
submersion
sudden infant death (SIDS)
superficial vena cava
superior mesenteric artery
superior vena cava
supine hypotensive (of pregnancy)
supravalvar aortic stenosis
supravalvular aortic stenosis
surdocardiac
suspended heart
Swan-Ganz
Swyer-James
syphilitic aorta
systemic inflammatory response
systolic click-late systolic murmur
systolic click–murmur
tachycardia-bradycardia
    (slang, tachy-brady)
taffy candy
Takayasu

syndrome *(cont.)*
　TAR (thrombocytopenia-absent
　　radius)
　Taussig-Bing
　Taussig-Snellen-Alberts
　Terry
　thoracic outlet
　thoracic outlet compression
　thrombocytopenia-absent radius
　　(TAR)
　thromboembolic
　Tietze
　tight-collar
　Townes-Brocks
　toxic shock
　transfusion
　transplant lung
　"trash foot"
　Treacher Collins
　trisomy 13(D)
　trisomy 13-15
　trisomy 18(E)
　trisomy 21 (Down)
　tropical eosinophilia
　Trousseau
　tuberous sclerosis
　turkish sabre
　Turner
　Turpin
　twiddler's
　Uhl
　Ullrich-Noonan
　unroofed coronary sinus
　upper-limb cardiovascular
　Upshaw-Schulman
　uremic cardiac
　vagal syncope
　vanishing lung
　Vaquez-Osler
　vascular
　vascular ring
　vasovagal

syndrome *(cont.)*
　VATER (vertebral anomalies, anal
　　atresia, tracheo-esophageal
　　fistula, radial and renal
　　anomalies)
　velocardiofacial (VCF)
　vena cava
　venous phlebitis-gangrene
　vertebral artery
　vertebral basilar artery
　visceral cholesterol embolization
　von Willebrand
　Von Rokitansky
　von-Hippel-Lindau
　VSD (ventricular septal defect) and
　　absent pulmonary valve
　Waardenburg
　WAGR (Wilms tumor, aniridia,
　　genitourinary involvement, and
　　retardation)
　wandering pacemaker
　Ward-Romano
　Waterhouse-Friderichsen
　Weber-Osler-Rendu
　Wegener
　Weingarten
　Weisenburg
　Weiss-Baker
　Werner
　wet lung
　white lung
　Willebrand (von Willebrand)
　Williams
　Williams elfin-facies
　Williams-Beuren
　Williams-Campbell
　Wilson-Mikity
　Winiwarter-Manteuffel-Buerger
　Wiskott-Aldrich
　Woakes
　Wolff-Parkinson-White (WPW)
　Wolf-Hirschhorn

syndrome *(cont.)*
  WPW (Wolff-Parkinson-White)
  X
  xiphoid process
  XO (Turner)
  XXXY and XXXXX
  Zeek
  Ziegler
  Synergyst DDD pacemaker
  synostosis
  synovial sarcoma of the heart
  synpneumonic empyema
  Synthaderm dressing
  synthetic patch angioplasty
  synthetic surfactant
  syphilis, cardiovascular
  syphilitic aneurysm
  syphilitic aorta syndrome
  syphilitic aortic regurgitation
  syphilitic aortitis
  syphilitic myocarditis
  syphilitic pericarditis
system
  Bard percutaneous cardiopulmonary
    support (CPS)
  cardiohemic
  CASE computerized exercise EKG
  Cenflex central monitoring
  CGR biplane angiographic
  Chemo-Port perivena catheter
  circumflex
  circumflex coronary
  codominant
  collateral
  conduction
  conductive (conduction)
  continuous-wave laser
  COROSKOP C cardiac imaging
  Desilets introducer
  dominant left coronary artery
  dominant right coronary
  Echovar Doppler

system *(cont.)*
  engorged collecting
  extracranial carotid
  Frank XYZ orthogonal lead
  greater saphenous
  Haemonetics Cell-Saver
  heart assist
  His-Purkinje (HPS)
  His-Purkinje conduction
  Hombach lead placement
  Innovator Holter
  kallikrein-kinin
  lesser saphenous
  Leukotrap RC (red cell) storage
  Mason-Likar 12-lead ECG
  MEDDARS cardiac catheterization
    analysis
  Medtronic Interactive Tachycardia
    Terminating
  Novacore left ventricular assist
    (LVAS)
  pacemaker tester
  PCA (patient-controlled analgesic)
  Probe balloon-on-a-wire dilatation
  pulmonary venous
  Q-cath catheterization recording
  Quinton computerized exercise
    EKG
  reticuloendothelial
  Rozanski lead placement
  saphenous
  SICOR (computer-assisted cardiac
    catheter recording)
  single-chamber cardiac pacing
    (PASYS)
  T (sarcolemma)
  Thora-Klex chest drainage
  transluminal lysing
  TRON 3 VACI cardiac imaging
  underwater chest drainage
  USCI Probe balloon-on-a-wire
    dilatation

system *(cont.)*
   vertebral artery
   V1-like ambulatory lead
   V5-like ambulatory lead
   Viagraph computerized exercise
      EKG
   water-seal drainage
systemic and topical hypothermia
systemic anticoagulation with heparin
systemic arterial circulation
systemic arterial oxygen desaturation
systemic arterial vasoconstriction
systemic AV O_2 difference
systemic blood
systemic carnitine deficiency
systemic circulation
systemic diastolic blood pressure
   (SDBP)
systemic disorders affecting heart
   function
systemic heparinization
systemic hypertension
systemic hypoperfusion
systemic inflammatory response
   syndrome
systemic lupus erythematosus
systemic mean arterial pressure
   (SMAP)
systemic necrotizing vasculitis
systemic oxygen saturation measured
   after balloon-occluding each
   collateral
systemic perfusion, diminished
systemic pressure
systemic-pulmonary artery anastomosis
systemic-pulmonary artery shunt
systemic resistance, vascular
systemic sclerosis
   fibrosing alveolitis associated with
   progressive
systemic sepsis

systemic vascular resistance (SVR)
systemic vascular resistance index
   (SVRI)
systemic vasculitis
systemic venous hypertension
systemic venous return
systole
   aborted
   atrial
   cardiac
   coupled premature
   electromechanical
   end of
   extra
   premature atrial
   premature junctional
   premature ventricular
   total
   ventricular
   ventricular ectopic
systolic anterior motion (SAM) of
   mitral valve
systolic anterior motion (SAM) on
   2-D echocardiogram
systolic blood pressure (SBP)
systolic bulge, late
systolic click (SC)
systolic click–murmur syndrome
systolic diameter (of LV)
systolic-diastolic blood pressure
systolic ejection click
systolic ejection murmur (SEM)
systolic ejection period (SEP)
systolic ejection sound
systolic fractional shortening
systolic gradient
systolic grating sound
systolic heart failure
systolic hypertension
systolic impulse
systolic mammary souffle

systolic murmur (SM), graded from
    1 to 6
systolic pressure
systolic pressure determination (SLP)
systolic pressure-time index
systolic prolapse of mitral valve
    leaflet
systolic reserve
systolic retraction

systolic retraction of apex
systolic S waves
systolic scratch
systolic thrill
systolic time interval (STI)
systolic trough
systolic upstroke time
systolic velocity-time integral

T, t

TAAA (thoracoabdominal aortic
    aneurysm) surgery
TA-30 autosuture
TA-30 4.5 mm staples
TA-55 stapling device
TA-90 stapler
tab, fibrous
tabagism (nicotinism)
table
    anterior
    posterior
table of the sternum
TAC atherectomy catheter
tachyarrhythmia
    atrial
    digitalis-induced
    drug-resistant
    ectopic
    lethal
    malignant ventricular
    paroxysmal
    paroxysmal ventricular
    supraventricular
    sustained ventricular
    ventricular
tachycardia
    accelerated idioventricular

tachycardia (cont.)
    acceleration of
    accessory pathway reentrant
        paroxysmal supraventricular
    antidromic
    antidromic AV reciprocating
    antidromic AV reentrant
    antidromic circus-movement
    antidromic reciprocating
    atrial
    atrial automatic
    atrial ectopic automatic
    atrial paroxysmal (APT)
    atrial reentrant
    atrial reentrant paroxysmal
        supraventricular
    atrial reentry
    atrioventricular junctional
    atrioventricular nodal (AVNT)
    atrioventricular nodal reentrant
        (AVNRT)
    atrioventricular node re-entry
    atrioventricular reciprocating
        (AVRT)
    atypical AV nodal re-entry
    automatic atrial
    automatic ectopic (AET)

501

tachycardia *(cont.)*
  AV (atrioventricular)
  AV nodal re-entrant
  AV nodal re-entrant paroxysmal
    supraventricular
  AV nodal re-entry
  AV reciprocating
  benign ventricular
  bidirectional ventricular
  bundle branch block (BBB)
  bundle branch reentrant ventricular
  chaotic atrial
  circus movement (CMT)
  concealed accessory pathway (AP)
  concealed bypass-type
  congenital ventricular
  double
  drug-refractory
  ectopic atrial
  ectopic supraventricular
  endless-loop
  exercise-aggravated ventricular
  exercise-induced ventricular
  fast-slow AV nodal reentrant
  focal ventricular
  hypokalemia-induced ventricular
  idiopathic ventricular
  idioventricular
  incessant
  incessant ectopic atrial
  incessant focal atrial
  inducible
  intra-atrial reentrant
  intractable ventricular
  junctional
  macro-reentrant
  malignant ventricular
  monomorphic
  monomorphic ventricular
  multifocal atrial (MAT or MFAT)
  multiform
  narrow-complex

tachycardia *(cont.)*
  nodal reentrant
  nodoventricular
  nonparoxysmal atrioventricular
    junctional
  nonparoxysmal automatic atrial
  nonparoxysmal AV junctional
  nonparoxysmal AV nodal
  nonparoxysmal reciprocating
    junctional (NPRJT)
  nonsustained monomorphic
    ventricular
  nonsustained polymorphic
    ventricular
  nonsustained ventricular
  NPJT (nonparoxysmal AV
    junctional)
  orthodromic
  orthodromic AV reentrant
  orthodromic reciprocating (ORT)
  orthodromic supraventricular
  orthostatic
  pacemaker-mediated
  parasystolic ventricular
  paroxysmal
  paroxysmal atrial (PAT)
  paroxysmal junctional (PJT)
  paroxysmal sinus
  paroxysmal supraventricular
    (PSVT)
  permanent reciprocating
    atrioventricular junctional
  pleomorphic
  polymorphic ventricular
  primary electrical ventricular
  rapid nonsustained ventricular
  reciprocating
  reciprocating atrioventricular
  reciprocating permanent
    atrioventricular junctional
  reentrant
  reentrant supraventricular

tachycardia *(cont.)*
  reflex
  refractory
  repetitive monomorphic ventricular
    (RMVT)
  repetitive paroxysmal ventricular
  resting
  runs of
  SA (sinoatrial) nodal reentry
  salvos of ventricular
  self-terminating
  sinoatrial (SA) reentrant
  sinus
  sinus reentrant
  slow retrograde
  slow-fast
  slow-fast atrioventricular node
    reentry
  slow-fast AV nodal reentrant
  supraventricular (SVT)
  sustained ventricular
  torsades de pointes ventricular
  ventricular (VT)
  wide QRS
  wide-complex
  Wolff-Parkinson-White reentrant
  WPW (Wolff-Parkinson-White)
tachycardia-bradycardia syndrome
tachycardiac, tachycardic
tachydysrhythmia
Tachylog pacemaker
tachypnea, transient
tachypneic breathing pattern
tacrolimus
Tactilaze angioplasty laser catheter
tactile fremitus
tactile precordial phenomena
TAD guide wire
taffy candy syndrome
tagged blood cells
tagging cine magnetic resonance
tagging, myocardial

TAH (total artificial heart)
TAH, electromechanical
tailored to fit
Takayasu aortitis
Takayasu arteritis, supra-aortic
Takayasu pulseless disease
Takayasu syndrome
takedown of adhesions
takedown of laryngostomy
takeoff
  artery
  high (of left coronary artery)
  takedown of Fontan operation
  takeoff of left anterior descending
    coronary artery
  takeoff of vessel
Takeuchi repair
taking down of adhesions
talc
talc plaque
talc pneumoconiosis
talc poudrage
talcum powder
tall right precordial R waves
tamborlike
tambour quality of A_2
tambour sound
tamponade
  cardiac
  chronic
  florid cardiac
  full-blown cardiac
  heart
  low-pressure cardiac
  medical cardiac
  pericardial
  pericardial chyle with
  subacute cardiac
  surgical cardiac
tandem lesion
Tandem cardiac device
tangential constriction

tangentially
tank respirator
tank-type body ventilator
tanned red cells (TRC) test
tantalum bronchogram
tantalum, knitted
tap (tapping), pericardial
TAP (transesophageal atrial pacing)
tape
  braided
  compression
  Dacron
  silastic
  umbilical
  vascular
  white cotton umbilical
tapering, abrupt
tapering doses
tapering occlusion
tapering off
tapering stenosis
tape ligature
TAPSE (tricuspid annular plane
  systolic excursion) score
TAPVC (total anomalous pulmonary
  venous connection)
TAPVR (total anomalous pulmonary
  venous return)
Tar symptoms
TAR (thrombocytopenia-absent radius)
  syndrome
Tardieu spot
tardive cyanosis
tardus et parvus, pulsus
tardus, pulsus
target heart rate
target lesion
TARP (total atrial refractory period)
T artifact
Tascon prosthetic valve
Ta segment (electrocardiography)

TAT (thrombin-antithrombin III
  complex)
TAT inhibitor
taurine deficiency
Taussig-Bing anomaly
Taussig-Bing congenital anomaly of
  heart
Taussig-Bing congenital malformation
Taussig-Bing double-outlet right
  ventricle
Taussig-Bing syndrome
Taussig-Snellen-Alberts syndrome
taut pericardial effusion
taut skin
TAV (transcutaneous aortovelography)
Tawara atrioventricular node
TB (tuberculin) skin test
TB (tuberculosis)
TBNA (transbronchial needle aspira-
  tion)
TBT (transcervical balloon tuboplasty)
TCBF (total cerebral blood flow)
T cells
TCL (tachycardia cycle length)
Tc 99m or ^{99m}Tc (technetium)
TDI (toluene diisocyanate)
TDI sensitivity
T/D (thickness to diameter of
  ventricle) ratio
TD2 torque device
TE (echo delay time)
TE (thromboembolic) stroke
team, donor
tear
  eccentric
  intimal
  linear
  splint-type
tearaway sheath
tear in ascending aorta
tear in descending aorta

tearing, plaque
teased off
tea-taster's cough
TEB (thoracic electrical bioimped-
    ance)
teboroxime cardiac scan for
    myocardial infarction
TEC (transluminal extraction catheter)
TEC atherectomy device
technetium (see *contrast medium*)
technetium bound to DTPA
technetium bound to serum albumin
technetium bound to sulfur colloid
technetium pyrophosphate scanning
technician, pump
technique (see also *method,
    operation, procedure*)
    acquisition
    adjunctive
    Amplatz
    anterior sandwich patch closure
    aseptic
    Bentall
    Bentall inclusion
    Blalock-Hanlon
    bronchoscopic shuttle
    button
    Carpentier
    Carrel
    clamp-and-sew
    Damus-Kaye-Stansel (DKS)
    De Vega
    Dor
    dos Santos
    Dotter
    Dotter-Judkins
    double-umbrella
    double-wire atherectomy
    dye dilution
    ECG signal-averaging
    ECG-gated multislice MRI
    elephant-trunk

technique *(cont.)*
    equilibrium radionuclide
        angiocardiography
    esophageal balloon
    eversion
    extracorporeal carbon dioxide
    extrastimulus
    fat-suppressed breath-hold
    first-pass
    flow mapping
    Frouin
    gated
    Gruentzig angioplasty
    Gruentzig PTCA
    inclusion
    indicator-dilution
    J loop (on catheterization)
    Jerome Kay
    Judkins cardiac catheterization
    Judkins femoral catheterization
    Kawashima
    kissing atherectomy
    kissing balloon
    Lecompte
    Lown
    Mee
    modified Seldinger
    Müller and Dammann
    Mullins blade
    multiphasic multislice MRI
    multiple chord, center line
        echocardiogram
    multislice multiphase spin-echo
        imaging
    multislice spin-echo
    Nikaidoh
    noninvasive
    parachute (for distal anastomosis)
    Patrick-McGoon
    PCICO (pressure-controlled inter-
        mittent coronary occlusion)
    percutaneous

technique *(cont.)*
  percutaneous Judkins
  percutaneous puncture
  percutaneous transfemoral
  pharmacologic stress
  physiologic stress
  Potts
  pressure half-time
  radioenzymatic
  rapid thoracic compression
  Rashkind
  recanalization
  Reed annuloplasty
  reimplantation
  sandwich
  Schonander
  Seldinger
  Seldinger percutaneous
  serial cut film
  sheathless insertion
  silhouette
  Sones arteriography
  Sones brachial cutdown
  Sones cardiac catheterization
  Sones cineangiography
  Sones coronary arteriography
  Stewart-Hamilton cardiac output
  Stoney
  subclavian turndown
  swiss roll
  test and ablate
  thermal dilution
  thermodilution (for measuring
    cardiac output)
  Trusler aortic valve
  upgated
  Waldhausen
  Waterston-Cooley
  wraparound
  xenon computed tomography
    (XeCT)

TED, T.E.D. (thromboembolic
    disease)
  antiembolism stockings
  thigh-high stockings
tedious dissection
TEE (transesophageal echocardi-
    ography)
teeth-chattering chills
Teflon Bardic plug
Teflon catheter
Teflon felt bolster
Teflon felt pledget
Teflon-fluon fumes
Teflon graft or patch
Teflon intracardiac patch
Teflon pledget
Teflon-pledgeted mattress suture
Teflon suture
Tegaderm dressing
Teichholz ejection fraction in
    echocardiogram
Teichholz equation for left ventricular
    volume
Tektronix oscilloscope
telangiectasia
  cutaneous
  hereditary hemorrhagic
  Osler hereditary hemorrhagic
telangiectatic lesions
Telectronics defibrillator patches
Telectronics endocardial defibrillation
    (DF) lead system
Telectronics endocardial defibrillation/
    rate-sensing/pacing lead
Telectronics endocardial pacing lead
Telectronics Guardian ATP II ICD
Telectronics pacemaker electrode
Telectronics pacing lead
Telectronics PASAR antitachycardia
    pulse generator
telemetry

telephone monitoring of EKG
telephone transmission of EKG
Telfa pad
temperature
    core
    esophageal
    normothermic
temperature probe, nasopharyngeal
temperature-sensing pacemaker
temporal arteritis
temporal artery
temporal lobe syncope
temporary atrial pacing wire
temporary cardiac pacing
temporary pacing catheter
temporary percutaneous cardio-
    pulmonary support
temporary tracheostomy
tenacious bronchial exudate
tenacious mucus
tenacious secretions
tenacious sputum
tenderness
    calf muscle
    chest wall
    periumbilical area
tendineae
    chordae
    ruptured chordae
tendinosum, xanthoma
tendinous hiatus
tendon
    Krehl
    left ventricular false
    Todaro
tennis racquet cells
Tennis Racquet angiography catheter
tense pulse
Tensilon (prostigmin and edrophonium
    chloride) test

tension
    alveolar wall
    decreased inspired oxygen
    epicardial
    ventricular wall
tension pneumatocele
tension pneumopericardium
tension pneumothorax
tensionless anastomosis
tension-time index (TTI)
tensor apparatus
tent
    croup
    mist
tentative diagnosis
tented up
tent-shaped T waves
teratogenicity
teratoma
    cardiac
    malignant (of the heart)
terminal air sacs
terminal air space
terminal aortic thrombosis
terminal bronchioles
terminal crest of right atrium
terminal edema
terminal inversion
terminalis
    crista
    sulcus
terminal negativity of P wave
terminal, RNS
Terry syndrome (oxygen toxicity to
    retina)
tertiary spread of tumor
Terumo sheath
tesla
test (see also *assay, analysis, testing*)
    acid-fast
    Adson
    Allen

test *(cont.)*
Allen circulator
ANA (antinuclear antibody)
Anderson-Keys total serum
    cholesterol
antihyaluronidase
antistreptolysin-O titer
antistreptozyme (ASTZ)
Apt
APTT clotting
ASO titer
ASTZ (antistreptozyme)
atrial pacing
atrial pacing stress
Bactec culture
Bernstein acid infusion
bicycle ergometer
bicycle ergometer exercise
bicycle exercise
blood culture
Brodie-Trendelenburg (for varicose
    veins)
bronchial provocation
C3a serum level
capillary fragility
capillary resistance
cardiokymographic (CKG)
carotid sinus
coccidioidin
cold agglutinins
cold pressor (Hines and Brown)
cold pressor exercise
collagen vascular screen
collateral circulation
contraction stress (CST)
Coombs
costoclavicular
^{11}C palmitate uptake
^{11}C propranolol uptake
Crampton
creatine phosphokinase (CPK)
cuff

test *(cont.)*
culture and sensitivity
cytological
Dehio
dehydrocholate
diaphragmatic stimulation
dipyridamole echocardiography
dipyridamole handgrip
dipyridamole infusion
dipyridamole thallium stress
direct Coombs
Donath-Landsteiner
DPT-positive skin prick
drop (for pneumoperitoneum)
Duke
dynamic exercise
electrophysiologic
equivocal exercise
ergonovine provocative
erythrocyte sedimentation rate
    (ESR)
euglobulin lysis
exercise
exercise stress
exercise thallium-201 stress
exercise tolerance (ETT)
Fisher exact
flat-hand
fungal
Gibbon and Landis
Goethlin
graded exercise tolerance
graded treadmill
handgrip exercise
handgrip stress
hanging drop (for pneumo-
    peritoneum)
HDM (house dust mites) bronchial
    provocation
head-up tilt
Henle-Coenen
Hess capillary

test *(cont.)*
Hines and Brown
Howell
hydrogen
hyperabduction
hyperemia
hyperventilation
[123]I heptadecanoic acid uptake
indirect Coombs
inhalation bronchial challenge
injection (for pneumoperitoneum)
intermediate tuberculin
isometric exercise
isometric exercise stress
isometric stress
Kobert
Korotkoff
Kveim
lactate dehydrogenase (LDH)
Landis-Gibbon
Levine
Lewis and Pickering
Liebermann-Burchard
Mantoux
Master two-step (2-step) exercise
Matas
match
maximal exercise
meniscus of saline (for pneumoperitoneum)
methacholine bronchial provocation
mirror
Moschowitz
multiple-puncture tuberculin
Newman-Keuls
niacin
noninvasive
nonstress (NST)
Northern blot
one-stage clotting
one-stage prothrombin time
pacemaker threshold

test *(cont.)*
Pachon
PaO_2
partial thromboplastin time
passive tilt
Paul-Bunnell
Pearson chi-squared (calculation
   used for artificial heart)
Perthes
Phalen stress
plantar ischemic
plasma renin activity (PRA)
Plesch
polymerase chain reaction (PCR)
positive skin
positive tilt
postmyocardial infarction exercise
postural stimulation of aldosterone
PPD (purified protein derivative)
primed lymphocyte (PLT)
prothrombin
prothrombin consumption
prothrombin-proconvertin
provocative
PT/PTT
pulmonary function (PFT)
Quick
Quick one-stage prothrombin time
Reflotron bedside theophylline
R-lactate enzymatic monotest
Salkowski
Salzman
Sandrock
scalene
Schiff
Schlichter
Schultze
Sclavo PPD
sickle cell
sickling
skin-prick
Snider match

test *(cont.)*
  Southern blot hybridization
  Southwestern blot
  SPECT thallium
  Sterneedle tuberculin
  spirometric
  streptokinase resistance
  stress
  Stypven time
  submaximal treadmill exercise
  symptom-limited maximal exercise
  TB (tuberculin)
  teichoic acid antibody
  thallium stress
  thallium-201 exercise
  tilt
  tine tuberculin
  tolazoline
  tourniquet
  treadmill (TMT)
  treadmill exercise (TET)
  treadmill stress (TMST)
  Trendelenburg
  Tris-buffer infusion
  tuberculin (TB)
  Tuberculin Mono-Vacc
  Tuberculin Tine (old)
  Tubersol
  Tuffier
  two-step exercise
  Valsalva
  ventilation
  von Recklinghausen
  Waaler-Rose
  Western blot
  Williamson
  Zwenger
test and ablate technique
test battery
testing (see also *test*)
  extrastimulus (EST)
  mycobacteria susceptibility

testing *(cont.)*
  nuclear gated blood pool
  serial electrophysiologic (SET)
  stress
  upright tilt-
  test-occluded, vessel was
  test of vasomotor function
  test result
    false negative
    false positive
  TET (treadmill exercise test)
  tethered ventricular assist device
  tetrad spells
  tetrahedron chest
  tetralogy of Fallot (TOF)
    atypical
    pink
  tetralogy of Fallot plus atrial septal
    defect
  tetrapolar esophageal catheter
  tetrodotoxin effect
  tetrodotoxin potential
  tet (tetralogy of Fallot) spell
  Tevdek suture
  TGA (transposition of great arteries)
  thalassemia
    alpha
    beta
  thalassemia major
  thalassemia minor
  thalassemia–sickle cell disease
  thallium clearance
  thallium defect
  thallium imaging
  thallium injection
  thallium myocardial perfusion imaging
  thallium perfusion study
  thallium, regional myocardial uptake of
  thallium scintigraphy
  thallium SPECT (thallium-201 single-
    photon emission computed tomo-
    graphic) imaging

thallium stress test
thallium treadmill
thallium uptake
thallium washout
thallium-201 myocardial imaging
thallium-201 myocardial scintigraphy
thatched roof worker's lung
thebesian circulation
thebesian foramen
thebesian valve
thebesian vein
Theden method
T-helper lymphocyte alveolitis
theophylline toxicity
theorem
   Bayes (exercise stress testing)
   Bernoulli
therapeutic blood level of drug
therapeutic embolization
therapeutic intervention
therapeutic modality
therapeutic phlebotomy
therapeutic pneumothorax
therapeutic range (of drug)
therapeutic thoracentesis
therapeutic trial
therapy
   adjunctive
   adjuvant
   aerosol
   anthelminthic
   antianginal
   antibacterial
   antibiotic
   anticoagulant
   antihypertensive
   antimicrobial
   antitachycardiac pacing
   antiviral
   aspirin
   beta-adrenergic blocker

therapy *(cont.)*
   bronchodilator
   cardiac rehabilitation
   chemical ablation (for arrhythmia)
   concomitant antiarrhythmic
   continuous lateral rotation
   continuous nebulization (CNT)
   dietary
   diuretic
   drug
   empiric, empirical
   exercise
   fibrinolytic
   immunosuppressive
   intracoronary thrombolytic
   lipid-lowering
   multidrug
   palliative
   quinidine
   radiofrequency ablation
   respiratory
   respiratory physical
   salvage
   step-care hypertensive
   supportive
   thrombolytic
   tiered
   tiered tachyarrhythmia
   transfusion
   transplacental drug
   triple-drug
   updraft
   vitamin K antagonist
   weight loss
therapy, abort
therapy zones
thermal compression
thermal dilution technique
thermal memory stent
Thermetics cardiac device
thermistor catheter

thermistor electrode
thermistor plethysmography
Thermoactinomyces sacchari
Thermocardiosystems left ventricular
    assist device
thermodilution balloon catheter
thermodilution cardiac output
thermodilution catheter
thermodilution ejection fraction
thermodilution method for determining
    cardiac output
thermodilution method of cardiac
    output measurement
thermodilution Swan-Ganz catheter
thermography, blood vessel
thermophilic actinomycete
Thermopolyspora (fungi)
Thermos pacemaker
THI needle
thiamine deficiency
thiazide diuretics
thick border of lung
thick echo
thick mucus secretions
thick sputum
thick yellowish-green discharge
thickened adventitia
thickened alveolar septa
thickened degenerated intima, friable
thickened mitral valve
thickened pericardium
thickened secretions
thickened valvular leaflets
thickening
    diffuse pleural
    focal intimal
    intimal
    mottled
    pleural
thickening of arterial intima, diffuse
thickening of valve
thickening of valve leaflets

thickening of ventricular wall
thick mucus secretions
thick sputum
thick yellowish-green discharge
thickness
    interventricular septal (IVST)
    IVS wall
    posterior LV wall
    posterior wall (PWT)
    septal
    septal wall
    ventricular free wall
    wall
thickness of sputum
thick sputum
thick-walled ventricle
thick yellowish-green discharge
thigh claudication
thigh-high antiembolic stockings
thigh-high TEDs (thromboembolic
    disease) (hose or stockings)
thin border of lung
thin fibrous cap
thin-walled atrium
thiocyanate blood level
thiocyanate toxicity
thionamides
third-degree atrioventricular (AV)
    block
third-generation device (first-, second-,
    fourth-, etc.)
third heart sound, physiologic
third intercostal space
third left interspace
third order chordae
third space sequestration
30° position
30° right anterior oblique
    projection
Thomas Allis forceps
Thompson carotid artery clamp
Thomsen disease

thoracentesis
  diagnostic
  therapeutic
thoracentesis needle
thoracic aneurysm
thoracic aorta
thoracic aorta aneurysm
thoracic aorta, descending
thoracic aorta-femoral artery bypass
  graft
thoracic aortic dissection
thoracic aortography
thoracic asymmetry
thoracic cage configuration
thoracic catheter
thoracic cavity
thoracic deformity
thoracic duct
thoracic empyema
thoracic fistula
thoracic gas volumes
thoracic inlet
thoracic kyphosis, loss of
thoracicoabdominal fistulectomy
thoracicoabdominal incision
thoracicogastric fistulectomy
thoracicointestinal fistulectomy
thoracic outlet compression syndrome
thoracic outlet syndrome
thoracic outlet, widened
thoracic pain
thoracic trauma, blunt
thoracic wall
thoracoabdominal aneurysm
thoracoabdominal aorta
thoracoabdominal aortic aneurysm
  (TAAA) surgery
thoracoabdominal approach
thoracoabdominal nerves
thoracoabdominal wall
thoracoepigastric vein
thoracoepigastric vein periphlebitis

thoracofemoral conversion
thoracolaparotomy
thoracoplasty, Schede
thoracoport
thoracoscopic implantation
thoracoscopic resection, video-assisted
thoracoscopy
  transpleural
  video-assisted (VAT)
thoracostomy, tube
thoracotomies, bilateral staged
thoracotomy
  anterolateral
  anterolateral muscle-sparing lateral
  bilateral anterior
  closed tube
  left lateral
  left posterolateral
  posterolateral
  resuscitative
Thora-Klex chest drainage system
thorascopic apical pleurectomy
thorascopic talc pleurodesis
Thoratec BVAD (biventricular assist
  device)
Thoratec cardiac device
Thoratec RVAD (right ventricular
  assist device)
Thoratec VAD (ventricular assist
  device)
thorax
  asymmetrical
  cylindrical
  squared off
  symmetrical
Thorel bundle of muscle fibers in
  heart
Thorel pathway
thready pulse
threatened vessel closure post-PTCA
three-antigen recombinant immunoblot
  assay

three-block claudication
3-D (three-dimensional)
3-D echocardiography
3DFT magnetic resonance angio-
    graphy (3-dimensional Fourier
    transform)
3-D reconstruction
3-D time of flight magnetic resonance
    angiographic sequences (3DTOF
    MR angiographic sequences)
3-D transesophageal echocardiography
three-pillow orthopnea
3 sign
three-step test
3:2 block ("three to two")
three-turn electrode
three-vessel coronary disease
three-vessel runoff
three-way stopcock connector
thresher's lung
threshing fever
threshold
    anaerobic
    capture
    defibrillation (DFT)
    high pacing
    implant
    lead
    myocardial
    pacemaker
    pacemaker stimulation
    pacing
    pain
    satisfactory
    sensing
    sensitivity
    stimulation
threshold current
threshold for arrhythmia
threshold load training
threshold of activation
threshold rate of excretion

thrill
    aneurysmal
    aortic
    apical
    arterial
    basal precordial
    crescendo-systolic
    dense
    diastolic
    diastolic apical
    faint
    palpable
    parasternal systolic
    precordial
    presystolic
    purring
    supramanubrial systolic
    suprasternal notch
    systolic
    vibratory
throat
    inflamed
    irritated
    raw
    scratchy
    strep
    swollen
throbbing pain
thrombectomy
thrombi (pl. of thrombus)
thrombin
    coil soaked in
    topical
thrombin-antithrombin III complex
    (TAT)
Thrombinar
thrombin inhibitor
thrombin time
thromboangiitis obliterans,
    Winiwarter-Buerger
thromboarteriectomy
thromboatherosclerotic process

thrombocytopenia
  heparin-induced
  Werlhof autoimmune
thrombocytopenia-absent radius (TAR)
  syndrome
thrombocytopenic purpura
  primary
  secondary
thrombocytosis, essential
thromboembolectomy
thromboembolic disease (TED)
thromboembolism
  aortic
  catheter-induced
  deep venous
  pulmonary
  venous
thromboembolization
thromboendarterectomized
thromboendarterectomy
  aortoiliofemoral
  carotid
  femoral
  transaortic renal
thrombogenesis
thrombogenic, thrombogenicity
thromboglobulin plasma level
thrombolysis
  antistreplase
  eminase
  intracoronary
  intravenous coronary
  rt-PA (recombinant tissue plasmino-
    gen activator)
  streptokinase
  t-PA (tissue plasminogen activator)
  urokinase
thrombolytic agent or drug
thrombolytic enzymes
thrombolytic therapy
thrombolytic treatment of coronary
  thrombosis

thrombo-obliterative process
thrombopathia
thrombophlebitis
  anterior chest wall
  breast
  femoral
  iliofemoral
  migratory
  Mondor
  postpartum
thrombophlebitis cerulea dolens
thromboplastic material into the
  circulation
thromboplastin
thromboresistance
thrombosed graft
thrombosis (see also *thrombus*)
  abdominal aorta
  acute aortic
  agonal
  aortic
  aortoiliac
  arterial
  atrial
  atrophic
  axillary vein traumatic
  capsular
  cardiac
  cavernous sinus
  central splanchnic venous (CSVT)
  cerebral
  coronary arterial
  coronary artery
  creeping
  deep venous (DVT)
  dilatation
  effort
  femoropopliteal
  hepatic vein
  iliofemoral vein
  infective
  intracardiac

thrombosis *(cont.)*
  intravascular
  intraventricular
  left atrial
  left ventricular
  Lian-Siguier-Welti venous
  limb-threatening
  luminal
  marantic
  marasmic
  mesenteric arterial
  mesenteric venous
  migrating
  mural
  necrotizing
  nonpyogenic
  plate
  platelet
  portal vein
  postangioplasty mural
  postoperative
  propagating
  puerperal
  pulmonary
  pulmonary artery
  renal vein
  Ribberts
  septic
  stent
  superficial venous
  terminal aortic
  traumatic
  venous
thrombosis in pulmonary vessels
thrombosis in situ of pulmonary
  arteries
thrombosis of aortic aneurysm,
  induced
thrombotic gangrene
thrombotic microangiopathy
thrombotic thrombocytopenic purpura

thrombus (pl. thrombi) (see also
  thrombosis)
  adherent
  agonal
  agony
  annular
  antemortem
  apical
  ball
  ball valve
  blood plate
  blood platelet
  calcified
  calf vein
  coral
  currant jelly
  fibrin
  fibrin-rich
  hyaline
  infective
  intra-arterial
  intracardiac
  intravascular
  laminated
  laminated intraluminal
  laser desiccation of
  lateral
  luminal
  marantic
  marasmic
  migratory
  mixed
  mobile
  mural
  nonocclusive luminal
  obstructive
  occluding
  occlusive
  occlusive arterial
  organized
  pale

thrombus *(cont.)*
  parietal
  pedunculated
  pericatheter
  plate
  platelet
  platelet-rich
  postmortem
  primary
  propagated, propagating
  propagation of
  red
  remodeling of
  saddle
  stratified
  traumatic
  white
thrombus formation
thrombus inhibitor
thrombus nidus
thrombus propagation, prevention of
thrombus stripper, Dunlop
through-and-through injury
through-and-through sutures
through-the-wall mattress sutures
Thruflex PTCA balloon catheter
thrust
  apical
  brief anterior
  cardiac
  double systolic outward
  left ventricular
  presystolic outward
thrusting ventricles
thumping of heart in chest
thump, precordial
thumpversion (striking patient's chest)
thymoma of the heart
thymus gland
  blood supply of
  lymph vessels of
  veins of

thyrocardiac disease
thyroid artery
thyroid cartilage
thyroid hormone deficiency
thyroid hormone excess
thyroid studies
thyrotoxic heart disease
thyrotoxicosis, neonatal
thyrotoxicotic cardiomyopathy
TIA (transient ischemic attack)
tibial artery disease
tibial in situ bypass
tibial outflow tracts, blind
tibial-peroneal trunk
tibioperoneal occlusive disease
tick-borne protozoa
tick-tack sound
Ti-Cron suture (also Tycron)
tidal breathing
tidal expiratory flow, peak
tidal flow, midexpiratory
tidal inspiratory flow-volume
tidal volume, decreased
tidal volume of 10 mL/kg
tidal wave of carotid arterial pulse
tie
  free
  plastic
  tracheotomy
tie gun
tiered tachyarrhythmia therapy
tiered therapy for ventricular fibrilla-
    tion, defibrillation, and bradycardia
    pacing
tiered-therapy ICD
tiered-therapy programmable cardio-
    verter-defibrillator (PCD)
Tietze syndrome
tigering
tight-collar syndrome
tightener, wire
tight lesion

tightness of chest
tilt table protocol
tilt test
  head-up
  positive
timbre metallique
time
  acceleration
  activated partial thromboplastin
    (APTT)
  aortic ischemic
  arm-to-tongue
  atrial activation
  atrioventricular
  bleeding
  cardiopulmonary bypass
  carotid ejection
  circulation
  conduction
  corrected sinus node recovery
    (CSNRT)
  cross-clamp
  deceleration
  diastolic perfusion
  donor heart-lung
  donor organ ischemic
  Duke bleeding
  echo delay
  ejection (ET)
  insensitive
  ischemic
  isovolumic contraction
  isovolumic relaxation (IVRT)
  Ivy bleeding
  left ventricular ejection (LVET)
  maximum inflation
  maximum walking (MWT)
  mean pulmonary transit (MTT)
  myocardial contrast appearance
    (MCAT)
  pain-free walking (PFWT) (on
    treadmill)

time (cont.)
  partial thromboplastin (PTT)
  perfusion
  prothrombin (PT)
  pulmonary transit (PTT)
  pulse reappearance
  pump
  reaction recovery
  relaxation
  right ventricle-to-ear
  sinoatrial conduction (SACT)
  sinus node recovery (SNRT)
  systolic upstroke
  T1 relaxation (in MRI)
  T2 relaxation (in MRI)
  total cross-clamp
  total ischemic
  two-stage prothrombin
  venous filling (VFT)
  venous return (VRT)
  ventricular activation (VAT)
  ventricular isovolumic relaxation
time activity curve of contrast agent
time of heartbeat
time-out, ventriculoatrial
time to peak contrast (TPC)
time to peak filling rate (TPFR)
timed imaging
TIMI (thrombolysis in myocardial
  infarction) classification
TIMI grading system for patency
TIMI II, IIA, IIB protocol
timothy grass
tine tuberculin test
tined atrial J pacing/defibrillation lead
tined lead
tined lead pacemaker
tinkling rales
tinnitus, pulsatile
tip
  Andrews suction
  catheter

tip *(cont.)*
  directable (of bronchoscope)
  Frazier suction
  leaflet
  mitral valve leaflet
  tonsil suction
  valve
  Yankauer suction
Tissot spirometer
Tissucol fibrin-collagen material for
  hemostasis
tissue
  apical
  cone of apical
  cryopreserved homograft
  devitalized
  gangrenous
  granulation
  hematopoietic
  indurated
  subadventitial
  subcutaneous
  tuberculosis granulation
tissue active
tissue borne
tissue breakdown
tissue contrast
tissue expander
  PMT AccuSpan
  Silastic H.P.
  T-Span
tissue factor pathway inhibitor
tissue inflow valve
tissue-interface barrier, Vitacuff
tissue migration, mesenchymal
tissue outflow valve
tissue perfusion
tissue plasminogen activator (t-PA)
tissue thromboplastin
tissue veil
tissue viability

titer
  antistreptolysin-O (ASO)
  cold agglutinin
  Mycoplasma antibody
titrated dose or dosing
titration of dosage
Titrator
TKO (to keep open), intravenous
TKO-type I.V. (to keep open [the
  vein])
Tl (thallium) myocardial imaging
^{201}Tl (thallium-201)
^{201}Tl stress imaging
TLC (total lung capacity)
TLC (total lymphocyte count)
TLC (triple-lumen catheter)
T loop (vectorcardiography)
T (thymus-dependent) lymphocytes
TMST (treadmill stress test)
TMT (treadmill test)
TNB (Tru-Cut needle biopsy)
to-and-fro murmur
Todaro tendon resection
Todaro, triangle of
Todd units for ASO titer
toe ulceration
toenails, thickened
toes, purple
TOF (tetralogy of Fallot)
toilet (toilette)
  aggressive pulmonary
  pulmonary
  tracheal
  tracheostomy
tolazoline test
tolerance, exercise
Tom Jones closure
tomogram, -graph (x-ray)
  single-slice long-axis
  stacked
tomographic slices

tomography
  biplanar cardiac blood pool
  computerized axial (CAT)
  exercise thallium-201
  GE single-photon emission
    computerized
  myocardial perfusion
  positron emission (PET)
  rapid acquisition computed axial
    (RACAT)
  seven-pinhole
  single photon emission computed
    (SPECT)
  slant-hole
  SPECT (single photon emission
    computed)
tomoscintigraphy
T_1 heart sound (tricuspid valve
  closure)
T1 relaxation time (in MRI)
T1-weighted image
tone, postural
tongue
  chicken heart
  geographic
tongue of vein material
toothed Adson tissue forceps
toothpaste shadows
top normal limits in size
topical antimicrobial prophylaxis
topical cold saline
topical cooling of heart with saline
topical cooling with ice slush
topical drugs
topical ice
topical lavage
topical lidocaine spray
topical myocardial hypothermia
topically cooled
topographic
topographical

topography
  arterial
  vessel
Torcon catheter
Torcon NB selective angiographic
  catheter
Toronto SPV aortic valve
Toronto SPV bioprosthesis
torque, constant clockwise (of electrode tip)
torque response
torr pressure
torsades de pointes ventricular tachycardia
torsades de pointes-type ventricular
  tachycardia
torsemide
tortuosity and elongation
tortuosity of blood vessel
tortuosity of superficial veins
tortuosity of veins
tortuosity precluding catheter passage
tortuous aorta
tortuous emptying
tortuous veins
tortuous vessel
torus aorticus
Toshiba echocardiograph machine
total absence of pericardium
total alternans
total anomalous pulmonary venous
  connection
total anomalous pulmonary venous
  drainage
total anomalous pulmonary venous
  return
total anomalous venous return
total artificial heart (TAH) (see *artificial heart* and *heart*)
total atrial refractory period (TARP)
total body heparinization

total body water
total cavopulmonary connection
total heart replacement, orthotopic
total lung capacity (TLC)
total peripheral resistance (TPR)
total valvectomy
totalis, situs inversus
tour de force
tourniquet
  caval
  Esmarch
  Medi-Quet surgical
  rotating (for pulmonary edema)
  Rumel myocardial
  vena caval
tourniquet inflated to 300 mm Hg
tourniquet test for collateral circulation
Townes-Brocks syndrome
toxemia of pregnancy
toxic appearance
toxic fumes
toxic gas inhalation
toxic insult
toxic myocarditis
toxic pneumonia
toxic shock
toxic shock syndrome
toxic vapor inhalation
toxicity
  cyanide
  cyclosporine
  digitalis
  oxygen
  pulmonary
  theophylline
  thiocyanate
Toxocara canis infection
toxoplasmosis, recrudescent
toxoplasmotic myocarditis
TP segment on EKG

t-PA (tissue plasminogen activator)
t-PA thrombolysis
TPA (thrombotic pulmonary
  arteriopathy)
TPC (time to peak contrast)
  (myocardial)
TPFR (time to peak filling rate)
T-piece oxygen
TPM (turning-point morphology)
TPR (temperature, pulse, and
  respiration)
TPR (total peripheral resistance)
TPR (total pulmonary resistance)
TQ segment
TR (repetition time)
TR (tricuspid regurgitation)
trabecula (pl. trabeculae)
trabecula septomarginalis
trabeculae carneae cordis
trabeculated atrium
trabeculation, endocardial
trace edema
trace hematest positive
Trace vein stripper
tracer (see *radioisotope*)
tracer activity
tracer dose
trachea
tracheal anastomosis
tracheal aspiration through artificial
  airway
tracheal aspiration through natural
  airway
tracheal bifurcation
tracheal bronchial lavage
tracheal caliber
tracheal cartilage
tracheal deviation
tracheal displacement, anterior
tracheal hook
tracheal injury, concomitant

tracheal rales
tracheal ring
  first
  second
  third
tracheal stenosis
tracheal toilet
tracheal tug
tracheitis
  acute
  catarrhal
tracheobronchial fistula
tracheobronchial lavage
tracheobronchial lymph nodes
tracheobronchial secretions
tracheobronchial tract
tracheobronchial tree
tracheobronchial tuberculosis
tracheobronchitis
tracheobronchomalacia, acquired
tracheobronchomegaly
tracheoesophageal fistula
tracheoesophageal fistulectomy
tracheomalacia
tracheostomy
  mediastinal
  temporary
tracheostomy stoma
tracheostomy toilet
tracheostomy tube
tracheotomizing
tracheotomy
tracheotomy ties
tracing
  electrocardiographic
  flat
  monitor lead
  postexercise
  pulmonary capillary wedge
track valve
trackability
Tracker catheter

tracking limit
tract, tracts
  aberrant AV bypass
  atrio-His
  atrio-Hisian (atriohisian) bypass
  atriofascicular
  atriofascicular bypass
  atrionodal bypass
  blind tibial outflow
  Breckenmacher
  bypass
  fasciculoventricular bypass
  free-wall
  inflow
  internodal
  James atrionodal bypass
  James intranodal
  left ventricular inflow
  left ventricular outflow (LVOT)
  nodoventricular bypass
  outflow
  pulmonary conduit outflow
  pulmonary outflow
  respiratory
  right ventricular bypass
  right ventricular inflow
  right ventricular outflow (RVOT)
  tracheobronchial
  ventricular flow
  ventricular outflow
traction suture
tractotomy, pulmonary
training
  threshhold load
  ventilatory muscle
trajectory, missile
tramlines shadow
transabdominal left lateral retroperitoneal maneuver
transaminase, glutamic oxaloacetic
transannular patching
transaortic approach

transaortic endarterectomy
transaortic extraction endarterectomy
transaortic gradient
transaortic radiofrequency ablation
transaortic renal thromboendarterectomy
transapical endocardial ablation
transarterial pacemaker insertion
transatrial approach
transatrial surgical approach
transbronchial biopsy
transbronchial lung biopsy
transbronchial needle aspiration
  (TBNA)
Trans-Scan
transcatheter ablation
transcatheter embolization
transcatheter His bundle ablation
transcatheter knife blade atrial
  septostomy
transcatheter occlusion of ASD with
  button device
transcatheter radiofrequency modification
transcatheter sclerotherapy
transcervical balloon tuboplasty (TBT)
transcranial Doppler sonography
transcranial Doppler ultrasonography
transcrural
transcutaneous drive lines
transcutaneous extraction catheter
  atherectomy
transcutaneous femoral artery puncture
transdermal nitroglycerin
transdiaphragmatic approach
transdiaphragmatic implantation
transducer
  arterial line
  Bentley
  Diasonics
  epicardial Doppler flow

transducer *(cont.)*
  Gould Statham pressure
  Hewlett-Packard
  M-mode
  Millar catheter-tip
  pressure
  Statham strain-gauge
  strain-gauge
  Ultramark 8
transect, transected
transection
  beveled
  traumatic aortic
  transection of aorta
transesophageal Doppler color flow
  imaging
transesophageal echocardiographic
  probe
transesophageal echocardiography
  (TEE), biplane
transesophageal imaging
transesophageal pacing
transesophageal transducer
transfemoral arteriogram
transfemoral endovascular stented
  graft procedure
transfemoral Fogarty embolectomy
transfixion suture
transfusion, transfusions
  autogenous blood
  autologous blood
  homologous blood
  intraoperative autologous (IOAT)
  massive blood
  multiple blood
  twin-to-twin
transfusional hemosiderosis
transfusion syndrome
transfusion therapy
transient apnea
transient cerebral ischemia
transient decrease of consciousness

transient ECG changes
transient ectopic pulsation
transient infiltrate
transient infiltrations of lungs
transient ischemic attack (TIA)
  crescendo
  ipsilateral hemispheric carotid
  limb-shaking
transient ischemic carotid insufficiency
transient left ventricular dilation
transient loss of consciousness
transient monocular blindness
transient perfusion defect
transient repolarization changes
transient tachypnea, newborn
transient tricuspid regurgitation of
  infancy
transient ventricular tachycardia (VT)
transition zone
transitional cells
transitional rhythm
transitory symptoms
transitory weakness
translingual nitroglycerin
translocation of coronary arteries
translucent depression in interatrial
  septum
translumbar aortography
transluminal angioplasty, percutaneous
transluminal balloon angioplasty
transluminal coronary artery angioplasty complex
transluminal extraction catheter (TEC)
transluminally placed stented graft
transluminal lysing system
transmedial plane
transmediastinal pacemaker electrode
  insertion
transmitral flow
transmitral gradient
transmitted carotid artery pulsations
transmucosal nitroglycerin

transmural cryoablation
transmural infarct
transmural myocardial infarction
transmural steal
transmyocardial perfusion pressure
transnasal approach
transnasally
transoral approach
transorally
transpectoral approach
transperitoneal approach
transplacental drug therapy
transplant, transplantation
  allogeneic
  cardiac
  heart
  heart and lung
  heart-lung
  heterotopic
  heterotopic heart
  kidney
  Lower-Shumway cardiac
  lung
  orthotopic heart
  piggy-back cardiac
  single-lung
  syngenesioplastic
  valved venous
transplant lung syndrome
transpleural thorascoscopy
transport, mucociliary
transport of cholesterol by lipoproteins
transposed aorta
transposition
  atrial
  carotid-subclavian
  congenitally corrected
  corrected great arteries
  great arteries
  great vessels
  Jatene
  Mustard procedure for

transposition *(cont.)*
　partial (of great vessels)
　Senning procedure for
　ventricular
transposition of great arteries (TGA)
　complete
　corrected (CTGA)
　anterior-aorta
　posterior-aorta
　side-by-side
transposition of great vessels
transposition of pulmonary veins
transpulmonary echo ultrasound
　reflectors
transpulmonary pressure (P_{TP})
transpulmonic gradient
transseptal angiocardiography
transseptal approach
transseptal cardiac catheterization
transseptal left heart catheterization
transseptal perforation
transseptal puncture
transseptal radiofrequency ablation
transstenotic pressure gradient
transtelephonic ICD interrogation
transtelephonic monitoring
transthoracic approach
transthoracic echocardiography (TTE)
transthoracic imaging
transthoracic needle aspiration biopsy
transthoracic needle aspiration,
　ultrasound-guided
transthoracic pacemaker electrode
　insertion
transtracheal aspiration
transtricuspid approach
transudates
transudation of fluid
transudative pericardial fluid
transvalvar gradient
transvalvular gradient
Transvene electrode

Transvene lead system
transvenous approach
transvenous defibrillation
transvenous electrode
transvenous electrode stimulation of
　atrium
transvenous endomyocardial biopsy
transvenous implantation
transvenous insertion of vena caval
　filter
transvenous lead defibrillator
transvenous pacemaker insertion
transvenous pacing
transvenous ventricular demand
　pacemaker
transventricular aortic valvotomy,
　closed
transventricular approach
transventricular dilator
transverse aortic arch hypoplasia
transverse aortotomy
transverse arch
transverse arteriotomy
transverse diameter
transverse heart
transverse pericardial sinus
transverse plane
transverse submammary incision
transverse venotomy
transversus thoracic muscle
transxiphoid approach for pacemaker
　lead
trap
　embolus
　Lukens
trapdoor incision
trapdoor-type aortotomy
trapezius muscle
Trapper catheter exchange device
trapping, air
"trash foot" (blue toe syndrome)
Traube murmur

Traube aortic regurgitation sign
trauma
  blunt chest
  blunt thoracic
traumatic aortic transection
traumatic emphysema
traumatic pericarditis
traumatic pneumothorax
traumatic tap
traumatic thrombus
traumatic tricuspid incompetence
trauma to heart
  nonpenetrating
  penetrating
Travenol pump
Treacher Collins–Franceschetti
  syndrome
Treacher Collins syndrome
treadmill
  Astrand
  Borg exertion scale on
  Ellestad
  exercise
  motorized
  Q-Stress
treadmill exercise stress test
treadmill exercise test (TET)
treadmill inclination, incremental
  increases in
treadmill slope
treadmill speed, incremental increases
  in
treadmill stress test (TMST)
treadmill testing
treatment (see also *therapy*)
  adjunctive
  conjunctive
  empiric
  IPPB
  nebulizer
  prenatal corticosteroid
  updraft

Tredex powered bicycle
tree
  arterial
  bronchial
  coronary
  coronary artery
  iliocaval
  tracheal-bronchial
  tracheobronchial
tree-in-winter appearance (on x-ray)
trefoil balloon catheter
Treitz ligament
Trendelenburg excision of varicose
  veins
Trendelenburg position
Trendelenburg test for valve
  competency
Trendelenburg test for varicose veins
trendscriber
Treponema pallidum infection
treppe ("staircase") phenomenon of
  Bowditch
triad
  acute compression
  adrenomedullary
  Beck
  classical (of symptoms)
  Grancher
  Kartagener
  Oster
trial (see also *study*)
  BARI
  BASIS (Basel Antiarrhythmic
    Study of Infarct Survival)
  CABG-Patch (prophylactic ICD
    implantation with coronary
    artery bypass grafting)
  CAVEAT II (directional coronary
    atherectomy versus PTCA)
  Circadian Anti-Ischemic Progress
    in Europe (CAPE)
  GISSI-2 thrombolytic

trial *(cont.)*
  Leiden Intervention
  Lipid Research Clinics Coronary
    Primary Prevention
  MADIT (Multicenter Automatic
    Defibrillator Implantation)
  MIAMI (intravenous metoprolol in
    acute myocardial infarction)
  Multicenter Unsustained
    Tachycardia (MUSTT)
  Multiple Risk Factor Intervention
    (MRFIT)
  PROMISE
  San Francisco Arteriosclerosis
    Specialized Center of Research
    (SCOR) Intervention
  SAVE (Survival and Ventricular
    Enlargement)
  SWIFT (Should We Intervene
    Following Thrombolysis)
  TAMI (Thrombolysis and Angio-
    plasty in Myocardial Infarction)
  Urokinase Pulmonary Embolism
    (UPET)
triangle
  Burger scalene
  cardiohepatic
  carotid
  Einthoven
  femoral
  Garland
  Gerhardt
  internal jugular
  Koch
  Korányi-Grocco
  Scarpa
  supraclavicular
  Todaro
triangular area of dullness
triangulation of Carrel
triatriatum, cor
triatriatum dextrum, cor

tributary (pl. tributaries), venous
Trichinella myocarditis
Trichinella spiralis infection
trichinosis
trichinous embolism
tricuspid aortic valve
tricuspid atresia
tricuspid incompetence
tricuspid murmur
tricuspid orifice regurgitation
tricuspid regurgitation
tricuspid stenosis
tricuspid valve (TV)
tricuspid valve abnormalities
tricuspid valve annuloplasty
tricuspid valve annulus
tricuspid valve anomaly
tricuspid valve closure
tricuspid valve converted to bicuspid
tricuspid valve deformity
tricuspid valve disease
tricuspid valve incompetence
tricuspid valve insufficiency
tricuspid valve obstruction
tricuspid valve regurgitation
tricuspid valve repair, Danielson
  method of
tricuspid valve stenosis
tricuspid valvuloplasty
tricyclic antidepressants
trifascicular block
trifascicular heart block
trifid precordial motion
trifoil balloon
trifurcates
trifurcation
  patent
  popliteal
trigeminal pattern
trigeminus distention of neck veins
trigeminy
triggered activity

triggered by physical exertion
triggering mechanism
trigger, recognizable
triggering ventricular contraction
triglycerides (neutral fat)
   serum
   familial elevated
trigone
   fibrous
   left fibrous
   right fibrous
trigonum caroticum
Triguide guide catheter
triiodothyronine
trilayer appearance
trileaflet
triloculare biatriatum, cor
trilogy, Fallot
trimelittic anhydride pneumonitis
trimmed on the bias
Trios M pacemaker
triphasic
triphasic contour of QRS complex
triple-drug therapy
triple extrastimuli
triple-lumen catheter
triple-lumen central venous catheter
triple-lumen line
triple rhythm
triple ripple
triplet beat
tripod position
tripolar electrode catheter
tripolar tined endocardial lead
tripolar transvenous screw-in electrode
trisomy 13(D) syndrome
trisomy 13-15 syndrome
trisomy 18(E) syndrome
trisomy 21 (Down) syndrome
Triumph VR pacemaker
trivial mitral regurgitation

trocar
   Davidson thoracic
   Hurwitz thoracic
   Nelson thoracic
trocar cannula
TRON 3 VACI cardiac imaging
   system
trophic skin changes
tropical endomyocardial fibrosis
tropical eosinophilia
tropical eosinophilia syndrome
tropical eosinophilic lung
tropomyosin
troponin T test
troubleshooting
trough level of drug
trough of venous pulse
trough
   systolic
   X
   Y
Trousers, Medical Anti-Shock
   (MAST)
Trousseau dilator
Trousseau phenomenon
Trousseau sign of superficial thrombophlebitis
Trousseau syndrome
true lumen
true polycythemia
true posterior wall myocardial
   infarction
true truncus arteriosus
true vocal cords
truncal artery
truncal valve
truncated atrial appendage
truncated exponential simultaneous
   monophasic waveforms
truncation of peak flow
truncular congenital vascular defect

truncular vascular defects
truncular venous defects
truncular venous malformations
truncus arteriosus
  common
  persistent
  true
truncus arteriosus communis
trunk
  brachiocephalic
  common
  peroneal-tibial
  pulmonary
  saphenous
  single arterial
  supra-aortic
  tibial-peroneal
  twin
  vagus
trunk of atrioventricular bundle
Trusler repair
Trusler rule for pulmonary artery
  banding
Trusler technique to reconstruct aortic
  valve
Trypanosoma cruzi
trypanosomiasis, African
TS (tricuspid stenosis)
T-Span tissue expander
tsutsugamushi disease
TSV (total stroke volume)
T system (sarcolemma)
TTE (transthoracic echocardiography)
TTI (tension-time index)
TTM (transtelephonic electrocardio-
  gram monitoring)
T2 relaxation time (in MRI)
T2-weighted image
TU wave
Tubbs dilator
Tubbs mitral valve dilator

tube
  Andrews Pynchon suction
  angled 24F pleural
  angled pleural
  Argyle chest
  Argyle Sentinel Seal chest
  bilateral pleural
  Bivona tracheostomy
  Broncho-Cath endotracheal
  chest
  cuffed endotracheal
  double-lumen endobronchial
  endotracheal
  Endotrol tracheal
  fenestrated
  Frazier suction
  Haldane-Priestley
  Hi-Lo Jet tracheal
  Holter
  J-shaped
  large-caliber
  Lindholm tracheal
  Lo-Pro tracheal
  nasogastric
  nasotracheal
  oroendotracheal
  Pleur-evac suction
  pleural
  polyethylene
  Rehfuss
  right-angle chest
  rubber
  Sarns intracardiac suction
  Shiley tracheotomy
  Silastic
  straight chest
  suction
  Thora-Klex chest
  tracheostomy
  water-seal chest
  Yankauer suction

tube drainage
tube graft (see *graft*)
tube guide
tube thoracostomy
tubercle
tubercle bacillus
tubercle of a rib
tubercles, noncaseating
tubercular empyema
tubercular infection
tuberculin reaction
tuberculin test, intermediate
tuberculosis (TB)
  acute
  adult
  aerogenic
  anthrocotic
  atypical
  avian (transmissible to humans)
  basal
  bovine (transmissible to humans)
  caseating
  cavitary
  cestodic
  childhood
  disseminated
  endobronchial
  extrapulmonary
  exudative
  fulminant
  hilus
  inhalation
  miliary
  multidrug-resistant (MDR-TB)
  open
  postprimary
  primary
  pulmonary
  reinfection
  tracheobronchial
tuberculosis infection, atypical
tuberculosis of bronchial glands

tuberculosis of serous membranes
tuberculosis reactivation, corticosteroid-
  administration-related
tuberculous bronchiectasis
tuberculous constrictive pericarditis
tuberculous pericarditis
tuberculous pneumothorax
tuberosa, chorditis
tuberosum simplex, xanthoma
tuberous sclerosis syndrome
tubing, extension
tubular breath sounds
tubular breathing
tubular graft, horseshoe
tubular lesion
tubular segment
tubular stenosis
tubular ventricle
Tuffier rib spreader
Tuffier test
tumor
  alveolar cell
  benign bronchial
  benign peripheral
  carcinoid (of bronchus)
  friable
  granular cell (of the heart)
  juxtaglomerular cell
  mediastinal
  metastatic myocardial
  metasynchronous
  mobile pedunculated left atrial
  Purkinje cell
  renin-secreting
  vascular
  Wilms
tumor embolism
tumor embolization, cardiac
tumorlike shadow
tumor necrosis factor alpha (TNFa)
tumor of heart
tumor of neural crest origin

tumor plop sound
tumor prolapsed through mitral valve
    orifice
tunica adventitia
tunica intima
tunica media
tunnel
    aortic-left ventricular
    aortico-left ventricular
    aortopulmonary
    baffled
    retroperitoneal
    subaortic stenosis
    subcutaneous
tunnel operation
tunnel repair
tunnel subaortic stenosis
tunnel subvalvular aortic stenosis
tunnel (verb), tunneled
tunneler, hollow
tunneling instrument
tunneling, retroperitoneal
Tuohy-Borst introducer
Tuohy-Borst Y adapter
turbid effusion
turbid fluid
turbinates, nasal
turbulence
turbulent blood flow
turbulent intraluminal flow
turbulent signal
turgor
Turkish sabre syndrome
Turner syndrome
turning-point morphology (TPM)
turnover
    erythrocyte iron (EIT)
    plasma iron (PIT)
    red blood cell iron (RBC IT)
Turpin syndrome
tussive fremitus

tussive syncope
Tuttle thoracic forceps
TV (tricuspid valve)
T vector
T wave, T waves
    biphasic
    broadened
    depressed
    diphasic
    enlarged
    flattened
    flipped
    hyperacute
    inverted
    inverted in V_1 and V_3
    ischemic
    Pardee
    persistently upright
    pseudonormalization of inverted
    tall
    tent-shaped
    upright
T wave amplitude, increased
T wave changes
T wave deflection
T wave flattening
T wave inversion, terminal
12-lead electrocardiogram
24-hour urine creatinine concentration
24-hour urine potassium concentration
24-hour urine sodium concentration
24-hour urinary secretion of VMA
    (vanillylmandelic acid)
twiddler's syndrome
twinned beats
twin-to-twin transfusion
twin trunk
twister, wire
2+ pitting edema
2-D (two-dimensional)
2-D echocardiogram, -graphy

2-D format
two-frame gated imaging
two-pillow orthopnea
two-stage prothrombin time
two-stage venous cannulation
two-step exercise test
two-turn electrode
two-vessel runoff
Tycron suture (also Ti-Cron)
Tygon catheter
tympanitic percussion note
tympanitic sound
tympany, Skoda
"tynoid" (see *phthinoid*)
type A dissections
type A personality
type B dissections

type B personality
type I (supracristal) ventricular septal
    defect
type II (infracristal) ventricular septal
    defect
type III (canal type) ventricular septal
    defect
type IV (muscular) ventricular septal
    defect
typhoid endocarditis
typhoid pleurisy
typhus, scrub
typical angina
typing, HLA
tyramine response
"tysis" (see *phthisis*)

U, u

ubiquitous sound
UCG (ultrasonic cardiography)
Uhl anomaly
Uhl syndrome
ulcer
  atheromatous
  craterlike (with jagged edges)
  decubital
  decubitus
  heel
  hypertensive ischemic
  indolent
  ischemic skin
  penetrating atherosclerotic aortic
  stasis
  stress
  toe
  varicose
  venous stasis
ulcerated atheromatous plaque
ulcerated lesion
ulcerated plaque
ulceration
  arteriolar ischemic
  ischemic
  penetrating

ulceration *(cont.)*
  penetrating aortic
  penetrating atherosclerotic
  toe
ulcerative endocarditis
ulcerative pharyngitis
ulcerative rhinitis
ulcus varicosum
Ullrich-Noonan syndrome
ulnar pulse
U loop
ULP (ultra low profile) catheter
Ultracor prosthetic valve
ultrafast imaging
ultrafast train pacing
ultrafiltration, extracorporeal
Ultraflex self-expanding stent
ultra-low profile fixed-wire balloon
  dilatation catheter
Ultramark 8 transducer
ultrarapid pacing
ultrasonic aortography
ultrasonic cardiogram (UCG)
ultrasonic nebulizer (USN)
ultrasonic scalpel
ultrasonic tomographic image

ultrasonography (also *ultrasound*)
  B-mode
  compression
  continuous wave
  Doppler
  duplex B-mode
  endovascular
  fetal
  gray-scale
  Hewlett-Packard
  intracoronary
  intravascular (IVUS)
  Irex Exemplar
  pulsed Doppler
  real-time
  transcranial Doppler
  transthoracic
  VingMed
ultrasound (see *ultrasonography*)
ultrasound-guided transthoracic needle
  aspiration
ultrasound nebulizer
  DeVilbiss
  Varic
ultrathin bronchoscope
Ultravent nebulizer
umbilical artery
umbilical artery catheterized
umbilical tape
umbilical vein, Biograft stabilized
  human
umbilical vein catheterized
umbilical vein graft, modified human
umbilical venous approach
umbrella
  atrial septal
  Bard Clamshell Septal
  Bard PDA
  Mobin-Uddin
umbrella closure of patent ductus
  arteriosus, percutaneous
umbrella filter, Mobin-Uddin

UMI catheter
UMI dilator (*not* Humi)
UMI needle
unbuttoning of device
uncomplicated convalescence
uncomplicated, non-Q-wave
  myocardial infarction
uncomplicated pneumothorax
uncomplicated Q-wave myocardial
  infarction
unconscious, unconsciousness
uncontrolled bronchospasm
uncooperative patient
under fluoroscopic guidance
underdetection
underdrive pacing
underdrive termination
underloading, ventricular
underperfused, underperfusion
undersensing of pacemaker
underventilation
underwater seal and suction
underwater-seal drainage
undulant impulse
undulating or scalloped contour
uneven murmur
uneventful recovery
unfavorable prognosis
ungrafted vessels
unicommissural aortic valve
unicommissural valves
unicusp
unicusp with central raphe
unicuspid aortic valve, stenosis of
unidirectional lead configuration
unifascicular block
unifocal
unifocalization operations
unilateral aortofemoral graft
unilateral emphysema
unilateral hyperlucent lung
unilateral loss of pulse

unilateral overinflation
unilateral pulmonary emphysema
UNILINK anastomotic device
Unilith pacemaker
unimodal
unipolar coil electrode
unipolar lead
unipolar limb lead
unipolar mode
unipolar pacemaker
unipolar pacing
unipolar programmable rate-response
　　pacemaker generator
unit
　　acute coronary care
　　BICAP
　　coronary care (CCU)
　　critical care (CCU)
　　progressive care (PCU)
　　stepdown
　　Wood (of pulmonary vascular
　　　　resistance)
univariate logistic regression
univentricular heart
universal biocompatibility protection
universal pacemaker
universal pacing mode
universal precautions
universale, angiokeratoma corporis
　　diffusum
University of Akron artificial heart
University of Wisconsin solution for
　　donor heart preservation
unloaded hyperpnea
unmasked by ductus arteriosus closure,
　　pulmonary hypoperfusion
unmitigated (unrelieved)
unmodulated radiofrequency current
unmodulated sine wave
Unna boot
unoxygenated blood

unrelenting pain
unreliable marker
unremitting pain
unresponsive
unresponsive hypotension
unresponsive programming
unroof
unroofed coronary sinus syndrome
unsaturated fats
unsaturation
　　arterial blood oxygen
　　oxygen
unstable angina
unstable blood pressure
unstable lesion
untoward event
untreated hypertension
up-biting biopsy cup forceps
updraft therapy
updraft treatment
upper airway neoplasm
upper airway obstruction, foreign
　　body
upper and lower extremities blood
　　pressure discrepancy
upper extremity in situ bypass
upper-limb cardiovascular syndrome
upper lobe vein prominence on chest
　　x-ray
upper rate behavior
upper rate interval
upper rate limit
upper respiratory infection (URI)
upper respiratory tract disease
upright T wave
upright tilt-testing electrocardiogram
upright U wave
Upshaw-Schulman syndrome
upsloping ST segment
upsloping ST segment depression
upstairs-downstairs heart

upstream sampling method
upstroke
  brisk carotid
  carotid pulse
  weak carotid
upstroke and falloff
upstroke phase of cardiac action
  potentials
uptake
  ^{11}C (C-11) palmitate
  diffuse myocardial
  increased lung
  increased RV
  localized myocardial
  observed maximal oxygen
  predicted maximal oxygen
upward retraction of left costal margin
urea nitrogen, blood (BUN)
uremic cardiac syndrome
uremic pericarditis
uremic pneumonitis
ureteral stent placed prior to surgery
URI (upper respiratory infection)
urinary creatinine
urinary metanephrine

urine creatinine concentration, 24-hour
urine potassium concentration, 24-hour
urine sodium concentration, 24-hour
urokinase thrombolysis
urticaria
USAFSAM treadmill exercise protocol
USCI angioplasty guiding sheath
USCI angioplasty Y connector
USCI arterial sheath
USCI Bard catheter
USCI guide wire
USCI guiding catheter
USCI Mini-Profile balloon dilatation
  catheter
USCI Probe balloon-on-a-wire
  dilatation system
USCI Sauvage EXS side-limb
  prosthesis
USCI sheath
USCI shunt
USN (ultrasonic nebulizer)
Utah TAH (total artificial heart)
uvulopalatopharyngoplasty
U wave inversion
U wave, prominent

V, v

V (lung volume)
V (ventilation)
V (ventricular)
V (volts)
V_A (alveolar ventilation)
VA (ventriculoatrial)
VA block cycle length
vaccine
  flu
  influenza
  pneumonia
V-A conduction
Vacor Rat Killer
V_2-A_2 curve
Vacutainer
VAD (ventricular assist device)
vagal carotid sinus syncope
vagal influence
vagal reaction
vagal reflexes
vagal response
vagal stimulation
vagal syncope syndrome
vago-vagal syncope
vagus nerve
vagus pulse

vagus trunk
V-A interval
Vairox high compression vascular
  stockings
Valdes-Cruz method
valley fever
Valsalva maneuver
Valsalva release
Valsalva sinus aneurysm
Valsalva strain
Valsalva test for pneumothorax
valvar aortic stenosis
valvar congenital aortic stenosis
valve (see also *prosthesis*)
  absent pulmonary
  Angell-Shiley bioprosthetic
  Angell-Shiley xenograft prosthetic
  Angiocor prosthetic
  annuloplasty
  anterior semilunar
  aortic (AV)
  aortocoronary
  artificial cardiac
  atrioventricular (AV) left or right
  atrioventricular (mitral and
    tricuspid)

valve *(cont.)*
  ball
  ball-and-cage prosthetic
  ball and seat
  ball-cage
  ball-occluder
  Baxter mechanical
  Beall prosthetic
  Beall prosthetic mitral valve
  Beall-Surgitool ball-cage prosthetic
  Beall-Surgitool disk prosthetic
  bileaflet tilting-disk prosthetic
  bicommissural aortic
  bicuspid
  bicuspid aortic
  bicuspid atrioventricular
  bicuspid pulmonary
  bileaflet
  billowing mitral
  Biocor prosthetic
  biological tissue
  bioprosthetic
  Bio-Vascular prosthetic
  Björk-Shiley convexo-concave disk
    prosthetic
  Björk-Shiley monostrut prosthetic
  Björk-Shiley prosthetic aortic
  Björk-Shiley prosthetic mitral
  bovine heart
  Braunwald-Cutter
  Braunwald-Cutter ball prosthetic
  butterfly heart
  caged ball occluder prosthetic
  caged disk occluder prosthetic
  calcification of mitral
  calcified
  calcified aortic
  Capetown aortic prosthetic
  CarboMedics
  cardiac
  Carpentier-Edwards aortic

valve *(cont.)*
  Carpentier-Edwards bioprosthetic
  Carpentier-Edwards glutaraldehyde-
    preserved porcine xenograft
    bioprosthesis
  Carpentier-Edwards mitral annulo-
    plasty
  Carpentier-Edwards pericardial
  Carpentier-Edwards porcine
    prosthetic
  Carpentier-Edwards Porcine
    SupraAnnular (SAV)
  C-C (convexo-concave) heart
  cleft mitral
  commissural pulmonary
  competent
  composite aortic
  conduit
  congenital absence of pulmonary
  congenital anomaly of mitral
    (CAMV)
  congenital bicuspid aortic
  congenitally bicuspid aortic
  congenitally quadricuspid aortic
  congenital unicuspid
  convexo-concave (C-C) disk
    prosthetic
  Cooley-Cutter disk prosthetic
  Coratomic prosthetic
  Cross-Jones disk prosthetic
  cryopreserved allograft heart
  Cutter-Smeloff heart
  DeBakey prosthetic
  DeBakey-Surgitool prosthetic
  Delrin frame of
  disc-type
  doming of
  Duromedics aortic
  Duromedics prosthetic heart
  dysplastic
  early opening of

valve *(cont.)*
eccentric monocuspid tilting-disk
  prosthetic
echo-dense
Edmark mitral
Edwards-Duromedics bileaflet
Edwards-Duromedics prosthetic
eustachian
extirpation of
fibrotic distortion of
fibrotic mitral
flail mitral
flexible cardiac
floppy
floppy aortic
floppy mitral
glutaraldehyde-tanned porcine heart
Gott shunt/butterfly heart
Guangzhou GD1 prosthetic
Hall-Kaster disk prosthetic
Hall prosthetic heart
hammock
hammocking of
hammock mitral
Hancock aortic prosthetic
Hancock bioprosthetic
Hancock mitral prosthetic
Hancock pericardial prosthetic
Hancock porcine heterograft
Hancock porcine prosthetic heart
Hancock prosthetic mitral
Hancock II porcine prosthetic
Harken prosthetic
healed
Hemex prosthetic
heterograft
hockey-stick tricuspid
Holter
Hufnagel prosthetic
hypoplastic
incompetent

valve *(cont.)*
intact Medtronic xenograft
Intact xenograft prosthetic
Ionescu-Shiley bioprosthetic
Ionescu-Shiley bovine pericardial
Ionescu-Shiley heart
Ionescu-Shiley low-profile prosthetic
Ionescu-Shiley pericardial
  xenograft
Ionescu-Shiley standard pericardial
  prosthetic
Ionescu trileaflet
Jatene-Macchi prosthetic
Kay-Shiley disk prosthetic
Kay-Shiley mitral
Kay-Suzuki disk prosthetic
leaky
left semilunar
Lillehei-Kaster disk prosthetic
Lillehei-Kaster pivoting-disk
  prosthetic
Lillehei-Kaster prosthetic mitral
Liotta-BioImplant LPB prosthetic
low-profile prosthetic
Magovern-Cromic ball-cage
  prosthetic
mechanical
Medtronic prosthetic
Medtronic-Hall heart
Medtronic-Hall monocuspid tilting
  disk
midsystolic buckling of mitral
midsystolic closure of aortic
mitral (MV)
Mitroflow pericardial prosthetic
monocusp
narrowed
native
native aortic
neo-aortic
notching of pulmonic

valve *(cont.)*
Omnicarbon prosthetic heart
Omniscience prosthetic heart
parachute mitral
Pemco prosthetic
porcine heart
posterior semilunar
premature closure of
premature mid-diastolic closure
of mitral
prosthetic heart
Puig Massana-Shiley annuloplasty
pulmonic; pulmonary (PV)
quadricuspid pulmonary
regurgitation of mitral
rheumatic mitral
right atrioventricular
right semilunar
semilunar (aortic and pulmonary)
Smeloff-Cutter ball-cage prosthetic
Sorin prosthetic
Starr-Edwards prosthetic aortic
Starr-Edwards prosthetic mitral
Starr-Edwards Silastic
Stellite ring material of prosthetic
stenosis of mitral
stenotic
stent-mounted allograft
stentless
stentless porcine aortic valve
St. Jude bileaflet prosthetic
St. Jude Medical bileaflet
straddling atrioventricular
Surgitool prosthetic
synthetic
systolic anterior motion of mitral
Tascon prosthetic
thebesian
thickened mitral
tilting-disk valve
Toronto SPV aortic

valve *(cont.)*
track
tricuspid (TV)
tricuspid aortic
trileaflet aortic
truncal
Ultracor prosthetic
unicommissural
unicommissural aortic
vegetation of
Vascor porcine prosthetic
venous
Wada-Cutter disk prosthetic
Wessex prosthetic
xenograft
Xenomedica prosthetic
Xenotech prosthetic
valve area
valve calcification
valve coaptation site
valvectomy, total
valve cusps
valved conduit
valve dehiscence
valved venous transplant
valve excision
valve function, pulmonary and
tricuspid
valve incision
valve incompetence
valve leaflets
valve of coronary sinus
valve of foramen ovale
valve of Vieussens
valve outflow strut
valve plane
valve pockets
valve prosthesis (see *valve*)
valve replacement
valve scarring
valve strut

valve thickening and scarring
valve tip
valviform
valvotome
    expanding
    spade-shaped
valvotomy
    aortic
    balloon
    balloon mitral
    closed transventricular aortic
    double-balloon
    mitral
    open
    percutaneous balloon aortic
    percutaneous balloon pulmonary
    percutaneous mitral balloon (PMV)
    pulmonary
    single-balloon
    transventricular aortic
    transventricular closed
valvular aortic insufficiency
valvular aortic stenosis
valvular apparatus
valvular atresia
valvular cardiac defect
valvular damage
valvular disease
valvular dysfunction
valvular heart disease
valvular incompetence
valvular opening
valvular orifice
valvular pneumothorax
valvular pulmonic stenosis
valvular pulmonic stenosis murmur
valvular regurgitant lesion
valvular regurgitation
valvular stenosis
valvulitis
    chronic
    rheumatic

valvuloplasty
    aortic
    bailout
    balloon
    balloon aortic
    balloon mitral
    balloon pulmonary (BPV)
    Carpentier tricuspid
    catheter balloon (CBV)
    double-balloon
    Kay tricuspid
    percutaneous aortic (PAV)
    percutaneous aortic balloon
    percutaneous balloon
    percutaneous balloon aortic
    percutaneous mitral balloon (PMV)
    prosthetic valve
    pulmonary
    pulmonary balloon
    retrograde simultaneous double-
        balloon
    retrograde simultaneous single-
        balloon
    single-balloon
    tricuspid
valvulotome
    Gerbode mitral
    Himmelstein
    Leather venous
    Mills pulmonary
valvulotome in intraluminal Hall valve
    disruption technique
valvulotomy (valvotomy)
valvutome (see *valvulotome*)
VAN (vein, artery, nerve)
Van Andel catheter
van den Bergh test of concentration of
    bilirubin in blood
vanillylmandelic acid (VMA)
vanishing lung
vanishing lung syndrome (on x-ray)
Van Praagh symbolic convention

Van Tassel pigtail catheter
vaporization of abnormal blood vessels
vaporization of atheromatous plaque
vaporization of plaque material
vapor massage
Vaquez-Osler syndrome
variability
    beat-to-beat
    peak flow
variable intensity
variable murmur
variable response rate
variant angina pectoris
variant
    electrocardiographic
    Kussmaul-Maier
    Loeffler (Löffler)
    orthostatic hypotension
varices (pl. of varix)
    aneurysmal
    arterial
    arteriovenous
    bilateral saphenous
    esophageal
    pelvic
    saphenous
    scrotal
    sublingual
    vulval
varicography
varicose aneurysm
varicose bronchiectasis
varicose veins
    familial
    primary
varicosity (pl. varicosities)
varicosum, ulcus
Varic ultrasound nebulizer
Variflex catheter
variola (smallpox)
Varivas R denatured homologous vein

varix (pl. varices)
varying P-R interval
vasa vasorum (of artery)
Vas-Cath
Vascor porcine prosthetic valve
vascular anastomosis
vascular atrophy
vascular attachments
vascular bed, pulmonary vascular
vascular bud
vascular bundle
vascular catastrophe
vascular channels, aberrant
vascular cirrhosis
vascular clamp, atraumatic
vascular compromise
vascular congestion
vascular dementia
vascular disease, peripheral
vascular engorgement
vascular graft (see also *graft*)
vascular hemophilia
vascular heterograft
vascular impedance
vascularis, plexus
vascularity
    decreased
    lung
vascular ligation, selective
vascular lumen
vascular markings
vascular nephritis
vascular network
vascular obstruction
vascular pedicle
vascular plexus
vascular redistribution
vascular resistance
    coronary
    increased pulmonary
    raised

vascular ring
vascular ring syndrome
vascular sling
vascular spasm
vascular syndrome
vascular systemic resistance
vascular tape
vascular tone
vascular wall damage
vascular xenograft
vasculature
   pulmonary
   splanchnic
vasculitis (pl. vasculitides)
   allergic
   hypersensitivity
   leukocytoblastic
   livedo
   necrotizing
   nodular
   polyarteritis-like systemic
   postperfusion pulmonary
   renal
   segmented hyalinizing
   systemic
   systemic necrotizing
   toxic
vasculopathy
Vascutek gelseal vascular graft
Vascutek knitted vascular graft
Vascutek woven vascular graft
vasoactive medication
vasoactive response
vasoconstriction
   hypoxic pulmonary
   peripheral
   peripheral circulatory
   peripheral cutaneous
   pulmonary arteriolar
   spontaneous transient
   systemic arterial

vasoconstrictor response
vasoconstrictors
vasodepressive
vasodepressor carotid sinus syncope
vasodepressor reaction (VDR)
vasodepressor response
vasodepressor syncope
vasodilatation or vasodilation
   breakthrough
   judicious
vasodilate
vasodilation or vasodilatation
vasodilator, peripheral
vasodilatory effect
vasodilatory response
vasomotion, coronary
vasomotor paresthesia
vaso-occlusive angiotherapy (VAT) in
   congenital vascular malformations
vasopressor
vasoreactivity, pulmonary
vasorelaxation of epicardial vessels
vasorum, vasa (of artery)
vasospasm
vasospastic angina
vasovagal arrest
vasovagal attack
vasovagal bradyarrhythmia
vasovagal episode
vasovagal orthostatism
vasovagal phenomenon
vasovagal syncope, malignant
vasovagal syndrome
Vas recorder
vastus medialis muscle
VAT (vaso-occlusive angiotherapy)
VAT (ventricular activation time)
VAT (video-assisted thoracoscopy)
VATER (vertebral anomalies, anal atresia, tracheoesopahgeal fistula, radial
   and renal anomalies) syndrome

VATS (video-assisted thoracic surgery)
Vaughn Williams classification of
   antiarrhythmic drugs
VC (vital capacity)
VCB (ventricular capture beat)
VCF (ventricular contractility function)
VCG (vectorcardiogram)
VCO_2 (venous CO_2 production)
VD (valvular disease)
VDD pacing mode
VDI (venous distensibility index)
VDR (vasodepressor reaction)
VEA (ventricular ectopic activity)
VEB (ventricular ectopic beat)
vector
   mean cardiac
   mean QRS
   P
   QRS
   ST
   T
   T wave
vectorcardiogram, -graphy
   Frank
   frontal plane
   sagittal plane
   spatial
   transverse plane
vector EKG
vector lead
vector loop
Veg. (vegetation)
vegetation
   bacterial
   friable
   necrotic fibrinoid
   valvular
vegetation of valve
vegetative endocarditis
vegetative symptoms
veil, tissue

Veillonella
vein, veins
   antecubital
   anterior cardiac
   autogenous
   azygos
   blind percutaneous puncture of
      subclavian
   Boyd perforating
   brachiocephalic
   cannulated central
   capacious
   cephalic
   communicating
   congenital stenosis of pulmonary
   cutdown over cephalic
   deep
   dilated
   distended neck
   distention of neck
   Dodd perforating group of
   engorged
   external jugular
   familial varicose
   feeder
   flat neck
   great cardiac
   great saphenous
   harvested
   hemiazygos
   iliofemoral
   inferior pulmonary
   inferior thyroid
   infradiaphragmatic
   innominate
   intercostal
   internal jugular
   internal thoracic
   jugular
   leaking
   lesser saphenous

vein *(cont.)*
  lobe of azygos
  marginal
  Marshall
  middle cardiac
  parent
  peroneal
  posterior interventricular
  pulsating
  renal
  reversed greater saphenous
  saphenous
  scimitar
  small cardiac
  small saphenous
  soleal
  subclavian
  subcutaneous
  superficial
  superficial femoral
  superior intercostal
  superior pulmonary
  thebesian
  Thebesius
  thoracoepigastric
  tortuous
  varicose
  vertebral
  visibly distended external jugular
vein graft
  ankle brachial systolic pressure
    index monitoring of
  blood flow patterns in
  color-flow duplex imaging of
  stenosis of
  thrombosis
  patency of
vein graft failure
vein graft occlusion
vein nodularity
vein patch angioplasty
vein patch closure

vein patency
veins distended at 45°
veins elevated at 90°
vein sign
vein stripping operation
Velcro rales
velocardiofacial (VCF) syndrome
velocimetry, Doppler
velocity
  blood flow
  closing
  coronary blood flow (CBFV)
  decreased closing
  diastolic regurgitant
  fiber-shortening
  forward
  maximal transaortic jet
  mean aortic flow
  mean posterior wall
  mean pulmonary flow
  meter per second (m/sec)
  peak aortic flow
  peak flow
  peak pulmonary flow
  peak systolic
  peak transmitted
  regurgitant
velocity-encoded magnetic resonance
  imaging
velocity mapping, phase
velocity-time integral of early diastole
velocity-time integral of late diastole
velocity waveforms (VWFs)
velour collar prosthesis
vena cava (pl. venae cavae)
  inferior (IVC)
  superior (SVC)
vena cava clip, Adams-DeWeese
vena cava (or caval) filter
  bird's nest
  Gianturco-Roehm bird's nest
  Greenfield

vena cava filter (cont.)
  Kimray-Greenfield
  Mobin-Uddin
vena caval sieve
vena caval to left atrial communication
vena caval tourniquet
vena cava syndrome
venae cavae (pl. of vena cava)
venae cordis minimae
venarum, sinus
Vena Tech percutaneous LGM filter
VenES II Medical Stockings
Venflon cannula
venipuncture site
venoarterial admixture
venoarterial cannulation
venoarterial shunt
venoarterial shunting
venodilators
venofibrosis
venogram, -graphy
  contrast
  isotope
  lower limb
  radionuclide
  radionuclear
  technetium 99m
veno-occlusive disease (VOD)
venostasis
venosus defect, sinus
venosus, plexus
venotomy, transverse
venotripsy
venous access
venous angioma
venous anomaly
venous backflow
venous blood, arterialization of
venous blood gas values
venous cannula (see cannula)

venous cannulation
venous capillaries
venous catheter (see catheter)
venous circulation
venous claudication
venous congestion
venous cutdown
venous decompensation
venous defects
venous distention
venous Doppler exam
venous dysplasias of infant
venous embolus
venous engorgement, bilateral
venous excursion
venous filling
  early
  late
venous gangrene
venous hum (nun's murmur)
venous hyperemia
venous hypertension
venous insufficiency
venous junction
venous ligation at femoral level
venous malformation (VM)
venous motion, discernible
venous murmur (see murmur)
venous obstruction
venous oxygen content
venous phlebitis-gangrene syndrome
venous pooling
venous pressure, elevated
venous pressure increased, inspiratory
venous pulsations 3 cm above the
  sternal angle
venous pulse
  diastolic collapse
  trough of
venous refill time (VRT)
venous reservoir

venous return
  anomalous pulmonary
  total anomalous
venous segment, nonfilling
venous sinus
venous spasm
venous stasis
venous thromboembolism
venous thrombosis (see *thrombosis*)
venous ulcer
venous valve construction
venous valves
venous vascular malformation
venovenous cannulation
vent
  aortic
  intracardiac
  left atrial
  left ventricular
  pulmonary arterial
  slotted needle
Ventak AICD (automatic implantable
  cardioverter-defibrillator) pacemaker
Ventak ECD (external cardioverter-
  defibrillator)
Ventak ICD (internal cardioverter-
  defibrillator) pacemaker
Ventak P2 pulse generator
Ventak PRx defibrillation system
Ventak PRx pulse generator
Ventak PRx transvenous ICD
Ventak pulse generator
vented-electric HeartMate LVAD
ventilation
  airway pressure release
  alveolar (V_A)
  assisted
  continuous mechanical
  continuous positive pressure
    (CPPV)
  controlled

ventilation *(cont.)*
  excessive
  high minute
  intermittent mandatory (IMV)
  low-frequency positive-pressure
  mask
  maximal voluntary (MVV)
  mechanical
  minute
  positive-pressure
  pressure-cycled
  reduced
  reduced alveolar
  synchronized intermittent mandatory
    (SIMV)
  time-cycled
  volume-controlled inverse ratio
  volume-cycled
  wasted
  weaned off
ventilation equivalent
ventilation lung scan
ventilation-perfusion (V/Q)
ventilation-perfusion defect
ventilation-perfusion imbalance
ventilation-perfusion, impaired
ventilation-perfusion inequality
ventilation-perfusion lung scan
ventilation-perfusion maldistribution
  and hypoxemia
ventilation-perfusion ratio
ventilation-perfusion scan
ventilation pneumonitis
ventilation test
ventilator
  Bear Cub
  Bennett PR-2
  Bourns-Bear
  Bourns infant
  Harvard
  high-frequency jet

ventilator *(cont.)*
 high-frequency oscillation
 MA-1
 Monaghan
 pressure-controlled
 Puritan-Bennett
 tank-type body
 Siemens Servo
ventilator/resuscitator, pneuPAC
ventilatory and perfusion lung scan
ventilatory assistance
ventilatory capacity
ventilatory capacity-demand imbalance
ventilatory defect, restrictive
ventilatory dysfunction
ventilatory effort
ventilatory failure, acute
ventilatory inefficiency
ventilatory muscle training protocol
ventilatory responsiveness
ventilatory support
ventilometric measurements
venting
venting aortic Bengash-type needle
venting of left heart
ventral aorta
ventral branch
ventricle
 akinetic left
 apex of left
 atrialized
 augmented filling of right
 auxillary
 common
 double-inlet
 double-inlet left
 double outlet left (DOLV)
 double-outlet right (DORV)
 dual
 dysfunctional left
 hypokinetic left
 hypoplastic

ventricle *(cont.)*
 hypoplastic heart
 hypoplastic left
 left (LV)
 Mary Allen Engle
 parchment right
 primitive
 right (RV)
 rudimentary right
 single
 thick-walled
 thrusting
 tubular
Ventricor pacemaker
ventricular aberration
ventricular activation time (VAT)
ventricular actuation, direct
 mechanical (DMVA)
ventricular afterload
ventricular aneurysm
ventricular apex
ventricular assist device (VAD)
 Abiomed BVS
 BioMedicus pump
 electrically conditioned and driven
  skeletal muscle
 fully implanted
 HeartMate implantable
 Hemopump
 left
 mechanical
 Novacor
 Penn State
 Pierce-Donachy
 Pierce-Donachy Thoratec
 right
 tethered
 Thermetics
 Thoratec
ventricular asynchronous pacemaker
 (VOO)
ventricular burst pacing

ventricular capture beat
ventricular cavity
ventricular cineangiogram
ventricular compliance
ventricular contraction
ventricular contraction pattern
ventricular couplets
ventricular D-loop
ventricular decompensation
ventricular demand inhibited
    pacemaker
ventricular demand triggered
    pacemaker
ventricular depolarization
ventricular depression
ventricular dilatation
ventricular disproportion
ventricular dysfunction
ventricular dysrhythmias, malignant
ventricular ectopy
ventricular effective refractory period
    (VERP)
ventricular ejection friction
ventricular elastance, maximum
    (EMAX)
ventricular electrical instability
ventricular enlargement
ventricular escape mechanism
ventricular extrastimulation
ventricular fibrillation
    idiopathic
    refractory
ventricular fibrillation pacing
ventricular fibrillation therapy
ventricular filling
ventricular filling sound (third heart
    sound)
ventricular free wall thickness
ventricular function, compromised
ventricular function curve
ventricular function parameters

ventricular fusion beats
ventricular gallop
ventricular gallop rhythm
ventricular gallop sound
ventricular gradient
ventricular hypertrophy
ventricular hypoplasia
ventricular intracerebral hemorrhage
ventricular inversion
ventricular irritability
ventricular lead
ventricular left-handedness
ventricular myocardium
ventricular myxoma
ventricular obstruction, intraventricular
    right
ventricular overdrive pacing
ventricular paced (V_P) beat
ventricular paced cycle length
ventricular pacing
ventricular paroxysmal tachycardia
ventricular perforation
ventricular pre-excitation
ventricular premature contraction
ventricular premature contraction
    couplets
ventricular premature depolarization
    (VPD)
ventricular pressure, right
ventricular pseudoperfusion beats
ventricular rate
ventricular refractoriness
ventricular refractory period
ventricular repolarization
ventricular response
    atrial fibrillation with high-rate
    fast
    moderate
    rapid
    slow
ventricular rhythm disturbance

ventricular right-handedness
ventricular segmental contraction
ventricular sensed (V_S) event
ventricular septal (VS)
ventricular septal aneurysm
ventricular septal defect (VSD)
  flap valve
  juxta-arterial
  juxtatricuspid
  perimembranous
  Swiss cheese
ventricular septal rupture
ventricular septal summit
ventricular septum
  intact
  overriding (of aorta)
ventricular single and double
  extrastimulation
ventricular standstill
ventricular status
ventricular stiffness
ventricular synchrony
ventricular systole
ventricular tachyarrhythmia
  malignant
  transient
  reversible
ventricular tachycardia (VT, V tach)
  monomorphic
  nonsustained monomorphic
  nonsustained polymorphic
  polymorphic
  recurrent intractable
  refractory
  salvos of
  torsades de pointes
ventricular tachycardia detection
ventricular tachycardia reversal
ventricular tachycardia therapy
ventricular transposition
ventricular wall motion
ventricular wall tension

ventricularization of left atrial
  pressure pulse
ventricularization of pressure
ventricularized morphology
ventriculoarterial conduit
ventriculoarterial connections,
  discordant
ventriculoarterial discordance
ventriculoatrial (VA) conduction
ventriculoatrial effective refractory
  period
ventriculoatrial time-out
ventriculogram, -graphy
  axial left anterior oblique
  bicycle exercise radionuclide
  biplane
  digital subtraction
  dipyridamole thallium
  exercise radionuclide
  first-pass radionuclide
  gated blood pool
  gated nuclear
  gated radionuclide
  LAO (left anterior oblique)
    projection
  left (LVG)
  radionuclide (RNV)
  RAO (right anterior oblique)
    projection
  retrograde left
  single plane left
  ventriculography
  xenon 133
ventriculoinfundibular fold
ventriculoplasty, Dor remodeling
ventriculoradial dysplasia
ventriculorrhaphy
  linear
  Reed
ventriculotomy
  encircling endocardial
  endocardial

ventriculotomy *(cont.)*
   map-guided partial endocardial
   paracoronary right
   partial encircling endocardial
   transmural
Ventritex Cadence ICD
Ventritex Cadence pulse generator
Ventritex defibrillation leads
Venturi effect
Venturi mask for oxygen administration
venule, venules
   high endothelial
   postcapillary
vera, polycythemia
Verbatim balloon catheter
verification of ASD occlusion by echo
   Doppler studies
Veriflex cardiac device
Veriflex guide wire
vernal edema
vernix membrane
VERP (ventricular effective refractory
   period)
verrucous carditis
verrucous endocarditis
   atypical
   nonbacterial
verrucous hemangioma
verrucous nodules
Versatrax pacemaker
Versatrax pulse generator
Verstraeten bruit
vertebral arterial dissection
vertebral artery
vertebral artery syndrome
vertebral artery system
vertebral-basilar arterial insufficiency
vertebral-basilar artery syndrome
vertebral-basilar ischemia
vertebrobasilar insufficiency
vertebral column

vertebral part of medial surface of
   lung
vertebral pleural reflection
vertebral vein
vertebral venous plexus
vertical heart
vertical long-axis slice
vertiginous syncope
vertigo, laryngeal
very low-density lipoproteins (VLDL)
vesicles, pulmonary
vesiculae pulmonales
vesicular block
vesicular breath sounds
vesicular breathing
vesicular emphysema
vesicular rales
vessel
   angiographically occult
   anomalous
   arcuate
   atherectomized
   brachiocephalic
   caliber of
   circumflex
   codominant
   collateral
   contralateral
   cranial
   cross-pelvic collateral
   culprit
   diminutive
   disease-free
   dominant
   eccentric
   great
   infrapopliteal
   intercostal
   interlobular
   lymphatic
   nondominant
   occipital

vessel *(cont.)*
  patent
  peripelvic collateral
  peripheral
  peroneal
  plump
  posterior lumbar
  runoff
  splanchnic
  tortuous
  transposition of
  wraparound
vessel caliber
vessel closure, abrupt
vessel cutoff of contrast material
vessel loop
Vesseloops rubber band
vessel rupture
vessel test-occluded
vessel topography
VEST ambulatory function monitor
vestibule, laryngeal
vestigial commissure
vestigial left sinoatrial node
VF, V fib (ventricular fibrillation)
VFT (venous filling time)
VG synch period
V-H interval
viability, tissue
viable myocardium
Viagraph computerized exercise EKG
vibrating pulse
vibration
vibratory systolic murmur
vicious cycle
Vicor pacemaker
Vicryl suture
video-assisted thoracoscopic resection
video-assisted thoracoscopy (VAT)
videoangiography, digital
videodensitometry

videoendoscopic surgical equipment
VideoHydro laparoscope
videolaseroscopy
Vieussens
  circle of
  isthmus of
  limbus of
  loop of
  ring of
  valve of
view
  anterior
  apical and subcostal four-chambered
  apical four-chamber (echocardio-
    gram)
  apical two-chamber
  biplane orthogonal
  caudal
  cineradiographic
  cranial angled
  four-chamber apical
  hemiaxial (x-ray)
  hepatoclavicular
  ice-pick M-mode echocardiogram
  LAO (left anterior oblique)
  LAO-cranial
  left anterior oblique (LAO)
  long axial oblique
  long-axis parasternal
  parasternal long-axis
  parasternal long-axis echocardio-
    gram
  parasternal short-axis
  RAO (right anterior oblique)
  RAO-caudal
  right anterior oblique (RAO)
  right ventricular inflow
  short-axis
  short-axis parasternal
  sitting-up
  spider x-ray

view *(cont.)*
  steep left anterior oblique
  subcostal four-chamber (echo-
    cardiogram)
  subcostal long-axis (echocardio-
    gram)
  subcostal short-axis (echocardio-
    gram)
  subxiphoid (echocardiography)
  suprasternal notch (echocardiogram)
  weeping willow x-ray
Vigilon dressing
vigorous manual massage
Vineberg cardiac revascularization
  procedure
Vineberg operation for collateral
  circulation
VingMed ultrasound
violaceous hue
violent sneezing spells
VIPER PTA catheter
viral bronchitis
viral infection
viral myocarditis
viral pericarditis
viral pharyngitis
viral pneumonia
viral tonsillitis
viral toxicity
Virchow perivascular space
Virchow-Robin perivascular space
Virchow thrombosis triad
Virchow triad
viremia
viremic shock
viridans streptococcal infection
viridant streptococci
virology studies
virulent atherosclerosis
virus
  adenovirus
  causative

virus *(cont.)*
  coxsackie A
  coxsackie B
  cytomegalovirus
  Epstein-Barr (EB)
  Four Corners
  parainfluenza
  respiratory syncytial (RSV)
virus bronchopneumonia
virus-infected cells
visceral cholesterol embolization
  syndrome
visceral embolus
visceral heterotaxy
visceralis, pleura
visceral layer
visceral pericardium
visceral pleura, silicotic
visceral pleurisy
visceral rotation incision
visceral situs abnormalities
visceral situs solitus
viscerum inversus, situs
viscid sputum
viscosity
  blood
  increased blood
  plasma
  sputum
viscous sputum
viselike pain
visible anterior motion
visibly distended external jugular
  veins
Vista pacemaker
visual disturbance
visualization, inadequate
visualization of the small vessels
visuomotor response
Vitacuff dressing
Vitacuff tissue-interface barrier
vital capacity (VC)

Vital Cooley microvascular needle-
holder
Vitalcor venous catheter
Vital Ryder microvascular needle-
holder
vital signs, stable
vitamin B complex deficiency
vitamin B_{12} (or B12) deficiency anemia
vitamin B_{12} (or B12) injections
vitamin K antagonist therapy
vitamin K deficiency
Vitatrax pacemaker
Vitatron catheter electrode
Vitatron Diamond ICD (internal
cardioverter-defibrillator)
Vitatron pacemaker
VLDL (very-low-density lipoprotein)
VLDL-TG (VLDL-triglyceride)
VLDL-TG/HDL-C ratio
V_1-like ambulatory lead system
V_5-like ambulatory lead system
VLP (ventricular late potential)
VMA (vanillylmandelic acid))
VO_2 (oxygen consumption per unit
time)
VO_2 (ventilatory oxygen consumption)
VO_2 (whole body oxygen consumption)
VO_2 max (maximum oxygen consumption)
vocal fremitus
vocalis muscles
VOD (veno-occlusive disease)
Voda catheter
void, signal
Volkmann retractor
voltage
battery
increased (on EKG)
low (on EKG)
precordial
pulse
R

voltage criteria
volts (V)
volume
adequate stroke
alveolar
atrial emptying
augmented stroke
blood
cavity
central blood
chamber
circulating blood
circulation
closing
decreased stroke
decreased tidal
determination of lung
diastolic atrial
diminished lung
Dodge area-length method for
ventricular
end-diastolic
end-expiratory lung
endocardial
end-systolic (ESV)
end-systolic residual
epicardial
expiratory reserve (ERV)
extracellular fluid
forward stroke (FSV)
increased extracellular fluid
inspiratory reserve (IRV)
left ventricular chamber
left ventricular end-diastolic
left ventricular inflow (LVIV)
left ventricular outflow (LVOV)
left ventricular stroke
LV (left ventricular) cavity
mean corpuscular (MCV)
mean corpuscular red cell
minute
pericardial reserve

volume *(cont.)*
  plasma
  prism method for ventricular
  pulmonary blood
  pyramid method for ventricular
  radionuclide stroke
  reduced plasma
  reduced stroke
  regurgitant
  regurgitant stroke (RSV)
  residual (RV)
  respiratory
  right ventricular
  right ventricular end-diastolic
  right ventricular end-systolic
  Simpson rule method for
    ventricular
  stroke (SV)
  systolic atrial
  Teichholz equation for left
    ventricular
  thermodilution stroke
  total stroke (TSV)
  ventricular end-diastolic
  von Recklinghausen test
volume-controlled inverse ratio
  ventilation
volume-controlled ventilator
volume-dependent hypertension
volume depletion
  intravascular
  profound
volume infusion
volume loss
volume overload
volume regulation
voluntary coughing
voluntary hyperventilation, eucapnic
vomitus
von Hippel-Lindau syndrome
Von Rokitansky syndrome

von Willebrand bleeding disorder
von Willebrand blood coagulation
  factor
von Willebrand disease
von Willebrand factor
von Willebrand syndrome
VOO pacemaker
Vorse-Webster clamp
voxel
VPB (ventricular premature beat)
VPC (ventricular premature complex)
VPC (ventricular premature contrac-
  tion)
VPD (ventricular premature depolar-
  ization)
V peak of jugular venous pulse
VPT (ventricular paroxysmal
  tachycardia)
V/Q (ventilation-perfusion)
V/Q imbalance
V/Q scan
VRT (venous refill time)
VRT (venous return time)
VS (ventricular septal)
VSD (ventricular septal defect)
VSD and absent pulmonary valve
  syndrome
VSR (vulcanizing silicone rubber)
VT (ventricular tachycardia)
V tach (ventricular tachycardia)
VTED (venous thromboembolic
  disease)
V_1 through V_6 (precordial EKG leads)
VT/VF (ventricular tachycardia/
  ventricular fibrillation)
vulcanizing silicone rubber
vulnerable myocardium
vulval varices
V_1–V_2 curve
VVI/AAI pacemaker
VVI pacemaker

VVI pacing mode
VVT pacemaker
V wave, augmented
v wave in jugular venous pulse with
tricuspid incompetence
v wave of jugular venous pulse
V wave of right atrial pressure
V wave pressure on left or right atrial
catheterization

V wave (blood pressure measurement
by cardiac catheterization)
V wave on catheterization
V wave on pulmonary capillary
wedge tracing
VWFs (velocity waveforms), Doppler
V-Y atrioplasty

W, w

W (whoop)
Waaler-Rose test
wafer of endocardium
WAGR (Wilms tumor, aniridia, genitourinary involvement, and retardation)
waist in the balloon
Wakabaushi shunt
waking, breathlessness on
waking with chest tightness
Waldhausen and Nahrwold technique
wall akinesis
wall hypokinesis
wall, left anterior chest wall
wall motion, ventricular
wall thickness
Wallstent (made by Schneider)
Wallstent biliary endoprosthesis
Wallstent spring-loaded stent
wand, programmer
wandering atrial pacemaker (WAP)
wandering pacemaker syndrome
waning pain
WAP (wandering atrial pacemaker)
Ward-Romano syndrome
warm blood cardioplegic induction (WBCI)

warm continuous retrograde cardioplegia
warmed heelstick for neonates
Warthin sign of increased pulmonary sounds in acute pericarditis
washed clot
washed red cell autotransfusion
washings
  bronchial
  cell
washings and brushings
washout
  delayed xenon
  lung
  nitrogen
washout phase
wasted ventilation
wasting, potassium
water-hammer pulse
water retention
water, total body
Waterhouse-Friderichsen syndrome
watershed area in lung transplantation
watershed region
Waterston anastomosis
Waterston anastomosis for congenital pulmonary stenosis

Waterston-Cooley anastomosis
Waterston groove
Waterston shunt
waterwheel bruit
watery sputum
watt-second
wave (electrocardiogram)
  A
  A larger than V
  alpha
  augmented V
  C
  constant tilt
  CV
  depolarization
  depolarizing
  dicrotic
  F (fibrillary)
  H
  inverted T
  J
  notched P
  P
  Osborn (hypothermia)
  palpable A
  Q
  Q (in the right precordial leads)
  R
  rapid filling
  recoil wave
  regurgitant CV
  retraction
  S
  slow filling
  standardization
  stationary arterial
  systolic S
  T
  Ta
  tidal
  Traube-Hering
  U

wave (electrocardiogram) *(cont.)*
  V
  ventricular
wave (jugular venous pulse)
  a
  c
  cannon
  cannon a
  f
  giant a
  h
  intermittent cannon a
  v
  x
  y
wave form
  monophasic shock
  truncated exponential simultaneous
    monophasic
wax, bone
waxing and waning pain
waxing pain
weak carotid upstroke
weak signal
weakened arteries
weakness
  profound
  respiratory muscles
  transitory
wean, difficult to
weaned from cardiopulmonary bypass
weaned from IABP
weaned off bronchodilators
weaned off ventilation
weaning from ventilator
Weavenit (and New Weavenit)
  Dacron prosthesis
web
  laryngeal
  lateral
Weber-Osler-Rendu syndrome
Weber protocol (exercise stress testing)

Webster needle holder
Webster orthogonal electrode catheter
Weck clip
wedged
wedge position, pulmonary capillary
wedge pressure, pulmonary venous
wedge resection of lung
wedge-shaped density
wedge-shaped hemorrhagic area
wedge-shaped lobe
Wegener granulomatosis
Wegener syndrome
weight loss therapy
weight on the chest
weight reduction
Weil disease or syndrome
   (Adolf Weil)
Weill sign of pneumonia in infant
   (Edmond Weill)
Weinberg-Himelfarb syndrome
Weingarten syndrome
Weingarten tropical pulmonary
   eosinophilia
Weisenburg syndrome
Weiss-Baker syndrome
welder's lung
welder's siderosis
well-preserved ejection fraction
Wenckebach AV (atrioventricular)
   block
Wenckebach incomplete atrio-
   ventricular (AV) heart block
Wenckebach phenomenon
Wenckebach secondary atrioventricu-
   lar heart block
Wenckebach upper rate response
Werlhof autoimmune thrombocyto-
   penia (ATP)
Werlhof disease
Werlhof idiopathic thrombocytopenic
   purpura (ITP)
Werner syndrome

Westermark sign
Western blot test
Westcott scissors
wet cough
wet lung syndrome
wet pleurisy
Wexler catheter
wheal (weal), skin
Wheat procedure
Wheatstone bridge
wheeze, wheezes
   asthmatoid
   end-expiratory
   end-inspiratory
   expiratory
   fine
   inspiratory
wheezing
   audible
   breathless when
   diffuse inspiratory and expiratory
   grossly audible
   localized
   paroxysmal
wheezing audible without a stethoscope
wheezing in chest
wheezing respirations
wheezy
whining, expiratory
whispered pectoriloquy
whispering pectoriloquy
whistling rales
whistling respirations
whistling rhonchi
white-appearing blood pool
white blood cell count shift to the left
white clot syndrome
white cotton umbilical tape
white lung syndrome
white-noise artifact
white silk suture
white sound

whitish sputum
whole blood infusion
whole blood monoclonal antibody
whole body inflammatory response
Wholey Hi-torque modified J wire
Wholey wire
whoop (W)
    late systolic
    musical
whooping cough
whooping murmur
whorled appearance
whorls
wide-based blunt-ended right-sided
    atrial appendage
wide-bore needle
widely split second sound
widened heart shadow
widened mediastinum
widened respiratory splitting
widened S_1 or S_2 splitting
widened thoracic outlet
widening, mediastinal
wide pulse
wide splitting of first heart sound
wide splitting of second heart sound
width, pulse
Wiktor coronary stent
Wiktor stent
Wilcoxon rank-sum test (calculation
    for artificial heart)
Willebrand disease (von Willebrand)
Willebrand factor (von Willebrand)
Willebrand syndrome
Williams-Beuren syndrome
Williams-Campbell syndrome
Williams cardiac device
Williams elfin-facies syndrome
Williamson sign or test
Williams sign
Williams syndrome

Willis, circle of
Wilms tumor
Wilson-Mikity syndrome
window
    aorticopulmonary
    aortopulmonary
    apical
    esophageal
    gastric
    parasternal
    pericardial
    subcostal
    suprasternal
window ductus
windsock aneurysm
Winiwarter-Buerger disease
Winiwarter-Buerger thromboangiitis
    obliterans
Winiwarter-Manteuffel-Buerger
    syndrome
winter cough
Wintrich sign
Wintrobe hematocrit
Wintrobe sed(imentation) rate
wire
    deflector
    hydrophilic guide
    Hyperflex guide
    Hyperflex steerable
    magnum guide
    Microven nitinol
    pacing
    sensing
    Wholey Hi-torque modified J
wire-mesh self-expandable stent
wire tightener
wire twister
Wiskott-Aldrich syndrome
Wizard cardiac device
Woakes ethmoiditis
Woakes syndrome

Wolf-Hirschhorn syndrome
Wolff-Parkinson-White (WPW)
    syndrome
Wolman disease
Wolvek sternal approximation fixation
    instrument
wood asthma
Wood units of pulmonary vascular
    resistance
woody mass
Wooler annuloplasty
Wooler-type annuloplasty
woolsorter's inhalation disease
work, maximal capacity for
worn-out red cells
worsening of asthma, nocturnal
worthlessness
wound
    missile
    stab

woven Dacron gusset
woven Dacron tube graft
woven Teflon prosthesis
WPW (Wolff-Parkinson-White)
    syndrome
wracking cough
wraparound graft
wraparound technique
wraparound vessel
wrap-inclusion composite valve graft
    procedure, Bentall
wrapped aneurysmal sac
wrapping of graft
Wright nebulizer
Wright peak flow
wrinkled pleura
Wuchereria bancrofti infection
Wylie carotid artery clamp

X, x

xanthelasma
xanthoma
  eruptive
  palmar
  tendinous
  tuberoeruptive
  tuberous
xanthoma tendinosum
xanthoma tuberosum simplex
xanthomatosis-hypercholesterolemia
x depression of jugular venous pulse
x descent of "a" wave
x descent of jugular venous pulse
XeCT (xenon computed tomography)
X' descent
xenograft (heterograft) (see *graft*)
  glutaraldehyde-preserved porcine
  porcine
  vascular
xenograft valve
Xenomedica prosthetic valve
xenon chloride (XeCl) excimer
xenon computed tomography (XeCT)
Xenotech prosthetic valve
xenotransplantation
xiphisternal joint
xiphisternal region

xiphoid area
xiphoid cartilage
xiphoid, hypersensitive
xiphoid process syndrome
xiphoidalgia
xiphopubic midline incision
X-linked abnormality
XO (Turner) syndrome
x-ray
  baseline chest
  chest (CXR)
  cineradiographic views
  computerized tomography (CT)
    scan
  selective coronary arteriography
  tomograms
X syndrome
XT cardiac device
X trough
XXXY and XXXXX syndrome
x' wave pressure on right atrial
  catheterization
x waves (negative) on jugular venous
  pulse (JVP) wave tracing
XY plane
Xyrel pacemaker
XYZ lead system

Y, y

Yankauer suction tube
Yasargil artery forceps
Yasargil carotid clamp
yawning
Y configuration, inverted
Y connector, ACS angioplasty
y depression of jugular venous pulse
Y descent
y descent of a wave
y descent of jugular venous pulse
Y graft

Yeager formula
yellow plaque, fibrofatty
yellow sputum
Yersinia infection
young female aortic arch arteritis
Y-shaped graft
Y trough
Y wave pressure on right atrial
    catheterization
y waves (negative) on jugular pulse
    wave tracing

Z, z

Zahn
  lines of
  pockets of
Zeek syndrome
Zener diode
Ziegler syndrome
Zimmer antiembolism support
  stockings
zipper scar
Zitron pacemaker
Z lines
Z point
z point pressure on left (or right) atrial
  catheterization
Zoll defibrillator
Zoll NTP noninvasive temporary
  pacemaker
zone
  arrhythmogenic border
  basal
  clear
  convergence

zone *(cont.)*
  ischemic
  lipid
  midlung
  precordial transition
  pyramidal hemorrhagic
  rough
  sonolucent
  transition
zone of fibrosis
zone of hemorrhage
zone of ischemia
zone of necrosis
zone of slow conduction (ZSC)
ZSC (zone of slow conduction)
Zuckerkandl para-aortic bodies at
  bifurcation of aorta
Zucker and Myler cardiac device
Zucker #7 French catheter
Zwenger test
zygapophyseal articulation
ZY plane